Prenatal and Postnatal Care

Prenatal and Postnatal Care

Edited by **Gordon Hart**

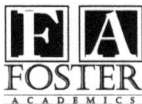

FOSTER
ACADEMICS

New Jersey

Published by Foster Academics,
61 Van Reypen Street,
Jersey City, NJ 07306, USA
www.fosteracademics.com

Prenatal and Postnatal Care
Edited by Gordon Hart

International Standard Book Number: 978-1-63242-329-0 (Hardback)

Printed in the United States of America.

Contents

Preface

This book focuses on providing information regarding prenatal and postnatal care. Obstetrics is growing at a rapid pace and holds high prominence for advancement in many other fields. This book imparts knowledge on the improvements in primary research and clinical practice. It also sheds light on recent problems related to this field, while discussing on preconception, pregnancy, labor and postpartum. This book guides the readers through difficult and complicated decisions in clinical administration. Moreover, it provides an insight into analytic knowledge of pathogenetic mechanisms involved in pregnancy and initiates more research by granting evidence of recent information and upcoming aspects in this area. Since the book is penned down by an elite group of knowledgeable authors from around the globe, it will definitely provide the readers with valuable knowledge for understanding maternal, paternal and fetal interactions as these are very necessary for a safe and successful birth.

This book is a result of research of several months to collate the most relevant data in the field.

When I was approached with the idea of this book and the proposal to edit it, I was overwhelmed. It gave me an opportunity to reach out to all those who share a common interest with me in this field. I had 3 main parameters for editing this text:

1. Accuracy – The data and information provided in this book should be up-to-date and valuable to the readers.
2. Structure – The data must be presented in a structured format for easy understanding and better grasping of the readers.
3. Universal Approach – This book not only targets students but also experts and innovators in the field, thus my aim was to present topics which are of use to all.

Thus, it took me a couple of months to finish the editing of this book.

I would like to make a special mention of my publisher who considered me worthy of this opportunity and also supported me throughout the editing process. I would also like to thank the editing team at the back-end who extended their help whenever required.

Editor

Who Selects Obstetrics and Gynecology as a Career and Why, and What Traits Do They Possess?

Bruce W. Newton
University of Arkansas for Medical Sciences
USA

1. Introduction

As the title implies, this chapter concerns the traits of students who select obstetrics and gynecology (OB/GYN) as a career, and the various factors which attract or inhibit them from entering a residency. Various professional organizations, medical students, residents and authors have differing opinions whether OB/GYN is considered a primary care residency, or a core surgical specialty (Indyk et al., 2011; Jacoby et al., 1998; Laube & Ling, 1999; McAlister et al., 2007). The reader needs to decide which definition is preferred. Regardless of the choice, the vast majority of these data can be applied to either definition. Although almost all studies collect data about OB/GYN vs. just obstetrics, these data can be applied to both designations. Finally, all data are gathered from the US unless otherwise indicated.

2. Personality traits of students and residents

There are numerous studies which examined the traits of students who enter the various medical specialties. This section will compare traits of students who desire to enter an OB/GYN residency with those who prefer another primary care residency, or a surgical residency. Specialties which are primary care are typified by a continuity of patient care and include OB/GYN, Family Medicine (FM; also known as Family Practice), Internal Medicine (IM), and Pediatrics (PED). Surgery (SURG) is not a primary care specialty, but along with FM, IM, PED and OB/GYN, SURG is considered a specialty that has a non-controllable lifestyle.

Obstetrics and gynecology, FM, IM, PED, and SURG can be contrasted with those specialties which are considered as having a controllable lifestyle, e.g., radiology, ophthalmology, pathology, and anesthesiology. A controllable lifestyle specialty is characterized by the physician controlling the number of hours spent on professional duties, leaving more time for personal activities. Increasingly, students are selecting residencies with a controllable lifestyle (Dorsey et al., 2005; Schwartz et al., 1990, 1989).

2.1 Medical students

In the 1970s, McGrath and Zimet (1977) studied the personality traits of male and female students vs. their specialty choice. Women were found to be more self-confident, autonomous and aggressive than men; whereas men displayed more nurturance than the normal population. Because females were the minority of medical students before and during the 1990s, it was postulated they had to be self-confident and aggressive in order to compete with their male peers.

In the 1980s, students entering medical school and considering OB/GYN were least depressed, highly motivated and exhibited feminine vs. masculine traits. They also exhibited large degrees of neuroticism, social anxiety, and public self-consciousness (Zedlow & Daugherty, 1991). By the 2000s, neuroticism, conscientiousness, openness, and agreeableness were prominent in students entering OB/GYN (Markert et al., 2008). Other studies in the 2000s, using various survey instruments, examined other medical student traits which influenced residency selection. Women who desired to enter an OB/GYN residency had the following traits in significantly greater amounts than men; sociability, a fondness for demanding and difficult work, agreeableness, conscientiousness, extraversion, openness, persistence, cooperativeness, and being reward-dependent. In contrast, men were significantly more aggressive/hostile, impulsive and sensation-seeking (Hojat & Zuckerman, 2008; Maron et al., 2007; Vaidya et al., 2004). Females exhibited slightly more neuroticism/anxiety than males when compared with other primary care specialties and SURG. On a positive note, male or female students entering into OB/GYN had the lowest neuroticism/anxiety tendencies (Hojat & Zuckerman, 2008; Maron et al., 2007).

In 2002, Borges and Savickas wrote a seminal paper reviewing studies, using the Myers-Briggs Type Indicator or the Five-Factor Model of Personality, on the personalities of students selecting the various medical specialties. Students entering an OB/GYN residency were extroverted, sensing-thinking-judging, highly conscientious, and achievement oriented. These students were less open to new experiences and less agreeable. When compared to students entering FM, OB/GYN students were less sympathetic, trusting, cooperative, and altruistic. However when compared to students entering IM or PED, the OB/GYN students were not as stiff, skeptical, extroverted, or neurotic, but were more conscientious and empathetic. Students entering SURG were much more open to new experiences and were more extroverted than those in primary care specialties.

The same trends were seen when the study by Doherty and Nugent (2011) found success in medical school was best predicted by a student who was conscientious and sociable. A survey of Swiss students affirmed the above and showed female students were more helpful, conscientious, and had greater intrinsic motivation than the males who expressed greater degrees of independence, decisiveness, and a desire for income and prestige. These personality differences showed females preferred specialties with a high degree of patient contact (e.g., OB/GYN), vs. males who were more interested in high-tech, instrument-driven specialties such as SURG (Buddeberg-Fischer et al., 2003).

Student academic achievement is another trait that influences residency selection. Jarecky and colleagues (1993) found that between 1964 and 1991 students who were elected into Alpha Omega Alpha (A US-based medical school honorary that includes only the very top students.) increasingly selected controllable lifestyle residencies, thereby reducing opportunities for students in the bottom 10% of their class from entering those residencies. Comparing data from 1964-1979 to 1980-1991, the number of top students who entered controllable lifestyle residencies increased from 21% to 36%, whereas students in the bottom

10% of their class who entered FM increased from 8% to 40%. Fortunately, for students entering OB/GYN, the trend was reversed with the number of top students increasing from 5% to 11% during the 1964-1979 to 1980-1991 timeframes. Conversely, the bottom 10% of students entering OB/GYN residencies fell from 10% to 5%, respectively.

Myles & Henderson, II (2002) found that students who failed Step I of the United States Medical Licensing Examination (USMLE; given at the end of the two basic science years of US medical education) were likely to fail the National Board of Medical Examiners (NBME) OB/GYN comprehensive exam given at the end of an OB/GYN clerkship. Thus, students who score at or below the 25th percentile on the USMLE Step I should be identified as in need of increased observation and training in the OB/GYN clerkship. This will help ensure a successful outcome and increase the potential number of students who may select an OB/GYN residency (Myles & Henderson, II, 2002). For students who had already indicated a prior interest in OB/GYN, it seems likely that earning a poor score on the NBME OB/GYN exam would discourage them from selecting an OB/GYN residency.

One undesirable trait, Machiavellianism (i.e., someone who avoids identifying with another's point of view, settles for less than the ideal, and isn't concerned for conventional morality), was found in 15% of students from four U.S. medical schools. (Merrill et al., 1993). Students who express this trait are authoritarian, shift blame to others when they have failed a patient, view the medical record and laboratory profile as more important than seeing the patient as a person, and find undiagnosable illnesses and unpredictable patient outcomes as offensive. Thankfully, students who select primary care specialties like OB/GYN (characterized by high patient-contact), exhibited the fewest Machiavellian traits; whereas, the low patient-contact specialties, e.g., anesthesiology, radiology and SURG exhibited the most Machiavellian traits. However, when the decreasing amount of empathy being expressed by students (cf. section 5) is combined with the emotional detachment characteristic of a Machiavellian, OB/GYN residents and faculty must always maintain highly professional, competent, patient/physician interactions (Konrath et al., 2011).

2.2 Practicing OB/GYNs

Female OB/GYNs from 1950 to 1989 were surveyed and their traits contrasted against female physicians in all other specialties (Frank et al., 1999). Like other female physicians, female OB/GYNs had equivalent amounts of home stress, and the same marital status and numbers of children. In contrast to other female physicians, women OB/GYNs spent less time on childcare, cooking and housework. They were more likely to be in a group practice and worked more clinical hours. Female OB/GYNs also had more on-call nights where they slept less, and were more likely to report they worked too much and had increased amounts of work-related stress. Female OB/GYNs counseled and screened more patients than most other female physicians because of their increasing role of having to act as a primary care physician. Their counseling and screening role was especially true for topics concerning breast cancer, hormone replacement therapy, HIV prevention, and the need for PAP smears and colonoscopies. It was revealing that traditional residency training inadequately prepared the residents for the realities of providing a substantial amount of non-OB/GYN primary care for many of their patients (Frank et al, 1999).

3. What do patients prefer in their OB/GYN?

There has always been a controversy over male physicians treating gynecologic and obstetric issues (Balayla, 2010). Even today there are considerable differences in the OB/GYN gender preference in patients within different age ranges. The shifting patient demographics, especially the increasing number of post-menopausal women, combined with the recent large influx of female OB/GYNs, has resulted in preference changes over the decades. In 1970, only 9% of medical students were female. This had increased to 45.7% by 2001 (as cited in Table 1; Johnson et al., 2005). From 1980 to 2000, the number of practicing female OB/GYNs increased from 12% to 32%. Between 1989 to 2002, the number of female OB/GYN residents rose from 44% to 74% (cf. refs. in Gerber & Lo Sasso, 2006). Projections indicate an expanding population of female OB/GYNs in the 2010s and beyond. For example, in 1980, females constituted 27.8% of the OB/GYN residents, and 12% of the physicians in practice. By 2001 those numbers increased to 71.8% and 39%, respectively (as cited in Table 1; Johnson et al., 2005).

It is clear from the studies cited below, that good bedside manner and professionalism are extremely important to patients. Plunkett and Midland (2000) found that "well-educated" Caucasians (from Chicago, Michigan, US) placed an emphasis on communication skills when selecting an obstetrician. In contrast, patients who were to undergo surgery decided the surgical reputation of the OB/GYN was more important than bedside manner. Over 90% of either set of patients wanted the OB/GYN to be responsive to their needs, exhibit professional behavior, and to be confident and knowledgeable. Only 38% of the patients thought that OB/GYN gender was an issue, and even fewer (15%) took the age of the OB/GYN into consideration. Of the 38% of patients who considered OB/GYN gender as important, 96% wanted a female obstetrician and 84% wanted a female gynecologist.

Plunkett et al. (2002) performed another study in Chicago, and included African-Americans, Hispanics, and individuals with varied levels of education. Less than one-half of the women (42%) considered OB/GYN gender as important. When seeing an obstetrician, bedside manner, office location, referral by another physician, and recommendations from friends and family were the four factors considered most important at 57%, 45%, 40% and 35%, respectively. When selecting a gynecologist, office location, recommendations from family and friends, bedside manner, and referrals by other physicians were the top four ranked attributes at 55%, 48%, 47% and 43%, respectively. When specifically asked if they preferred a male or female OB/GYN, 52.8% wanted a female, 9.6% wanted a male, and 37.6% had no preference.

There were similar findings in New York City, where 58% of patients preferred a female OB/GYN, while 7% wanted a male and 34% had no preference (Howell et al., 2002). Only 10% of patients thought the gender of their OB/GYN impacted their care. These patients thought female physicians would naturally understand more about "female issues" than would males. When asked to rank order important attributes patients desired in an OB/GYN, bedside manner, communication skills, and technical expertise were the dominant factors for selecting an OB/GYN — or leaving if they lacked any of these skills (Howell et al., 2002).

In a large study in Michigan, Mavis et al. (2005) found that OB/GYN gender mattered most to patients who were; underrepresented minorities, unmarried, less educated, and younger than 27. When asked what OB/GYN traits the patients wanted, the top five ranked selections all dealt with interpersonal communication; the OB/GYN is respectful, listens to me, explains things clearly, is easy to talk to, and is caring. These traits were considered more important than clinical expertise. Zuckerman et al. (2002) found striking gender preferences associated with patient religious practices in Brooklyn, New York. Female OB/GYNs were preferred by 56% of Protestants, 58% of Catholics and Jews, 74% of Hindus and 89% of Muslims. Yet patients indicated no gender difference in the quality of the care.

Johnson and colleagues (2005) found that in thirteen different sites in Connecticut, two-thirds of the patients had no gender preference for their OB/GYN, 6.7% preferred a male, and 27.6% preferred a female. Furthermore, the gender or age of the OB/GYN had no impact on the quality of care they received. The most important OB/GYN characteristics the women desired were an OB/GYN who was; attentive to their needs (69%), experienced (68%), knowledgeable (62%), had good technical skills (56%), and was accessible (53%). It is interesting to note that attributes dealing with communication skills and bedside manner were not expressly mentioned by patients in the Connecticut study.

3.1 Gender preferences outside the US

In Ontario, Canada, Fischer and colleagues (2002) found that 75% of patients had no gender preference, and only 21% strongly felt they desired a female OB/GYN, while 4% wanted a male OB/GYN. Various patient characteristics had no bearing on gender preference, e.g., single, pregnant, those with a history of abortion, STDs or sexual dysfunction. In Israel, Piper and colleagues (2008) found that 60.3% of patients expressed no gender preference for their OB/GYN. Women who had children had a predilection to prefer female OB/GYNs. The important factors for Israeli OB/GYN selection were; professional demeanor (98.9%), showing courtesy (96.6%), and being board certified (92%).

Studies performed in Iraq and the United Arab Emirates (UAE; Lafta, 2006; Rizk et al., 2005), showed that a high percentage of patients, 79% and 86%, respectively, preferred a female OB/GYN. Only 8% of Iraqi and 1.6% of UAE women preferred their OB/GYN to be a male. In either country, the preference for a female OB/GYN significantly increased as the educational level fell. Very few women in either country had no gender preference. It was clear that socio-cultural and religious traditions played a very significant role in preferring a female OB/GYN. In the UAE study, Muslim women did not accept a male OB/GYN, even in the presence of a female chaperone, and especially during Ramadan (Rizk et al., 2005). Another prominent barrier to accepting a male OB/GYN was feeling greatly embarrassed if they had to be examined by a male. Many patients (69%) felt that female OB/GYNs had a greater awareness of female reproductive issues, were more compassionate, and better listeners than male OB/GYNs. Younger women had a stronger preference for female OB/GYNs than older women. It seems clear that younger, less educated Muslim women view OB/GYN gender as a gateway requirement to care.

Additional data from the UAE study reveals that women look for the same positive traits in an OB/GYN of either sex, as the other aforementioned studies. They want their OB/GYN to show professionalism by being responsive to their needs, caring, empathetic, displaying a good bedside manner, and being a skilled communicator. Secondarily, they want their OB/GYN to be knowledgeable, experienced, and technically competent (Rizk et al., 2005).

Racz et al. (2008) examined the acceptability of involving Ontario-based medical students in OB/GYN care in two different patient groups: ages 17-85 and secondary school students with an average age of sixteen. Twenty-two percent of the older patients preferred a female student, increasing to 55% in the younger patients. Overall, the greater number of intimate examinations a patient had experienced, the less of a preference she had for OB/GYN gender. When the patients were asked about the presence of medical students in the examination room, there were significant differences expressed by the two age groups. The older patients were more accepting of having medical students of either sex participate in their care (73%) than the younger patients (32%). Over 36% of the younger patients said it would be "very embarrassing" or "unbearable" for a male medical student to perform an intimate examination. Because male medical students were rejected by younger patients to a much higher degree than by the older patients, it is advisable for clerkship directors to forewarn male medical students that younger patients may not want them in the examination room.

In conclusion, although many women may prefer a female physician, it has been demonstrated that physician gender is often not the most important attribute under consideration when patients select an OB/GYN. Clearly, good bedside manner and communication skills are essential in establishing an effective doctor/patient rapport. This is often followed by technical expertise and a good medical reputation. Before the 1970s, most patients had little say in the gender of their OB/GYN, but with the rapidly increasing number of practicing female OB/GYNs, patients now have a greater freedom to make gender a selection preference. Therefore, to maintain an adequate patient population, it will become even more important for male OB/GYNs to practice good bedside manners and empathic communication skills, as well as having technical expertise.

3.2 The influence of media on gender bias

A unique study by Kincheloe (2004) clearly found a physician gender bias when he examined six popular women's magazines over an 18 month period; *Cosmopolitan, Fitness, Glamour, Good Housekeeping, Ladies Home Journal* and *Redbook*. Kincheloe found that female physicians were 20 times more likely to have an identifying photograph as compared to males. Women OB/GYNs were interviewed 47-80% of the time, and female physicians from all other specialties accounted for 31-57% of the articles. When pronouns were used to describe an OB/GYN, a negative connotation was used 92% of the time for male OB/GYNs vs. 17% for females.

In five of the six magazines reviewed, physicians had their quoted gender changed from neutral to reflect female-specific pronouns. The exception was if the physician was portrayed negatively, and then the physician was significantly more likely to be identified as male (Kincheleo, 2004). Since attitudes are shaped by what we see, hear and read, women who buy these magazines seem to be influenced, whether purposefully or subliminally, to acquire a negative bias toward male physicians, in general, and male OB/GYNs specifically. Patients, and the physicians who refer patients, must be reminded to tell their patients that OB/GYN choice should be based on professionalism and clinical skills vs. using gender as a main deciding factor.

4. What is the ideal obstetrics/gynecologist physician and mentor?

Carmel and Glick did a study in 1996 where physicians were asked to rank six attributes of a "good" doctor. The physicians placed the following descriptions in rank order from highest to lowest; humane to patients, has good medical knowledge and skills, is devoted to helping their patients, has a good working relationship with the staff, can research and publish, and are good at management and administration. Carmel & Glick (1996) concluded that the rank order of these attributes was in contrast to the duties needed to get promoted in academia, i.e., research, publications, administrative duties and spending less time with each patient. Therefore, the current academic "system" does not reward being a "good" doctor. Medical students, after starting their clinical rotations, have slightly different priorities as compared to practicing physicians. Students felt that knowledge and skills were the most important factors, followed by being humane, intellectually competent, honest, and reliable (Notzer et al., 1988). It is understandable for students to place knowledge and skills as the most important qualities since they were in the initial stage of their career.

In light of the above, and despite the pressured academic environment in which physicians work, the ability to teach and mentor is viewed as extremely important by medical students. Therefore, faculty and residents must maintain a high degree of professionalism/humanism while still being technically competent. The same is true for residents being taught by faculty. Although patient care must take first priority, 62% of OB/GYN residents say finding time to look for "teachable moments" on the collection and interpretation of critical information in emergent situations is vital to the education of students and residents. Over 90% say you must find time to teach procedures (Gil et al., 2009). Faculty agree to a greater degree than residents that they need to be an appropriate role model, to be enthusiastic about patient care, and teach evidence-based medicine. Although residents still feel these are important skills, they are more pressured for time than faculty and are less likely to express these traits because of time constraints (Johnson & Chen, 2006).

Regardless of time constraints under which faculty and residents are placed, students appreciate constructive criticism given in a timely manner. Students have some ability to self-assess their progress, but specific, descriptive, written feedback is best for increasing student learning (Stalmeijer et al., 2010). In this regard, medical students say the ideal attending physician should spend more than 25% of their time teaching, with at least 25 hours of teaching per week occurring during rounds. Residents and faculty need to stress the importance of the doctor/patient relationship and emphasize the social aspects of medicine so that the patient is seen as an individual rather than an illness. Finally, students feel the faculty need to have served as chief resident in order to be a successful teacher (Wright et al., 1998).

5. Empathy in the doctor/patient relationship

Numerous studies have shown empathic physicians are better at maintaining a good doctor/patient relationship. This makes the patients more relaxed, confident in their physician, compliant, and less likely to sue for malpractice (cf. refs. cited in Newton et al., 2008). Accordingly, the American Association of Medical Colleges and the Accreditation Committee for Graduate Medical Education have emphasized the importance of promoting empathy and professionalism in the curriculum. Displaying empathy is counter to the natural tendency for medical students or physicians to distance themselves from disease and build an emotional detachment from the patient. Therefore, positive role models need to teach others how to deal with these conflicting emotions (Rosenfield & Jones, 2004).

Empathy is a multi-dimensional trait. Sociologists and psychologists break it down into two main categories; role-playing (cognitive) empathy and vicarious (innate) empathy (Hojat et al., 2009). There is an ongoing debate whether empathy is cognitive or emotional/vicarious (Spiro, 2009). Hojat defines cognitive empathy as, "Empathy is a predominately *cognitive* (rather than emotional) attribute that involves the *understanding* (rather than feeling) of experiences, concerns and perspectives of the patient, combined with a capacity to *communicate* this understanding." (Note: The words in italics and parentheses are part of the definition proposed by Hojat et al., 2009.) Vicarious empathy is defined by Mehrabian et al. (1988) as, "An individual's vicarious emotional response to perceived emotional experiences of others." In other words, vicarious empathy arises out of our own feelings and reactions; it happens when "you and I" becomes "I am you" or "I could be you" (Spiro, 2009).

Recently, a scale measuring cognitive empathy, the Jefferson Scale of Physician Empathy (JSPE), developed by Hojat and colleagues, is in wide use and shows that women have slightly higher JSPE scores than men (cf. ref. 6 in Hojat et al., 2002). The JSPE shows there are equivalent declines in cognitive empathy in male and female students as they progress through undergraduate medical school, with the largest drop occurring after completion of the first clinical year of training (Hojat et al., 2009). Specialties like FM, IM, PED and OB/GYN are "people-oriented", and students who entered these specialties had higher JSPE scores than those selecting "technology-oriented" specialties like SURG, radiology, anesthesiology, and pathology (Hojat et al., 2009).

Hojat and colleagues (2005) compared student JSPE scores, recorded in their first clinical year of training, to the clerkship director's subjective rating of their empathic behavior after their first year of residency. The results showed that residents who had higher JSPE scores as junior medical students were rated by the clerkship directors as being more empathetic than juniors who had lower JSPE scores. This implied that empathy remained stable during the senior year of medical school and into the first year of residency.

Hojat et al. (2002) also examined physician cognitive empathy which showed no significant gender differences. Psychiatrists had JSPE scores that were equivalent to PED, IM, and FM physicians. However, psychiatrists had significantly larger JSPE scores than OB/GYN, SURG, radiology, anesthesia and orthopedic physicians. For specialties with continuity of patient care, IM had the largest JSPE score, followed in rank order by PED, FM and OB/GYN. However, there were no significant differences in JSPE scores between these four specialties.

5.1 Vicarious/innate empathy in medical students

As previously described, empathy can be defined from an emotional vs. a cognitive standpoint. The Balanced Emotional Empathy Scale (BEES), developed by Dr. Albert Mehrabian (1996), was used by Newton and colleagues (2007; 2008) for a seven-year longitudinal study of undergraduate medical students at the University of Arkansas for Medical Sciences. Since the BEES is gender sensitive, the data revealed significant gender differences with women having higher BEES scores than men. Newton et al. (2007, 2008) separated the data into males and females who desired to enter "core" specialties which have continuity of patient care, i.e., IM, FM, OB/GYN, PED, and psychiatry or "non-core" specialties without continuity of patient care, e.g., radiology, pathology, emergency medicine, anesthesiology and SURG. Significant drops in vicarious empathy occurred in both sexes after the completion of the first and third years of undergraduate medical school. Those students who selected core specialties had a smaller drop in BEES scores compared to those whom selected non-core specialties. Females that selected core specialties had the smallest overall drop in BEES scores, while females selecting non-core specialties had the greatest overall decrease, with their BEES scores approaching the naturally lower BEES scores of males. These data suggest that females who desire to enter male-dominated specialties may be taking on the persona of the less empathic males (Newton et al, 2008).

When the BEES data from the final year of medical school were analyzed with respect to residency choice, students who entered core residencies had significantly higher BEES scores than students who entered non-core residencies (Newton et al., 2007). The average BEES score for the general population is 45. The top four residency BEES scores were OB/GYN (52.21), psychiatry (47.68), PED (46.30) and FM (39.00). The other core specialty, IM, had a BEES score of 33.02, and was ranked 9th out of 16 specialties. (All specialties with an n ≥ 8 students were considered as providing valid data.) In relation to the general population, the top four specialties had "average" vicarious empathy, while IM was "slightly low". Surgery had "moderately low" vicarious empathy (19.95), while plastic surgery (12.00) and neurosurgery (7.25) had "very low" empathy. However, the lowest two specialties did not have eight or more students entering the residencies over a seven-year period, so interpretive caution must be used since the aggregate BEES score may not be a true reflection of the vicarious empathy shown by this low number of medical students.

5.2 Empathy in non-US countries

Researchers outside of the US have used the JSPE to measure cognitive empathy. There are many similarities to the US data, but some differences are revealed. Italian physicians have lower empathy scores than US physicians and no gender differences were discovered. The JSPE scores for surgeons were no different from all other specialties, and it was suggested that all differences could be attributed to cultural differences (Di Lillo et al., 2009). In South Korea, no gender differences were found, and Korean student cognitive empathy was less than US empathy. It was proposed that the Korean empathy was lower because of the more authoritative role Korean physicians assume, combined with the less assertive nature of their patients (Roh et al., 2010). Female Japanese students had significantly larger JSPE scores than males. However, the overall mean JSPE score was significantly lower than those for US students. This difference may be cultural, since the Japanese show fewer emotions via facial expressions or gestures (Kataoka et al., 2009).

5.3 Maintaining empathy

Within the US, there are decreases in both cognitive and vicarious empathy as medical students progress through their undergraduate medical education. Various interventional measures were used to try to ameliorate empathic deterioration, but the results were variable, and if successful, empathic increases were usually short-lived. (cf. refs. in Newton et al., 2008). Newton (2008) proposed that the loss of innate empathy makes it difficult to maintain cognitive empathy. Thus, interventions to improve empathic behavior have to be taught on a repeated basis. Given that students who enter an OB/GYN residency have the highest BEES score, i.e., they better maintain their vicarious empathy than students entering other specialties, it is possible that interventions to improve empathic behavior may have a greater impact on these students as compared to those who enter other residencies. However, this suggestion must be weighed against cognitive empathy data that show students desiring an OB/GYN residency have JSPE scores which lie midway in the values for all specialty choices. It may be more desirable for students to have OB/GYN JSPE scores ranked near the top of the specialties, since having both high vicarious and cognitive empathy scores suggests a better outcome for interventions to improve empathy.

All students and physicians, whether in OB/GYN or not, must walk a fine line between being too emotionally attached to patients or being perceived as too aloof and emotionally detached. All humans are naturally repulsed by illness and death and tend to draw away from it (Rosenfield & Jones, 2004). Yet, physicians have selected a profession that deals with what is naturally repulsive. Therefore, it seems only natural that emotional conflicts arise. It is all too easy for a student or physician to depersonalize patients and transform them into a disease, or a cold list of laboratory numbers or physical findings in a medical record (Carmel & Glick, 1996). The increasing use of ever more sophisticated technology makes the depersonalization process all the more pernicious. Depending solely on "concrete numbers and images" hinders the ability to build a meaningful doctor/patient rapport. Spiro (2009) states, "Listening can create empathy – if physicians remain open to be moved by the stories they hear."

Despite decreases in student empathy as they progress through medical school, there are a number of suggested interventions to help improve empathy and, ergo, patient satisfaction. Mindfulness-based stress reduction, self-awareness training, Balint groups, and meaningful experience and reflective practice discussions have been suggested (cf. refs. in Neumann et al., 2011). Rosenfield and Jones (2004) suggested the dilemmas that erode empathy can be broken down into four different areas, each with a given solution:

1. "pathology vs. health" can be balanced with "get to know the whole person"
2. "not knowing vs. knowing too much" with "tolerate ambiguity and remain curious"
3. "vulnerability vs. denial" with "acknowledge the developmental stages you go through"
4. "reaction vs. inaction" with "know when to act"

Success in maintaining empathy depends on having faculty and residents exhibiting and promoting empathic behavior so that they can be role models for the students. Without a doubt, students entering into the clerkships will take on the persona of those to whom they are exposed.

6. The stability of the student and resident population selecting OB/GYN

Regardless of the country examined, most medical students will change their mind about what specialty they want to enter. This occurs between the times when they first matriculate to when they finally select a residency program. The exceptions are those students who are

100% sure they want to enter a particular specialty. In those rare cases, the cons of entering a specialty do not play a significant role in their decision making process. An eighteen-year longitudinal study (1975-1992) at an eastern US medical school revealed only 19% of students who showed an initial interest in OB/GYN, actually entered an OB/GYN residency program. The students who left OB/GYN, usually went into IM (19%) or SURG (17%). In comparison to OB/GYN data, 40% of students stayed with IM, 39% for FM and 22% for PED (Forouzan & Hojat, 1993). Compton and colleagues (2008) sampled the graduating class of 2003 at fifteen US medical schools, and found that at matriculation, 40 out of 942 students indicated an interest in OB/GYN. Of those, ten students (25%) placed into an OB/GYN residency, four (10%) changed their mind after going through the OB/GYN clerkship, five (13%) switched to another primary care residency and twenty-one (53%) switched to a non-primary care residency. In contrast to the OB/GYN data, 15% stayed with PED, 17% with IM and 23% with FM. In all of these cases, those who decided not to enter PED, IM, or FM also switched to non-primary care residencies.

Jeffe et al. (2010) looked all US graduates from 1997 to 2006, and found that the number of students desiring a primary care residency dropped within that time frame. Those desiring OB/GYN remained the most stable, but with low student interest. The numbers of graduates entering OB/GYN dropped from 8.2% to 6.1%. IM dropped from 15.7% to 6.7%. FM dropped from 17.6% to 6.9%, and PED dropped from 10.2% to 6.6%. Of those who entered an OB/GYN residency, 22.7% were male and 77.3% were female. In the UK, from 1974 to 2002, the number of male students who entered OB/GYN dropped from 2.6 to 1.1%. Meanwhile the female percentage dropped from 4.6 to 2%. Overall the number of UK graduates entering into OB/GYN dropped from 3.2 to 2.0% (Turner et al., 2006).

The gender disparity among students interested in OB/GYN was examined by a number of researchers. Gerber et al. (2006) reports that whereas the number of graduates entering OB/GYN residencies remained relatively stable from 1985 to 2000 (6% to 8%), the number of females practicing OB/GYN increased from 12% in 1980 to 32% in 2000. Accordingly, the number of female residents increased from 44% to 74%. Although the number of female OB/GYNs is steadily increasing, it must be remembered that the majority of patients have no gender preference in selecting an OB/GYN, and that only 14.7% of respondents in the study by Johnson and colleagues (2005) thought female OB/GYNs were better physicians than their male counterparts.

An unexpected consequence of the gender shift is that female OB/GYNs tend to work fewer hours than their male counterparts, and are only 85% as productive as full-time OB/GYNs (Pearse et al., 2001). This led the authors to conclude that increasing numbers of female OB/GYNs will lead to an aggregate decrease in OB/GYN productivity. This is occurring at a time when there are increasing numbers of women of all ages in the US, and that a workforce shortage would occur by 2010. (At the time this chapter was written, it's too early to tell if the prediction has come to fruition.)

6.1 How do US students select an OB/GYN residency and what attracts them?

Before the question posed by the section heading can be answered, we must first consider what factors medical students use to select a residency. It appears that for many students the selection of a specialty is somewhat haphazard. Allen (1999) found that UK students are given improper advice on what it means to be an MD. Counseling students on specialties is spotty and often anecdotal. There are few good role models (especially female) to emulate, and faculty advice rarely takes into account medical student abilities and aptitudes. Students are not encouraged enough and are given menial tasks to perform while on the clerkships. This discourages them from entering a particular specialty. Indeed, often a specialty choice is selected via the rejection of specialties until a few remain which are less onerous (Allen, 1999; Kassebaum & Szenas, 1995).

There are a large number of studies which have examined the reasons why entering medical students want to practice OB/GYN, especially if OB/GYN is considered a primary care specialty vs. a surgical subspecialty. Studies reveal that most students who enter into OB/GYN are from a cadre who had expressed a desire to practice in primary care. The remainder of this section summarizes these data, since many studies reveal similar findings.

Prior to the 1980s many of the top students selected IM or SURG residencies. This has steadily shifted to where top students desire residencies that have a controllable lifestyle, e.g., radiology, anesthesiology, pathology, vs. those specialties that are considered to have an non-controllable lifestyle, e.g., IM, FM, OB/GYN (Jarecky et al., 1993; Schwartz et al., 1990). Because of this shift, many students who selected non-controllable lifestyle, primary care residencies tend to have lower undergraduate science grades and lower medical school entrance exam scores, parents with a lesser amount of education, and a rural upbringing. Students who desire a primary care specialty usually state so upon matriculation, and are usually female, older, and a minority. These students have performed a greater amount of community service than the average applicant, espouse pro-social values, appreciate a broad scope of practice, and desire to ensure patients are counseled and educated on health-related issues (Bland et al., 1995; Owen et al., 2002; Reed et al., 2001; Schieberl et al., 1996). Schools which emphasize the importance of primary care, or whose mission is to produce primary care physicians, naturally have more graduates in OB/GYN, IM, FM and PED (Martini et al., 1994).

With special reference to OB/GYN, a series of seven studies, spanning 1991-2007, examined what influenced medical students to enter or reject an OB/GYN career (Fogarty et al., 2003; Gariti et al., 2005; Hammoud et al., 2006; McAlister et al., 2007; Metheny et al., 1991; 2005; Schnuth et al., 2003). Highly rated attractors common to five of the studies were; the student being female, having a positive OB/GYN clerkship experience, as well as being encouraged during the clerkship. (This latter finding was also found to be extremely important by Blanchard et al. (2005).) Expressing a strong desire to practice OB/GYN when entering medical school is also a good predictor. Also viewed as important attractors; were having continuity of patient care, seeing healthy patients, being devoted to patient education, disease prevention, and having strong opinions about reproductive health. Being exposed to a positive role-model was a variable attractor among these studies and influenced some students more than others.

The above seven studies also mention factors that discouraged students from considering OB/GYN. The issue of a non-controllable lifestyle was a variable factor, i.e., it mattered a great deal for some students, but was found to be of little or no concern for others. However, if a student was clearly devoted to entering OB/GYN, the issue of a non-controllable lifestyle, although known by the student, was not a significant detractor. It was very clear that a negative OB/GYN clerkship experience strongly deterred students from entering an OB/GYN residency. Some students felt a patient population restricted to women and/or female reproductive issues did not have a large enough variety of diseases and patients to provide job satisfaction. McAlister and colleagues (2007) found that Asians, Pacific Islanders, and students with no medical school debt, did not consider OB/GYN as a career. Two studies found that male students did not enter OB/GYN because of the perception that patients preferred a female OB/GYN, and/or, there were too many females in OB/GYN residencies so that males would constitute a minority (Hammoud et al., 2006; Schnuth et al., 2003).

Factors that were rated as neutral, were little concern over salary and medical school debt. The cost of malpractice insurance was an issue to a few students, but not a deciding factor if the person was determined to enter an OB/GYN career. Once again, those who were sure about entering an OB/GYN residency did not let the perceived detractors alter their choice. The opposite was true for those who had an initial interest in OB/GYN but were not resolved to practice it (Fogarty et al., 2003; Gariti et al., 2005; Metheny et al., 1991).

In 2005, both Blanchard and colleagues and Nuthalapaty et al. determined which non-medically-related factors were most important for students selecting an OB/GYN residency. There were similarities found in both studies. Many of the highly desirable residency traits were related to the "atmosphere/collegiality" of the residency program. For example, the degree of camaraderie between the residents was very highly rated, as well as how well the faculty cared about, and responded to, resident concerns. Faculty accessibility, commitment to resident education, and geographic location also played an important role for either gender. Females rated having family and friends in the area, the amount of primary care offered by the program, and the resident gender mix as significantly more important than the male's ratings. Males tended to view hospital facilities as more important than females. Males also rated salary and moonlighting opportunities as significantly more important than females, but the rank order of these two factors was near the bottom of the list, indicating that the other aforementioned factors played a much larger role in the decision making process. Results from a 1990 study by Simmonds and colleagues showed the same results. This demonstrated that what students are looking for in a residency has remained stable over a fifteen year period.

6.2 How do students in other countries select an OB/GYN residency?

A Canadian study found residency selection results that were similar to the US students, i.e., having OB/GYN as their first choice when entering medical school, being female, and desiring a narrow scope of practice were strong determinants for an individual to enter OB/GYN. Like US students, being exposed to a good clerkship experience and excellent mentors were very important influences for deciding to practice OB/GYN (Scott et al., 2010). It is important to note, that good mentors in other specialties can draw students away from OB/GYN (Bédard et al., 2006).

In non-North American countries, the reasons to enter OB/GYN vary. In Switzerland, being female, having an in initial desire to enter OB/GYN, being driven to succeed and being "people oriented" were positive attractors (Buddeberg-Fischer et al., 2006). In Germany, 10% of students are interested in OB/GYN because of its positive image, the ability to have a private practice and the variety of illnesses encountered (Kiolbassa et al., 2011). In the UK, having positive, active learning experiences in an OB/GYN clerkship was very important. Conversely, having a poor clerkship experience was a strong deterrent. Exposure to positive role models and having a good mix of medicine and surgery during the rotation were positive factors. Early career advice helped to keep students interested in OB/GYN (Tay et al., 2009). In Jordan, being female, the intellectual content of the specialty, and feeling confident in the specialty, were determining factors to enter OB/GYN (Khader et al., 2008). In Nigeria, material rewards, societal appreciation, and a quick response of patients to treatment, were motivating factors. Like other countries, positive, native, faculty role-models also inspired students to enter OB/GYN (Ohaeri et al., 1994).

6.3 Stability within residency programs

From 1997 to 2001, there was a 3.6% attrition rate for American OB/GYN residents, with female OB/GYNs 2.5 to 5 times more likely than males to leave because of family issues related to their spouses. Females who did leave an OB/GYN residency program were only half as likely to change to a different specialty (Moschos & Beyer, 2004). Most physicians left the OB/GYN residency during or right after their first postgraduate year (PGY) of training (63%), with 29% leaving in PGY2, and only 5% and 3% leaving in PGY 3 and 4, respectively. Gilpin (2005) had similar results with a resident attrition rate of 4.5% in 2003. Most residents left an OB/GYN program in PGY1 (49%), with 34% leaving in PGY2, 13% in PGY3, and 4% in PGY4. Of those who left, 60% went into another OB/GYN residency program, while equal numbers of the remainder selected controllable or non-controllable lifestyle residencies.

More recently, McAllister et al. (2008) looked at US data from 2001 to 2006. Of the 1,066 residents entering an OB/GYN program, 21.6% did not finish for various reasons. Of those who didn't finish, 58.3% switched to a different OB/GYN program, 32.9% left for another specialty, and 8.7% completely withdrew from graduate medical education. Over 90% of the females remained in OB/GYN, while only 41% of males stayed in an OB/GYN program. Residents that switched to a different specialty most often selected FM (18%), anesthesiology (15%), emergency medicine (9%), or PED (6%). Those who did not complete their residency training at their initial site were most often older, Asian, an underrepresented minority, or an osteopathic or international medical school graduate.

Overall, the trend to change OB/GYN residency programs or to leave OB/GYN altogether appears to be increasing. ACGME statistics show that from 1997 to 2005, the rate of departure has increased from 3.8% to 5.1% (cf. refs. McAlister et al., 2008). However, the likelihood of changing from the non-controllable lifestyle of an OB/GYN to a controllable lifestyle varies according to each study (Gilpin, 2005; McAlister et al., 2008; Moschos & Beyer, 2004).

6.4 What are specialty preferences in non-US countries

Table 1 shows there are considerable differences between choices in primary care and SURG in various countries. In all countries, except for Israel and Kenya, the percentage of females entering OB/GYN is larger than the male demographic. Iraq, Brazil and the UK have the greatest percentage of female OB/GYNs (19.1 - 9.6%). Norway, Turkey and Israel have <4%

of female students entering OB/GYN. Brazil, Israel and Kenya have the highest percentage of males entering OB/GYN (16 - 7.3%). Iraq, Turkey and Norway have the lowest numbers of males entering OB/GYN (1.5 - 1.1%).

Table 1 also shows the percentage of students entering into FM, IM, PED and SURG varies by country. More medical students enter one of the above specialties vs. OB/GYN for all countries examined. The IM specialty was most frequently selected in four countries; Brazil, Iraq, Israel and Switzerland. Surgery was most popular in the UK and Kenya, while PED was more popular in Turkey, and FM in Norway.

Country	OB/GYN		FM		IM		PED		SURG	
	M	F	M	F	M	F	M	F	M	F
Brazil (1)	16	16			18	23	14	30	15	6
Iraq (2)	1.5	19.1			20.6	8.8	16.2	8.8	25	0
Israel (3)	9.9	1.7	6.2	4.9	14.6	3.7	11.3	5.4	4.2	0.3
Kenya (4)	7.3	4.4	3.4	1.6	7.8	4.4	12.6	10.4	27.3	7.5
Norway (5)	1.1	3.2	48.1	46.4	10.2	9.1	2.0	3.6	9.8	8.1
Switzerland (6)	1.7	9.6	7.9	9.3	23.7	24.6	4.6	6.3	22.8	4.6
Turkey (7)	1.4	3.1	3.5	0.3	2.0	2.4	6.7	10.2	3.6	0.6
UK (8)	5	10					8	15	28	10

M = Male; F = Female; (1) Castro Figueiredo et al., 1997; (2) al-Mendalawi, 2010; (3) Reis et al. 2001; (4) Mwachaka & Mbugua, 2010; (5) Gjerberg, 2002; (6) Buddeberg-Fischer et al., 2006; (7) Dicki et al., 2008; (8) Lambert & Goldacre, 2002

Table 1. Percentages of students or residents entering into a specialty.

7. Why do residents and practicing OB/GYNs leave the profession?

Job satisfaction plays a large role in any occupation. It is then no surprise that physicians satisfied with their jobs will be more productive, get along better with their colleagues, and have a better mental attitude about job challenges and life in general. This section will explore job satisfaction among OB/GYN residents, faculty and those in private practice, and provide advice on how to enhance the OB/GYN experience.

Before job satisfaction is considered, generational differences on how people think and behave need to be taken into account, since each generation has an opinion on how the other generations behave. Drawing heavily from the publication by Phelan (2010), the "Silent Generation" (born between 1925 to 1942) is characterized as having heavily bureaucratic workplaces with clearly defined leaders, rules, policies and procedures. These individuals postponed gratification, are loyal to their jobs, detail-oriented, and respectful of the hierarchy. The "Baby Boomer Generation" (1943-1961) believes that vigorous competition is necessary to advance your career. They equate "work ethic" with their own "worth" to society and therefore, are driven and work long hours. The Baby Boomers miss many of their children's "firsts" and feel if they "pay their dues" they will eventually be rewarded with advancement.

"Generation X" (1962-1981) usually grew up in homes where both parents worked, or from single-parent homes. They are self-reliant, independent, resourceful and accepting of change.

They expect a balanced lifestyle, and are currently redefining the parameters of a "work week". These individuals saw the advent of personal computers and email. "Generation Y" (1982-2000) people are comfortable with technological advances and expect them to occur at ever increasing rates. *Importantly, GenYers are in a "continuous state of partial attention" due to growing up with cell phones, tweeting, texting, surfing the web and instant communication.* Accordingly, GenYers have difficulty filtering what they "say" because of the increasing amount of electronic vs. face-to-face communication, and this makes expressing empathy difficult (cf. section 5). The lack of verbal communication skills will contribute to their inability to form a trusting physician/patient bond. Furthermore, the speed of obtaining information is more important than dealing with the details, and where the information fits into the "big picture". Since data are only a web-search away, they do not feel the need to memorize large amounts of information. They see no need for knowing the history of a given subject.

For the medical profession, the infusion of Generation X and Y students and residents means they place a greater priority on lifestyle than the previous generations, and seek to have a more balanced work and home life. Thus, physicians born before Generation X and Y perceive these medical students and residents are not as dedicated to their work. Conversely, GenXers and GenYers see the Silent Generation and Baby Boomers working long hours, having too many demands on their time and having a limited or poor work-life balance. In order to maintain job satisfaction for all generations of OB/GYNs, each generation has to understand the other, and make attitudinal adjustments. It is vitally important to realize that although GenXers and GenYers do not desire to work as many hours as previous generations, they are still very dedicated to learning and being proficient. These individuals seek practice settings which provide them with professional satisfaction as well as personal growth. The GenXers and GenYers who seek flexibility in their work should not be considered as lazy or less committed (Phelan, 2010).

When examining all specialties, it is unfortunate that OB/GYN physicians are some of the least satisfied. Leigh and colleagues (2002) and Kravitz et al. (2003) found that only 34% of OB/GYNs were satisfied with their job, while 24% were dissatisfied. These data place OB/GYN physicians at next to last (30/31) for job satisfaction among all specialties. There are two main reasons for this disappointing statistic. Burnout and emotional exhaustion play the major roles which influence the remainder of the reasons for leaving an OB/GYN residency or career. Becker et al. (2006), reported 90% of OB/GYNs had moderate burnout, and 34% were clinically depressed. If a physician was dissatisfied in their profession, they were twice as likely to be depressed and suffer from emotional exhaustion. In addition, 96% of OB/GYN residents feared malpractice, which led 35% of them to pursue a fellowship for additional training. It's logical that depression, emotional exhaustion, and fear of malpractice are highly connected with job dissatisfaction.

Although not unique to OB/GYN, lack of sleep, especially while on call, also leads to burnout and job dissatisfaction. Only 10.8% of residents say they get more than four hours of sleep while on call, while 21.2% get less than one hour (Defoe et al., 2001). Many interns (77.6%) say they were fatigued when on call, while all residents reported negative medical experiences while sleep deprived. Sixty percent of residents feared a compromise of patient care because of a sleep-induced deterioration of clinical expertise. Additionally, a pernicious depersonalization of the patient may occur with sleep deprivation as professional traits are compromised by fatigue.

Perry and colleagues (2003) found that not only does the amount of sleep dramatically decrease after starting an OB/GYN residency, other lifestyle changes also occur which erode OB/GYN health. Residents are ill more often once they start an OB/GYN residency. The amount of time devoted to eating a proper diet and getting exercise drops. Time for religious activities and family interactions also decrease, with the latter causing residents to miss a greater number of "significant" events with the children and/or family. All of these detrimental factors contribute to burnout and emotional exhaustion. Fifty-nine and 61% of OB/GYNs report conflicts with colleagues and patients, respectively. This makes an OB/GYN more than twice as likely to suffer from emotional exhaustion (Yoon et al., 2010).

The traditional thought that working a long number of continuous hours has perceived benefits is not valid. In order to avoid burnout and emotional exhaustion, residents desire having some control over the number of hours worked. Allowing residents more personal time will help increase the current 48% of OB/GYNs that are currently satisfied with their life/work balance. Emphasizing the sense of personal accomplishment among the residents also helps to enhance career satisfaction (Keeton et al., 2007). A new type of practitioner, "The Laborist", can help alleviate the OB/GYN workload and reduce burnout and emotional exhaustion. The laborist is defined as a physician who is solely devoted to obstetric care and, therefore, releases the OB/GYN from being constantly on call when a patient is in labor. This allows the OB/GYN to perform other clinical and office duties without being interrupted until time for delivery. Weinstein (2003) explains the detailed roles of the laborist, and increasing numbers of hospitals are considering their use.

7.1 Why, or why not, practice academic medicine?

Those OB/GYNs that enter academic medicine do so because of their desire to carry out research and the intellectual stimulation that teaching in academia offers. Those that have completed an MD-PhD program are very likely to enter an OB/GYN department vs. entering private or group practice (cf. refs. in Straus et al., 2006). Furthermore, an academic setting is needed for the environment that provides opportunities for collaborative research, and the accommodation of equipment and animal care needs (if any) the research requires.

As residents progress through an OB/GYN program, interest in pursuing an academic career drops with each successive year of training (Cain et al., 2001; Straus et al., 2006). The reality of lower financial rewards and the burdensome bureaucracy associated with academia are, by far, the two primary reasons OB/GYN residents fail to enter academia. Another reason is residents feel they could not effectively balance the time needed to perform research and publish, do committee work, as well as address clinical duties. Cain and colleagues (2001) clearly pointed out the vital importance of good and consistent mentorship in trying to dispel student and resident misconceptions about academia. However, being realistic in addressing these issues is important.

8. Enhancing recruitment into OB/GYN residencies

Making effective teaching a priority in the clerkship or residency program is a must. Actually doing so, vs. giving education "lip service", shows students that an OB/GYN department is not under the sway of the "hidden curriculum" that abrogates teaching to a distant second place after the pursuit of clinical and research dollars (Hafferty, 1998). For example, when the University of Colorado Health Science Center restructured their clerkship to emphasize teaching and mentoring, they doubled the number of third year students interested in OB/GYN. Timely and constructive feedback from residents and faculty increased student satisfaction from 67% to 85%. There were highly significant increases in instructors being viewed as positive role models, being enthusiastic about teaching, and contributing to student professional development (Dunn et al., 2004).

In concert with good teaching, is good mentoring that adequately describes the duties of an OB/GYN physician, e.g., explaining the pros and cons of a private practice vs. an academic appointment. Furthermore, it is advantageous to let students know what to expect in the clerkship or residency, and to develop and nurture a professional rapport. Engaging the students in active learning and problem solving, while providing timely constructive vs. destructive criticism, is deeply appreciated by students. Asking students or residents to self-reflect on the improvements they need to make, shows the students the clerkship cares about helping them to become competent OB/GYNs. Finally, avoid telling students or residents "how it was" when you were in their position — often with a verbalized or implied statement that it was tougher "back then". Students and residents are concerned about mastering their current educational challenges and are not interested in the past.

In 2005, Bienstock and Laube wrote an article about how to recruit medical students into OB/GYN. Foremost, they concluded that clerkships can be improved by writing clear learning objectives for each session. Further, the relative importance of each objective needs to be stated, and the assessment of each objective needs to be clearly explained. Having students exposed to good OB/GYN role models during their basic science years of medical training gives them an early, positive exposure to the discipline. Furthermore, instructors need to give very organized lectures which can be understood by undergraduate medical students who have no clerkship experience. All too often, the author of this chapter has seen faculty or residents (in any specialty) give the freshmen or sophomore students a lecture that was the equivalent of a grand rounds presentation. The lectures were too detailed and contained far too many PowerPoint slides to be shown in a 50 minute period. Student frustration was compounded by the lecturer not emphasizing key, important concepts.

The development of OB/GYN Student Interest Groups (SIGs) can help stir excitement in OB/GYN. Setting up an OB/GYN display during medical school orientation, which is manned by a dynamic resident or faculty member, attracts student attention to your discipline. If other specialties have these SIGs and your OB/GYN department doesn't, it is missing a valuable opportunity to influence interested medical students into sustaining their initial interest in OB/GYN. Furthermore, developing a well-structured OB/GYN elective will maintain student interest, and help sway those students who are considering OB/GYN, along with other specialties, to enter an OB/GYN residency.

9. The future

In 1998, Jacoby and colleagues accurately predicted that within the US, females would soon constitute the majority of OB/GYN physicians. This prediction is becoming reality in many nations. If the increasing number of patients in the aging population is combined with the decreased productivity of female OB/GYNs, especially in their child-bearing and child-rearing years, then there will be a shortage of OB/GYNs (Pearse et al., 2001). Laborists, midwives and FM physicians can only accommodate part of the increased obstetric load, and their use varies widely between countries (Jacoby et al., 1998; Scott et al., 2010; Weinstein, 2003). In addition, the predicted shortage of OB/GYNs will reduce the number of OB/GYN physicians many aging women use as their primary care provider. Therefore, OB/GYN residency programs must take into consideration the need for teaching various primary care skills (including geriatric issues) to their students so that every OB/GYN can be prepared for the aging female population (Frank et al., 1999).

10. Conclusions

There are several major points which need to be considered by OB/GYN residency programs. First, the student population is changing and there are increasing numbers of students who desire specialties with controllable lifestyles. Therefore, enticing students into an OB/GYN program, that is considered to have a non-controllable lifestyle, needs to be started early in their medical school career. Organizing OB/GYN SIGs which expose medical students to good role models is important. Ensuring that faculty and residents make a positive impression upon students in the OB/GYN clerkship will help overcome the decline in OB/GYN interest that occurs during undergraduate medical education. Furthermore, the recent perception that males are not welcome in the profession has to be aggressively overcome.

Second, students and residents must be made fully aware of the varied roles an OB/GYN may have to assume. These future OB/GYNs must be prepared for the obstetric, surgical and increasing primary care roles they may need to provide. Finally, departmental chairs must be aware of the burnout and emotional exhaustion suffered by many of their residents and faculty. Increasing career satisfaction by reducing burnout will be challenging.

Evidence that the empathy of students is declining needs to be taken into account. Therefore, OB/GYN residency programs need to ensure that good physician/patient communication skills are continually reinforced, and that cynicism will not be tolerated. Every academic institution needs to have a review board who addresses breeches in professionalism. Each OB/GYN program needs to ensure that every medical student and resident receives equal opportunities to practice skills and obtain career advice. In this regard, ensuring that OB/GYN departments are not overly dominated by a single gender or ethnic group will help guard against perceived discrimination, as well as provide the students and residents with role models they can emulate.

11. Acknowledgements

The author thanks Mark R. Hurd for editorial assistance and Paul Thorn for support.

12. References

Allen, I. (1999). Factors affecting career choices in medicine. *Baillier's Clin Obstet Gynaecol*, vol. 13, pp. 323-336.

Al-Mendalawi, M. (2010). Specialty preferences of Iraq medical students. *The Clinical Teacher*, vol. 7, pp. 175-179.

Balaya, J. (2010). Male physicians treating female patients: Issues, controversies and gynecology. *McGill J Medicine*, vol. 13, pp. 72-76.

Becker, J., Milad, M. & Klock, S. (2006). Burnout, depression, and career satisfaction: Cross-sectional study of obstetrics and gynecology residents. *Amer J Obstet Gynecol*, vol. 195, pp. 1444-1449.

Bédard, M., Berthiaume, S., Beaulieu, M. et al. (2006). Factors influencing the decision to practise obstetrics among Québec medical students: A survey. *J Obstet Gynaecol Canada*, vol. 28, pp. 1075-1082.

Bienstock, J. & Laube, D. (2005). The recruitment Phoenix: Strategies for attracting medical students into obstetrics and gynecology. *Obstet Gynecol*, vol. 105, pp. 1125-1127.

Blanchard, M., Autry, A., Brown, H. et al. (2005). A multicenter study to determine motivating factors for residents pursuing obstetrics and gynecology. *Amer J Obstet Gynecol*, vol. 193, pp. 1835-1841.

Bland, C., Meurer, L. & Maldonado, G. (1995). Determinants of primary care specialty choice: a non-statistical meta-analysis of the literature. *Acad Med*, vol. 70, pp. 620-641.

Borges, N. & Savickas, M. (2002). Personality and medical specialty choice: A literature review and integration. *J Career Assessment*, vol. 10, pp. 362-380.

Buddeberg-Fischer, B., Klaghofer, R., Abel, T. et al. (2006). Swiss resident's specialty choices – impact of gender, personality traits, career motivation and life goals. *BMC Health Services Research*, vol. 6, p. 137. <http://www.biomedcentral.com/1472-6963/6/137> Accessed July 15, 2011.

Buddeberg-Fischer, B., Klaghofer, R., Abel, T. et al. (2003). The influence of gender and personality traits on the career planning of Swiss medical students. *Swiss Med Weekly*, vol. 133, pp. 535-540.

Cain, J., Schulkin, J., Parisi, V. et al. (2001). Effects of perceptions and mentorship on pursuing a career in academic medicine in obstetrics and gynecology. *Acad Med*, vol. 76, pp. 628-634.

Carmel, S. & Glick, S. (1996). Compassionate-empathic physicians: Personality traits and social-organizational factors that enhance or inhibit this behavior pattern. *Social Sci Med*, vol. 43, pp. 1253-1261.

Castro Figueiredo, J., Lourdes Veronese Rodrigues, M., Almeida Troncon, L. et al. (1997). Influence of gender on specialty choices in a Brazilian medical school. *Acad Med*, vol. 72, pp. 68-70.

Compton, M., Frank, E. & Carrera, J. (2008). Changes in U.S. medical students' specialty interests over the course of medical school. *J Gen Intern Med*, vol. 23, pp. 1095-1100.

Defoe, D., Power, M., Holzman, G. et al. (2001). Long hours and little sleep: Work schedules of residents in obstetrics and gynecology. *Obstet Gynecol*, vol. 97, pp. 1015-1018.

Dikici, M., Yaris, F., Topsever, P. et al. (2008). Factors affecting choice of specialty among first-year medical students of four universities in different regions of Turkey. *Croatian Med J*, vol. 49, pp. 415-420.

Di Lillo, M., Cicchetti, A., Lo Scalzo, A. et al. (2009). The Jefferson Scale of Physician Empathy: Preliminary psychometrics and group comparisons in Italian physicians. *Acad Med*, vol. 84, pp. 1198-1202.

Doherty, E. & Nugent, E. (2011). Personality factors and medical training: A review of the literature. *Medical Education*, vol. 45, pp. 132-140.

Dorsey, E., Jarjoura, D. & Rutecki, G. (2005). The influence of controllable lifestyle and sex on the specialty choices of graduating U.S. medical students, 1996-2003. *Acad Med*, vol. 80, pp. 791-796.

Dunn, T., Wolf, D., Beuler, J. et al. (2004). Increasing recruitment of quality students to obstetrics and gynecology: Impact of a structured clerkship. *Obstet Gynecol*, vol. 103, pp. 339-341.

Fisher, W., Bryan, A., Dervaitis, K. et al. (2002). It ain't necessarily so: Most women do not strongly prefer female obstetrician-gynaecologists. *J Obstet Gynecol Canada*, vol. 24, pp. 885-888.

Fogarty, C., Bonebrake, R., Fleming, A. et al. (2003). Obstetrics and gynecology – To be or not to be? Factors influencing one's decision. *Amer J Obstet Gynecol*, vol. 189, pp. 652-654.

Forouzan, I. & Hojat, M. (1993). Stability and change of interest in obstetrics-gynecology among medical students: Eighteen years of longitudinal data. *Acad Med*, vol. 68, pp. 919-922.

Frank, E., Rock, J. & Sara, D. (1999). Characteristics of female obstetrician-gynecologists in the United States. *Obstet Gynecol*, vol. 94, pp. 659-665.

Gariti, D., Zollinger, T. & Look, K. (2005). Factors detracting students from applying for an obstetrics and gynecology residency. *Amer J Obstet Gynecol*, vol. 193, pp. 289-293.

Gerber, S. & Lo Sasso, A. (2006). The evolving gender gap in general obstetrics and gynecology. *Amer J Obstet Gynecol*, vol. 195, pp. 1427-1430.

Gil, K., Savitski, J., Bazan, S. et al. (2009). Obstetrics and gynaecology chief resident attitudes toward teaching junior residents under normal working conditions. *Medical Education*, vol. 43, pp. 907-911.

Gilpin, M. (2005). Residency attrition rate in obstetrics and gynecology: Are we losing more postgraduates today? *Amer J Obstet Gynecol*, vol. 193, pp. 1804-1806.

Gjerberg, E. (2002). Gender similarities in doctors' preferences – and gender differences in final specialisation. *Social Science & Medicine*, vol. 54, pp. 591-605.

Hammoud, M., Stanfield, R., Katz, N. et al. (2006). The effect of the obstetrics and gynecology clerkship on students' interest in a career in obstetrics and gynecology. *Amer J Obstet Gynecol*, vol. 195, pp. 1422-1426.

Hafferty, F. (1998). Beyond curriculum reform: Confronting medicine's hidden curriculum. *Acad Med*, vol. 73, pp. 403-407.

Hojat, M., Vergare, M., Maxwell, K. et al. (2009). The devil is in the third year: A longitudinal study of erosion of empathy in medical school. *Acad Med*, vol. 84, pp. 1182-1191.

Hojat, M. & Zuckerman, M. (2008). Personality and specialty interest in medical students. *Medical Teacher*, vol. 30, pp. 400-406.

Hojat, M., Mangione, S., Nasca, T. et al. (2005). Empathy scores in medical school and ratings of empathic behavior in residency training 3 years later. *J Social Psychology*, vol. 145, pp. 663-672.

Hojat, M., Gonnella, J., Nasca, T. et al. (2002). Physician empathy: Definition, components, measurement, and relationship to gender and specialty. *Amer J Psychiatry*, vol. 159, pp. 1563-1569.

Howell, E., Gardiner, B. & Concato, J. (2002). Do women prefer female obstetricians? *Obstet Gynecol*, vol. 99, pp. 1031-1035.

Indyk, D., Deen, D., Fornari, A. et al. (2011). The influence of longitudinal mentoring on medical student selection of primary care residencies. *BMC Med Educ*, vol. 11:27 <http://www.biomedcentral.com/1472-6920/11/27> Accessed July 15, 2011.

Jacoby, I., Meyer, S., Haffner, W. et al. (1998). Modeling the future workforce of obstetrics and gynecology. *Obstet Gynecol*, vol. 92, pp. 450-456.

Jarecky, R., Donnelly, M., Rubeck, R. et al. (1993). Changes in the patterns of specialties selected by high and low academic performers before and after 1980. *Acad Med*, vol. 68, pp. 158-160.

Jeffe, D., Whelan, A. & Andriole, D. (2010). Primary care specialty choices of United States medical graduates, 1997-2006. *Acad Med*, vol. 85, 947-958.

Johnson, A., Schnatz, P., Kelsey, A. et al. (2005). Do women prefer care from female or male obstetrician-gynecologists? A study of patient gender preference. *J Amer Osteopathic Assoc*, vol. 105, pp. 369-379.

Johnson, N. & Chen, J. (2006). Medical student evaluation of teaching quality between obstetrics and gynecology residents and faculty as clinical preceptors in ambulatory gynecology. *Amer J Obstet Gynecol*, vol. 195, pp. 1479-1483.

Kassebaum, D. & Szenas, P. (1995). Medical students' career indecision and specialty rejection: Roads not taken. *Acad Med*, vol. 70, pp. 937-943.

Kataoka, H., Koide, N., Ochi, K. et al. (2009). Measurement of empathy among Japanese medical students: Psychometrics and score differences by gender and level of medical education. *Acad Med*, vol. 84, pp. 1192-1197.

Keeton, K., Fenner, D., Johnson, T. et al. (2007). Predictors of physician career satisfaction, work-life balance, and burnout. *Obstet Gynecol*, vol. 109, pp. 949-955.

Khader, Y., Al-Zoubi, D., Amarin, Z. et al. (2008). Factors affecting medical students in formulating their specialty preferences in Jordan. *BMC Medical Education*, vol. 8. p. 32. <http://www.biomedcentral.com/1472-6920/8/32> Accessed July 18, 2011.

Kincheloe, L. (2004). Gender bias against male obstetrician-gynecologists in women's magazines. *Obstet Gynecol*, vol. 104, pp. 1089-1093.

Kiolbassa, K., Miksch, A., Hermann, K. et al. (2011). Becoming a general practitioner – which factors have most impact on career choice of medical students? *BMC Family Practice*, vol. 12, p. 25.
<http://www.biomedcentral.com/1471-2296/12/25> Accessed July 12, 2011.

Konrath, S., O'Brien, E. & Hsing, C. (2011). Changes in dispositional empathy in American college students over time: A meta-analysis. *Personality and Social Psychology Review*, vol. 15, pp. 180-198.

Kravitz, R., Leigh, J., Samuels, S. et al. (2003). Tracking career satisfaction and perceptions of quality among US obstetricians and gynecologists. *Obstet Gynecol*, vol. 102, pp. 463-470.

Lafta, R. (2006). Practitioner gender preference among gynecologic patients in Iraq. *Health Care for Women International*, vol. 27, pp. 125-130.

Lambert, T. & Goldacre, M. (2002). Career destinations and views in 1998 of the doctors who qualified in the United Kingdom in 1993. *Medical Education*, vol. 36, pp. 193-198.

Laube, D. & Ling, F. (1999). Primary care in obstetrics and gynecology resident education: A baseline survey of residents' perceptions and experiences. *Obstet Gynecol*, vol. 94, pp. 632-636.

Leigh, J., Kravitz, R., Schembri, M. et al. (2002). Physician career satisfaction across specialties. *Archives Internal Medicine*, vol. 162, pp. 1577-1584.

Markert, R., Rodenhauser, P., El-Baghdadi, M. et al. (2008). Personality as a prognostic factor for specialty choice: A prospective study of 4 medical school classes. *Medscape J Med*, vol. 10, p. 49. PMCID: PMC2270893. Accessed June 28, 2011.

Maron, B., Fein, S., Maron, B. et al. (2007). Ability of prospective assessment of personality profiles to predict the practice specialty of medical students. *Proceedings (Baylor University Medical Center)*, vol. 20, pp. 22-26.

Martini, C., Veloski, J., Barzansky, B. et al. (1994). Medical school and student characteristics that influence choosing a generalist career. *JAMA*, vol. 272, pp. 661-668.

Mavis, B., Vasilenko, P. & Schnuth, R. (2005). Female patients' preferences related to interpersonal communications, clinical competence, and gender when selecting a physician. *Acad Med*, vol. 80, pp. 1159-1165.

McAlister, R., Andriole, D., Brotherton, S. (2008). Attrition in residents entering US obstetrics and gynecology residencies: Analysis of national GME census data. *Amer J. Obstet Gynecol*, vol. 199, pp. 574.e1-574.e6.

McAlister, R., Andriole, D., Brotherton, S. et al. (2007). Are entering obstetrics/gynecology residents more similar to the entering primary care or surgery resident workforce? *Amer J Obstet Gynecol*, vol. 197, pp. 536.e1-536.e6.

McGrath, E. & Zimet, C. (1977). Female and male medical students: Differences in specialty choice selection and personality. *J Med Educ*, vol. 52, pp. 293-300.

Mehrabian, A., Young, A. & Sato, S. (1988). Emotional empathy and associated individual differences. *Current Psychology Research Reviews*, vol. 8, pp. 223-229.

Merrill, J., Camacho, Z., Laux, L. et al. (1993). Machiavellianism in medical students. *Amer J Med Sci*, vol. 305, pp. 285-288.

Metheny, W., Blount, H. & Holzman, G. (1991). Considering obstetrics and gynecology as a specialty: Current attractors and detractors. *Obstet Gynecol*, vol. 78, pp. 308-312.

Moschos, E. & Beyer, M. (2004). Resident attrition: Is gender a factor? *Amer J Obstet Gynecol*, vol. 191, pp. 387-391.

Mwachaka, P. & Mbugua, E. (2010). Specialty preferences among medical students in a Kenyan university. *Pan African Medical J*, vol. 5, p. 18. <http://www.panafrican-med-journal.com/content/article/5/18/full> Accessed, June 22, 2011.

Neumann, M., Edelhäuser, F., Tauschel, D. et al. (2011). Empathy decline and its reasons: A systematic review of studies with medical students and residents. *Acad Med*, vol. 86, pp. 996-1009.

Newton, B., Barber, L., Clardy, J. et al. (2008). Is there hardening of the heart during medical school? *Acad Med*, vol. 83, pp. 244-249.

Newton, B., Clardy, J., Barber, L. et al. (2007) Who has heart? Vicarious empathy vs. specialty choice. *11th Annual Meeting of the International Association of Medical Science Educators*, 2007 Annual Meeting, Cleveland, Ohio, USA. <http://iamse.org/conf/conf11/abstracts/s10.htm> Accessed July 16, 2011.

Notzer, N., Soffer, S. & Aronson, M. (1988). Traits of the 'Ideal Physician' as perceived by medical students and faculty. *Medical Teacher*, vol. 10, pp. 181-189.

Nuthalapaty, F., Goepfert, A., Jackson, J. et al. (2005). Do factors that are important during obstetrics and gynecology residency program selection differ by applicant gender? *Amer J Obstet Gynecol*, vol. 193, pp. 1549-1543.

Ohaeri, J., Akinyinka, O. & Asuzu, M. (1994). Beliefs and attitudes of interns at Ibadan General Hospitals concerning ten medical specialties. *African J Medical Science*, vol. 23, pp. 341-346.

Owen, J., Hayden, G. & Connors, A. (2002). Can medical school admission committee members predict which applicants will choose primary care careers? *Acad Med*, vol. 77, pp. 344-349.

Pearse, W., Haffner, W. & Primack, A. (2001). Effect of gender on the obstetric-gynecologic work force. *Obstet Gynecol*, vol. 97, pp. 794-797.

Perry, M. & Osborne, W. (2003). Health and wellness in residents who matriculate into physician training programs. *Amer J Obstet Gynecol*, vol. 189, pp. 679-683.

Phelan, S. (2010). Generational issues in the Ob-Gyn workplace. *"Marcus Welby, MD" Versus "Scrubs". Obstet Gynecol*, vol. 116, pp. 568-569.

Piper, I., Shvarts, S. & Lurie, S. (2008). Women's preferences for their gynecologist or obstetrician. *Patient Education Counseling*, vol. 72, pp. 109-114.

Plunkett, B., Kohli, P. & Milad, M. (2002). The importance of physician gender in selection of an obstetrician or a gynecologist. *Amer J Obstet Gynecol*, vol. 186, pp. 926-928.

Plunkett, B. & Milad, M. (2000). How a woman selects her gynecologic surgeon and obstetrician and which factors are important to her. *J Gynecol Surgery*, vol. 16, pp. 107-111.

Myles, T. & Henderson II, R. (2002). Medical licensure examination scores: Relationship to obstetrics and gynecology examination scores. *Obstet Gynecol*, vol. 100, pp. 955-958.

Racz, J., Srikanthan, A., Hahn, P. et al. (2008). Gender preference for a female physician diminishes as women have increased experience with intimate examinations. *J Obstet Gynaecol Canada*, vol. 30, pp. 910-917.

Reed, V., Jernstedt, G. & Reber, E. (2001). Understanding and improving medical student specialty choice: A synthesis of the literature using decision theory as a referent. *Teaching and Learning in Medicine*, vol. 13, pp. 117-129.

Reis, S., Goldfracht, M., Tamir, A. et al. (2001). Trends in medical specialty choice among Israeli medical graduates, 1980-1995. *Israeli Medical Assoc J*, vol. 3, pp. 973-977.

Rizk, D., El-Zubeir, A., Al-Dhaheri, A. et al. (2005). Determinants of women's choice of their obstetrician and gynecologist provider in the UAE. *Acta Obstet Gynecol Scand*, vol. 84, pp. 48-53.

Roh, M.-S., Hahm, B.-J., Lee, D. et al. (2010). Evaluation of empathy among Korean medical students: A cross-sectional study using the Korean version of the Jefferson Scale of Physician Empathy. *Teaching and Learning in Medicine*, vol. 22, pp. 167-171.

Rosenfield, P. & Jones, L. (2004). Striking a balance: Training medical students to provide empathic care. *Medical Education*, vol. 38, pp. 927-933.

Schieberl, J., Covell, R., Berry, C. et al. (1996). Factors associated with choosing a primary care career. *West J Med*, vol. 164, pp. 492-496.

Schnuth, R., Vasilenko, P., Mavis, B. et al. (2003). What influences medical students to pursue careers in obstetrics and gynecology? *J Obstet Gynecol*, vol. 189, pp. 639-643.

Schwartz, R., Haley, J., Williams, C. et al. (1990). The controllable lifestyle factor and students' attitudes about specialty selection. *Acad Med*, vol. 65, pp. 207-210.

Schwartz, R., Jarecky, R., Strodel, W. et al. (1989). Controllable lifestyle: A new factor in career choice by medical students. *Acad Med*, vol. 64, pp. 606-609.

Scott, I., Nasmith, T., Gowans, M. et al. (2010). Obstetrics and gynaecology as a career choice: A cohort study of Canadian medical students. *J Obstet Gynaecol Canada*, vol. 32, pp. 1063-1069.

Simmonds, IV, A., Robbins, J., Brinker, M. et al. (1990). Factors important to students in selecting a residency program. *Acad Med*, vol. 65, pp. 640-643.

Spiro, H. (2009). Commentary: The practice of empathy. *Acad Med*, vol. 84, pp. 1177-1179.

Stalmeijer, R., Dolmans, D., Wolfhagen, I. et al. (2010). Combined student ratings and self-assessment provide useful feedback for clinical teachers. *Advances in Health Science Education*, vol. 15, pp. 315-328.

Straus, S., Straus, C., Tzanetos, K. et al. (2006). Career choice in academic medicine. *J General Internal Medicine*, vol. 21, pp. 1222-1229.

Tay, J., Siddiq, T. & Atiomo, W. (2009). Future recruitment into obstetrics and gynaecology: Factors affecting early career choice. *J Obstet Gynecol*, vol. 29, pp. 369-372.

Turner, G., Lambert, T., Goldacre, M. et al. (2006). Career choices for obstetrics and gynaecology: national surveys of graduates of 1974-2002 from UK medical schools. *British J Obstet Gynaecol*, vol. 113, pp. 350-356.

Vaidya, N., Sierles, F., Raida, M. et al. (2004). Relationship between specialty choice and medical student temperament and character assessed with Cloninger Inventory. *Teaching and Learning in Medicine*, vol. 16, pp. 150-156.

Weinstein, L. (2003). The laborist: A new focus of practice for the obstetrician. *Amer J Obstet Gynecol*, vol. 188, pp. 310-312.

Wright, S., Kern, D., Kolodner, K. et al. (1998). Attributes of excellent attending-physician role models. *N Engl J Med*, vol. 339, pp. 1986-1993.

Yoon, J., Rasinski, K. & Curlin, F. (2010). Conflict and emotional exhaustion in obstetrician-gynaecologists: A national survey. *J Medical Ethics*, vol. 36, pp. 731-735.

Zeldow, P. & Daugherty, S. (1991). Personality profiles and specialty choices of students from two medical school classes. *Acad Med*, vol. 66, pp. 283-287.

Zuckerman, M., Navizedeh, N., Feldman, J. et al. (2002). Determinants of woman's choice of Obstetrician/Gynecologist. *J Women's Health & Gender-Based Medicine*, vol. 11, pp. 175-180.

2

Maternal Immunity, Pregnancy and Child's Health

Alexander B. Poletaev
P.K. Anokhin Research Institute of Normal Physiology Russian Acad. Med. Sci.,
Medical Research Ctr. "Immunculus", Moscow,
Russia

1. Introduction

Why do women live longer, than men? Is gender-connected lifespan related to woman's ability to give a new life and partly depend on persistence of fetal cells in maternal tissues (microchimerism) [O'Donoghue, 2008]? On opposite side, childlessness leads to shortening of an average lifespan of women (http://www.moscowuniversityclub.ru/home.asp ?artId=5742). Some believes, that pregnancy (if happens not too often) leads to mobilizing of the biologic reserves in woman organism and improves the general health state. The phenomenon could be related to positive influence of fetal and placental trophic factors, and besides, to receiving of fetal stem-cell powerful reparative-regenerative potencies. In any case, if result of pregnancy is appearance of a new life (child) and strengthening of the woman's health and longevity, then this phenomenon principally can not be considered from viewpoint of pathology. Accordingly, it seems quite incorrect to habitual using some of "fetal invasion", "maternal aggression", or similar terms, semantically associated with rather negative (pathological) events. Normal pregnancy should not be considered from confrontational positions, because such approach distort the biological sense of pregnancy. Maternal organism does not struggle against new life, but helps embryo with implantation, growth, development and maturation of the last. Moira Howes provides refined arguments for idea that maternal immune influences upon the fetus are principally lacking of aggressiveness, because during gestation mother and fetus are in essence not two but rather one complicated organism [Howes, 2007]. Pregnancy seems to be peculiar example of mutually beneficial co-assistance of two biological systems temporally functioning in frame of united super-organism.

Ideology of this kind may became very useful for explanation of many not yet explained facets of pregnancy, including immune phenomena related to maternal-fetal interactions. First of all, we should decline an habitual attitude to the pregnancy as situation of immune conflict between mother and fetus. From such point of view any forms of mutual aggression should be considered as the pathology which may lead to pregnancy losses.

Is any absurd in this view? Hardly so. Besides we have other bright and widespread phenomena, similar to some extend. For example, any healthy human organism together with its obligatory inhabitants (permanently presented variants of normal micro-flora:

"domestic" microbes) also may be considered as super-organism, whose biologically antigenic components function for mutual benefit. Commensal microflora of gut play principal role in digestion and utilization of food as well as in production of vitamins [Grubb et al., 1989]. It is worth mentioning, that only allied microorganisms provide us with vitamin B12, which plays a key role in the normal functioning of the brain and nervous system, and plays great role for the formation of blood. Vitamin B12 is normally involved in the metabolism of every cell of the body, especially affecting no only DNA synthesis and regulation, but also fatty acid synthesis and energy production [Lieberman, & Marks, 2008; Zaichik, & Churilov, 2008]. Interestingly, B12 can be produced only through bacterial fermentation-synthesis in digestive tract of animals and humans [De Baets et al., 2000].

Today we don't know the most of important details about mechanisms and principles of co-existence with our micro-inhabitants, in spite of fact that symbiotic microorganisms compose nearly 10% of human body weight [Levinson, & Jawetz, 2000]. Fortunately, genetic and antigenic foreignness of such "components" of our body per se, does not imply obligatory mutual struggle [Pradeu T., Carosella, 2006]. Moreover, biologic non-relative organism (normal microflora and host-organism), as well as partly relative (mother and fetus) components forms a new entity – quasi-united superorganism. Of special interest is the fact, that immune system provides the main instrument not for rejection, but for peaceful and mutually useful integration of different and autonomous organisms under the guidance of alive host super-organism [Parnes, 2004].

Due to the system mother-fetus could be considered as peculiar and specialized example of super-organism there is no immunological or any other conflict between integrated components (maternal and fetal compartments) *in normal condition*. In case of united superorganism there is no "foreignness" of integrated components. Nevertheless, in some pathological situations maternal-fetal interactions can become abnormal and can lead to pathology of pregnancy development. Unfortunately obstetricians meet with such pathological cases too often, and comprehension of the main aspects of maternal-fetal interactions from immunological point of view may be practically important.

2. Maternal immunity and pregnancy

Probably up to 40% of all desired pregnancies is interrupted spontaneously during initial 1-3 weeks after fertilization [Radhupathy, 1997]. Additionally 10-15% loss of pregnancies occurs later. Many pregnancies, interrupted at the initial stages, can be related to genetic aberrations [Balakhonov, 2001], but further losses seems related mostly to epigenetic reasons [Poletaev, 2008]. In general most of authors believe that genetic abnormalities are reasonable for nearly 5-13% of unfavorably results and nearly 90% of such cases is based upon other reasons, including changes in immune mechanisms [Radhupathy, 1997; Poletaev, 2008; Sukhikh & Van'ko, 2003]. Participation of the immune mechanisms in regulation of pregnancy is far from being fairly understood yet. However it should be noted that many of cytokines (interleukins, interferons, chemokines) and autoantibodies seem to be important factors involved in mechanisms of tissue's regeneration, growth and cells differentiation [Khaitov, 2002; Poletaev, 2010]. These observations may become a key for the future understanding of the issue from viewpoint of constructive (not destructive) impact of immunity in pregnancy development and fetus formation and maturation.

Historically, immunology emerged as a branch of applied microbiology, therefore "microbiological" approaches and accents have persisted for decades due to the fact that generations of specialists in immunology have been educated by microbiologists. From habitual (microbiological) point of view the pregnancy is a paradox. For solution of this puzzle more than half of century ago Peter Medawar proposed the hypothesis about inability to adequate recognize the "alien" fetus by the immune system of pregnant women – Medawar proposed that this phenomenon could be based upon combined mechanisms of maternal immune suppression and maternal-fetal immune tolerance [Medawar, 1953]. Unfortunately this speculation was too seriously perceived by many obstetricians as rather elevated activity of the immune system during pregnancy [Sacks et al., 1999; Kaštelan et al., 2010]. In his review Entrican specially noted, that pregnancy is accompanied by changes in different components of the immune system, but these changes should not be considered as signs of immune suppression [Entrican, 2002].

Evidently at early 50th Medawar could not think out of frames of traditional views – that is about activity of the immune system aimed to and restricted by searching and destruction of aliens. But now many immunologists re-evaluate the main predestination of the immune system. Nearly half of century ago Pierre Grabar proposed a homeostatic function of the immune system mediated by the natural autoantibodies [Grabar, 1968]. Some earlier, in thirtieths, an idea of the regulatory autoantibodies was mentioned by Karl Landsteiner [Landsteiner, Scher, 1936]. However the main prophet of the new immunological views became Elia Metchnikoff. He had claimed that it would be wrong to consider the immune system mainly as a gendarme of an organism. Its participation in a constant struggle Host-against-Parasite is no more a particular case of much more wide biological predestination of the immune system – dynamic participation in self-maintenance, self-reparation, self-optimization, and maintenance of organism' harmony state under the constant pressure of the Environment [Metchnokoff, 1901]. Not *War but Peace* – or providing general homeostasis or "harmony" in Mechnikoff terms seems to be the main feature the immune activity [Matzinger, 2002; Poletaev, 2010]. Developing fetus is not inspected by the immune system as something hazard and does not became an object for attack in spite of evident non-selfness, but is considered by maternal organism as an object for integration. In this connection active maternal immune recognition of the fetus is an important and necessary condition for normal development of pregnancy [Howes, 2007]. In opposite side, if "the rate of recognition" of embryo and fetus by maternal immune system is too low - it may be reason for pregnancy losses. The last is typical for women with immune suppression related to different causes [Nyukhnin, 2007]. Moreover frequency of miscarriages is directly related to intensity of maternal immune suppression [Poletaev & Morozov, 2000].

More often general immune suppression in fertile women can be induced by chronic opportunistic infections (such as *Herpes viridae, Chlamidia*, etc.), and besides – by prolonged usage of some medicines, chronic intoxications, and chronic psychogenic stresses [Poletaev, 2008]. Situation of immune suppression may be associated with incomplete or insufficient fetal recognition by maternal immune system and with pregnancy loss. Frequent miscarriages are also common for women with genetical similarities to her spouse (in cases of marriage between relatives) because excessive similarities in MHC genes between spouses do not permit maternal immune system to recognize clearly the fetal-paternal antigens [Roberts et al., 1996]. Thus (in case of similarities in MHC patterns of mother, father and fetus) women's immune system turns out to be lacking of full-fledged recognition of the fetus as well as an ability to provide an active maintenance for growth and development of the later.

3. Natural autoantibodies and the health state of the human organism

In recent twenty years clinical immunology was characterized by emerge of paradoxes *sui generis* contradicting to adopted positions of many physicians. As an example, puzzle of natural serum autoantibodies may be noted. The generation of autoantibodies against self-antigens is a common phenomenon in humans. Elevated autoantibody level earlier has been associated directly and exclusively with the pathogenesis of autoimmune diseases. Now it is common place that the rise of serum content of many autoantibodies also occur in the context of other diseases, not belonging to autoimmune ones, including strike, cancer, or complicated pregnancy [Backes et al., 2011; Poletaev, 2010]. Moreover, it was clearly demonstrated that natural a-Abs of IgG, and IgM classes against very different self-antigens had been permanently presented in the blood serum of any healthy person [Lacroix-Desmazes et al., 1998]. Experimental data indicates for roughly equal serum content of a-Abs with the same specificity in the vast majority of healthy individuals [Lacroix-Desmazes et al., 1998], and conversely, indicates notably deviations in production and serum content of particular a-Abs, related to primary molecular changes in the certain cell populations in different tissues and organs, accompanying the plurality of diseases [Poletaev & Churilov, 2010]. It is proved that production and secretion of natural a-Abs is regulated directly by the quantity/availability of respective antigens (by feed-back principle [Kovaliov & Polevaya, 1985]. It is based on the fact, that although expression/degradation rates of any cytoplasmic, membrane, or nuclear antigens in any specialized cells are individual, but at the same time they are similar and represent same relative level/pattern in any healthy person (with slight variation between individuals). Only minor variability in serum level of a-Abs with different specificity is typical for humans in the normal (healthy) state, but not for cases of pathology. Plurality of very different chronic diseases has been connected directly to steady abnormal changes in rates of apoptotic, necroptotic, or necrotic events, as well as to abnormalities in expression/secretion of multiple autoantigens. Such events lead to the changes in a-Abs serum content with according specificity (feed-back principle).

In other words versatile set of natural autoantibodies with different specificity, can be considered as immune fingerprints of molecular content of an entire organism, and mirrors the functional state of the different populations of cells. The general system of autoantibodies has been named earlier as "Immunologic Homunculus" [Cohen & Young, 1991], or "Immunculus" [Poletaev & Osipenko, 2003; Poletaev & Churilov 2010]. Immunculus can be considered as an internal image of the current functional-metabolic state of the body expressed in the terms (language) of quantitative alterations in the content of different autoantibodies. To some extent the Immunculus concept is similar to the concept of Neurological Homunculus, which is an internal image of the body's anatomical/physiological state reflected by the nervous system in the language of the spikes activity of the brain's neuronal nets [Cohen & Young, 1991]. However, in contrast to the dimensionally fixed and morphologically structured neuronal nets, the Immunculus is a dissipative system constructed not by the cellular but by the highly mobile molecular elements: very different autoantibodies presented in the blood, lymph, and interstitial fluid in any spatial compartment of the body. Therefore, the content of autoantibodies with the different antigenic specificity may be considered as roughly the same in various compartments of the bloodstream. This feature permits us (at least potentially) to evaluate the functional-metabolic state of any organ (the heart, brain, liver, etc.) by measuring the content of autoantibodies with respected AG specificity (directed against cordial, brain, or hepatic AGs), presented in the same sample of the serum. Besides natural autoantibodies interacting with molecular structures of the self organism, represent one of the main instruments by which the immune system takes part in the control upon organism's homeostasis [Poletaev & Osipenko, 2003; Poletaev & Churilov 2010]. That is reflected by set of autoantibodies not only as passive "mirror" of the organism's state, but also as an active participator in tuning of the different physiologic functions, including clearance of organism from excessive producing molecular components and debris of dying cells [Poletaev, 2010]. The active regulatory function of the Immunculus has been clearly demonstrated by its participation in the mechanisms of regeneration of injured tissues [Poletaev, 2010]. The control and "tuning" functions of the Immunculus have been visible also in the processes of cellular differentiation and morphogenesis during early (fetal) ontogenetic development [Poletaev, 2008]. Regulatory, reparatory, and/or managerial functions of the Immunculus are illustrated by positive effects of the IVIG therapy in different pathologies (oncology, infection diseases, intoxications, neurology diseases, etc.) [Poletaev, 2008]. This kind of treatment, based on massive administration to the patient of immunoglobulines (autoantibodies), obtained from thousands of healthy donors, leads to the correction of the homeostasis and mitigates very different metabolic and functional deviations.

Serum content of various different autoantibodies is maintained in relatively common ranges (different for autoantibodies with each defined antigenic specificity) in any healthy person – in men and women. In opposite side, constant abnormal elevation or decreasing of some autoantibodies may be secondary reflection of primary tissue or organ pathology and may be used for estimation of clearance effectiveness in injured organ [Poletaev & Churilov, 2010]. More rarely primary abnormal rise of definite autoantibodies may become the background for autoimmune disease [Poletaev, 2010].

Bearing in mind the systemic (not summative) organization of autoantibody Network (Immunculus), it may be easily to comprehend, how it may reflect innumerable multiplicity of functional states of whole organism and its compartments. In this way, we would assume that reflection-recognition process of changeable and innumerable "antigenic images" of the body is based not upon changes of independent elements, but upon the whole immune network (Immunculus). In this context I would like to appeal to only two of quotations: "...The initial paradigm "one autoantibody for one disease" does not appear to be useful any longer. An autoantibody profile does seem to offer more diagnostic and prognostic power than the determination of single autoantibody specificity. The consequence is the use of new assays to detect different autoantibodies" [Meroni et al., 2007]. Backes C. and other [2011] wrote: "Instead of allocating single antigens to a specific group of diseases and even to a specific disease, it appears more appropriate to allocate seroreactivity patterns". This idea identification of autoantibody reactivity patterns, also addressed as autoantibody signatures that are highly specific for various diseases as shown by us and others". The main question is: how soon we will begin to learn very specific language which used the immune system for telling the wonderful story of dynamic changes of ours bodies?

4. Embryotropic antibodies

Serum content of any "embryotropic" autoantibodies [Poletaev, 2008] in healthy women was restricted by narrow limits (as well as for any other regulatory molecules). But at least in 90% of women suffered from habitual miscarriages, still births, or other forms of pathology of pregnancy, these parameters were changed prominently, and more prominent deviations in autoantibodies accompanied more often and severe reproductive problems [Poletaev & Morozov, 2000; Poletaev et al., 2007]. This phenomenon was successfully used for prognosis of result of planned pregnancy [Poletaev, 2010]. Question is – which of maternal autoantibodies of IgG class should be analyzed first of all (between thousands presented)? In accordance to reproductive function, it seems that abnormal changes in serum content of very different (practically any?) maternal autoantibodies may be causal factors of infertility, miscarriages, or other forms of pregnant pathology. That is to say, that plurality of autoantibodies (with any antigenic specificity) synthesized in mother's organism could be considered as "embryotropic" if they belonged to IgG class. Nor IgM, nor IgA, or IgE penetrate the placental barrier [Landor, 1995]. However some of them could be more important.

Systemic autoimmune disorders, SLE in particular, are accompanied by prominent rise of infertility and pregnancy losses. The last phenomenon was so typical, that Gleicher as well as Sherer and Shoenfeld have recommended to consider the recurring miscarriages as indication for supposed autoimmune disorder yet undiagnosed in observed woman [Gleicher et al., 1995; Sherer & Shoenfeld, 2004]. Therefore obstetricians can't overlook such a common marker of SLE and other systemic autoimmune disorders as elevated production of autoantibodies against DNA. Lot of publications about negative influences of anti-DNA autoantibodies upon pregnancy development appears yearly. However it is clear now that situation of excess of anti-DNA autoantibodies is no more than particular example of pathogenic immune influences in pregnancy.

Soon after having described antiphospholipid syndrome (APS) as defined nosology form, attention of obstetricians was draw to autoantibodies against phospholipides (cardiolipin, phosphatidilserin, phosphoinisitol, etc.) and against phosplipid-binding serum protein β2-Glycoprotein I; antibodies against the last seemed to be the most informative marker of APS [Sherer & Shoenfeld, 2004; Roubey, 2006]. It should be noted, obstetricians had met APS long before the syndrome was described by G.R.V. Hughes. Because abnormal elevation of anti-cardiolipin autoantibodies was typical for patients with syphilis, and many years was used for diagnostic of syphilis (since 1906: Wasserman' reaction). On other hand, it was known for decades that maternal syphilis was accompanied with rise of still-birth and miscarriage frequency in affected patients [Borisenko et al., 1998].

Fertility is strictly dependent on serum autoantibody level against DNA or cardiolipin, but also depends on changes in autoantibodies against luteinizing hormone, FSH, prolactin [Talwar, 1997], chorionic gonadotropin [Shatavi et al., 2006]. Premature ovarian failure can be accompanied by excessive production of autoantibodies against specific ovarian antigens [Tuohy & Altunas, 2007] and also autoantibodies against chorionic gonadotropin [Shatavi et al., 2006]. Relation to pathology of pregnancy could be associated with autoantibodies against PSG (pregnancy-specific glycoproteins) [Finkenzeller et al., 2000], against Mater (Maternal Antigen that Embryos Require) [Tong et al., 2004; Tuohy et al., 2007], and many others.

If we will take in mind that autoantibodies are biologically active regulatory molecules it will be evident, not only excessive production, but also shortages in many (any?) autoantibodies could lead to multiple deviations in gestation process, miscarriages and still-birth formation [Poletaev, 2008].

5. Opportunistic microflora as a cause of deviations in serum content of embryotropic antibodies

A lot of wide spreading conditionally pathogenic or opportunistic viruses and bacteria does not belong to the friendly or normal microflora. These inhabitants of the human organism are the most common ground for deviations of the immune system activity and steady changes in production and serum content of embryotropic autoantibodies. Such microbial agents can activate the different clones of immune competent cells, because members of *Herpesviridae* family (Herpes simplex virus, Epstain-Barr virus, Cytomegalovirus, etc) may implement the role of co-stimulators for CD4+ T-cells, and in their turn, lead to polyclonal activation of antibody-producing B-lymphocytes. Such intracellular bacteria as *Chlamydia, Mycoplasmae* and other, may activate B-cells directly (T-cell independent activation) by using mechanism of superantigens [Khaitov et al., 2002]. On the other hand the same microbes in one woman will induce immune deviations nearly inevitably, but in other one microbial influence will be minimal or nearly absent. This difference probably depends on individual genetic background, in particular from individual set of MHC molecules [Poletaev, 2008]. Therefore the fact of revealing of Herpes simplex viruses, Cytomegaloviruses, or *Mycoplasma hominis*, etc., by serological methods or by PCR is not the cause for obligatory prescription of treatment, but revealing of infection agents combined with induced immune changes should be. The situation provided the possibility of monitoring for antiviral or antibacterial treatment effectiveness by dynamic measuring of embryotropic autoantibodies [Poletaev, 2008]. In accordance to clinical observations in women suffered from habitual miscarriages [Serova, 2000] treatment directed to etiology can be the most effective if combined with the control on embryotropic autoantibodies in blood; and improvement of according immune parameters indicates for efficacy and sufficiency of used therapy [Serova, 2000].

Opportunistic microbial flora may induce not only abnormal immune activation, but also become direct cause of pathologic immune suppression, due to usage by microbes multiple molecular instruments for declining general activity of the immune system as important component of strategy of survival in the host-organism [Mayanskiy, 1999]. In their turn prominent maternal immune suppression may influence negatively the pregnancy development and sometimes can be fatal for the fetus [Poletaev, 2010].

Changes in serum content of autoantibodies, if appeared transitory (up to 2-4 weeks), do not influence prominently the fetus development, but long-term or constant prolonged changes may interrupts the pregnancy. Constant abnormal changes in serum content of autoantibodies is typical feature of many women with unexplained infertility (nearly 80-90% of all cases), including ones repeatedly unsuccessfully used IVF [Poletaev, 2010]. In such cases the immune anomalies can interrupt zygote implantation, as well as embryo development. Besides abnormal elevation many of maternal autoantibodies may be reason of pathology in fetus and deviations in child health, because direct action of autoantibodies, or indirectly, by mechanism of maternal immune imprinting (see below) [Lemke & Lange, 1999].

As well as opportunistic viruses and bacteria presented in woman organism may trigger for abnormal production of embryotropic autoantibodies, successful anti-microbial treatment of women with chronic infection will lead to normalization the immune parameters in most cases. It is interestingly to note that nearly 30% of recently infertile women had become pregnant during the first six months after anti-bacterial or anti-viral treatment if therapy was accompanied by normalization of serum content of embryotropic autoantibodies [Serova, 2000]. These observations indicate: some women with "unexplained infertility" in essence are fertile, and their pregnancy may happens often but interrupts at early stages (usually before diagnosing) because severe but reversible immune deviations. This deviations has been reflected and may be detected by quantitative measuring of changes in blood serum content of embryotropic autoantibodies.

Obstetricians often arise the question, which seems to be difficult: why did some women with opportunistic infection suffer from repeated miscarriages and other reproductive problems, but reproductive functions of some other women with the same herpetic or mycoplasmic infection was not disturbed? Serova [2000], and Litvak [2001] in observed patients, and Cronise and Kelly [1999] in experiments with laboratory mice show clearly: the cause of opportunistic (potentially pathogenic) microbial factor does induce systemic immune deviations, such situation is usually associated with reproductive problems. On opposite, the situation usually does not influence negatively the pregnancy course if presence of the same microbial factor has not associates with notable immune changes. These empirical data and conclusions are close to aphoristic idea of the founder of the modern microbiology Louis Pasteur: "microbe is nothing, background (that is reactivity of the host-organism) is everything" [Mayanskiy, 1999]. In this context investigation of serum level of embryotropic autoantibodies may became a useful instrument for evaluation of individual risk of pathology in pregnancy if some viruses or bacteria persist in organism of woman. Such observing is suitable for decision on necessity or its contradictions of antimicrobial treatment before planned pregnancy in each individual case.

6. Human papilloma viruses and reproductive health

Numerous human papilloma viruses (HPV; *papovaviridae*) belong to DNA-viruses. All species of HPV induce typical changes in mitotic activity of flat epithelial cells, and lead to appearance of neoplasm in skin and mucosa. Some variants of HPV are high oncogenic, especially types 16, 18, 31, 33, some other also may induce rare malignancy. Oncogenic variants of HPV may be found in more then 50% of melanomas [Dréau et al., 2000].

Clinical consequences of HPV infection is not restricted by risk of malignancy and cosmetic problems, but by influence on gestation process. In abortions' tissues HPV can be found nearly in 60% of cases of spontaneous abortions, but in 20% of cases, if we have deal with medical abortions [Spandorfer et al., 2006]. HPV prominently decreases the successes of IVF [Spandorfer et al., 2006]. Besides, clinical problems, concerned to inborn malformations of the nervous system, described to be related with HPV. Frequency of neural defects (very different) is arisen 10-12 times in children born by HPV infected women [Poletaev, 2008].

Influence of HPV infection on embryo and fetus development is supposingly related to induction of elevated serum level of autoantibodies against S100 proteins by mechanism of molecular mimicry. Common epitopes in molecules of S100 and few viral antigens were described [Poletaev, 2008]. Two dozen proteins of S100 family take part in regulation of apoptosis, and maturation of primordial nervous system (fetal) [Poletaev, 2008]. Therefore antibody-dependent disturbances of according processes may be related to some forms of malignancy, embryo death cases as well as to malformation of the nervous tube. Consequently the investigation for serum content of autoantibodies against S100 and preventive treatment in necessity should be recommended before pregnancy to each woman with external marker signs of HPV infection (warts, condylomas with any location).

7. Non-infection causes of immune deviations in women of fertile ages

Bacterial and/or viral infection (acute as well as activation of opportunistic infection) probably is the most often reason of deviations in activity of the immune system of investigated person, monitored by changes in serum content of natural autoantibodies. However other reasons conditioned the long-term immune deviations negatively influencing upon general fertility state, conception, pregnancy course and fetal development may be also important. Tight functional interrelation and prominent mutual influences the immune and neuro-endocrine systems [Poletaev et al., 2002] provides effect of falling dominoes. Any changes in the nervous system or endocrine system will obligatory lead to functional changes in the immune system. For example stroke, or thyroidal pathology, or hypothalamic dysfunction, etc. will be accompanied by changes in production and serum content plurality of autoantibodies, sometimes prominent and long-lasting [Poletaev, 2010]. In this connection even chronic psychogenic stresses may became the reason for immune deviations, negatively influencing upon fertility state [Poletaev, 2010]. Corresponding cases may be effectively treated by specialist in psychotherapy with or without using of antidepressants or similar medicine. Different ecological pollutants also can influence upon the immune state and, mediately, the fertility of investigated patient. The same situation may be provoked by incompetent medication in a course of non-professional "self-treatment". All above mentioned factors indicate for necessity of careful analysis of patient anamnesis: clarification of the main reason(s) leading to immune deviations in observed woman may become the first step in correction of reproductive dysfunction in each individual case.

8. Maternal immune imprinting

The biological meaning of a maternal organism in the development of a fetus is exclusive and maternal influences upon child's phenotype, have a priority compared to the paternal ones. It is illustrated clearly by the phenomenon of the epigenetic maternal immune imprinting of a system: Mother–Fetus–Child. The essence of this phenomenon is the "inheritance" by the child's organism many of the individual traits of the immune state of the mother, but not the father [Poletaev, 2008]. As a result, specific features of a child's immunity/autoimmunity become more or less an accurate copy (imprint) of the maternal immune state.

The adaptive meaning of maternal immune imprinting is evident. This phenomenon is responsible for the resistance acquisition against infection diseases by any newborn before the first real contact with the widespread viruses and bacteria. A more pronounced anti-infection immunity in the mother provides more potent inborn resistance against the same infection in her child [Lemke & Landor, 1999]. Observations of such kind provide the ground for possible induction of the inborn resistance to infectious diseases in a child after an active immunization of the mother before her pregnancy. If such approaches will be introduced in medical practice, it should help to reject certain vaccinations or at least decrease their number and frequency for the babies [Poletaev, 2010].

Unfortunately, the Nature is lack of perfectness, and there is another (negative) side of the coin. If mother has been suffered from any kind of immune deviations, the undesirable effects can be produced upon her child directly, as well as indirectly by mechanism of maternal immune imprinting. For example systemic lupus erythematosus in the mother may lead to the development of newborn's lupus in babies at 4-8 months of the postnatal life [Poletaev, 2008]. Woman with abnormally elevated production of autoantibodies against insulin and/or insulin receptors can "imprint" these features in the immune state of her child. As a result, an abnormally elevated production of the same Autoantibodies may be revealed in a 4-6 years old child, and may become a risk factor for the early development of the diabetes mellitus [Budykina, 1998]. The elevated production of anti-thyroid autoantibodies may be revealed for years in children, whose mothers had thyroid problems, and may become the risk factor for the thyroid gland diseases in child [Poletaev, 2008]. Elevated rates of the same forms of pathology in children (endocrine, cordial, nephrological, etc.) which was presented in mothers during pregnancy course [Khlystova, 1987] may be directly related to the phenomenon of maternal immune imprinting.

The main mechanisms of the maternal immune imprinting remain obscure although, we can propose that the fact of antigenic specificity of the phenomenon implies the participation of specialized autoantibodies (probably anti-idiotypic autoantibodies) and/or AG-specific lymphocytes. Transferred trans-placentally maternal anti-idiotypic autoantibodies and/or memory lymphocytes can be the basic elements, which provide a specific activation and tuning of certain clones of the fetal T- and B-lymphocytes, and become main triggers of the inborn pre-formation of the Immunculus of the fetus-newborn-child (similar to maternal ones).

Future investigations of the maternal immune imprinting may provide the new approaches in prediction and treatment of a large group of inborn abnormalities. Besides, the comprehension of the phenomenon may serve as an impetus for the promotion of the fundamental research in the fields of maternal-fetal interactions.

9. ELI-P-complex method

Immune abnormalities reflecting changes in blood serum content of autoantibodies may be found in 85-95% of women suffering from habitual miscarriages or other complications of pregnancy. Long-lasting immune deviations do not necessarily lead to unsatisfactory pregnancy outcomes, but obligatory accompanied by sharp raise of probability of miscarriages, fetal deaths, or developmental malformations [Poletaev, 2008]. Another important issue is the influence of maternal immune deviations upon the health state of her future child. Abnormal maternal changes in serum autoantibodies content during pregnancy if not lead to fetal loss, practically always influence on the newborn health state by means of direct transplacental transfer and by means of maternal immune imprinting [Poletaev, 2008]. Accordingly, evaluation of embryotropic autoantibodies before planned pregnancy (especially in women with obstetrical complications in anamnesis) may became an important preventive measure aimed to decrease of unsatisfactory results of pregnancy.

Especially if predictive diagnosis was combined with treatment, run over under control of immune parameters. It should be noted - in opposite to genetic aberrations, the immune deviations may be effectively treated in the most cases.

Soon after Chernobyl disaster the specialized immunochemical methods for mass-scale investigation of the general health state as well as reproductive health state inhabitants of polluted areas were worked out in the former Soviet Union. These methods were generally named as ELI-Tests (from: Enzyme-Linked-Immune-Tests). One of these methods, just method ELI-P-Complex (abbreviation "P" – from Pathology in Pregnancy) was intended for preventive investigations of a fertile age women. Since 1994 the method ELI-P-Complex has been used successfully for prognosis of the development of planned pregnancy in general obstetrician practice in Russia. Method is intended for analysis of individual "profiles" (patterns) of twelve autoantibodies of IgG class in the sample of blood serum. It is based upon evaluation of partial changes in the contents of autoantibodies against choriogonadotropin, ds-DNA, β2-Glycoprotein I, collagen II type, Fc-fragment of IgG, insulin, thyroglobulin, S100, Spr-06, ANCA, TrM-03, and KiM-05 [Poletaev, 2010]. In spite of diagnostic and prognostic effectiveness of the method proved in thousands investigations, the detailed mechanisms mediating influence of immune deviations measured by ELI-P-Complex upon the gestation process should be elucidated. Nevertheless, there is basis for some propositions. For example, any long-lasting active infection process (viral or bacterial) may be etiologically related to antiphospholipid syndrome induction and accompanied, in particular, by abnormally elevated serum levels of autoantibodies against β2-Glycoprotein I and DNA [Poletaev, 2008]. The mentioned autoantibodies could be pathogenically related to changes in blood coagulation [Sherer & Shoenfeld, 2004] which, in turn, may cause vascular problems in placenta and affect the gestation process. Relative surplus of anti-collagen II autoantibodies may indicate inborn or acquired defects of the connective tissue and active adhesion process. Changes in serum autoantibodies against S100 are typical for some women with still-births and fetal/newborns neural malformations in anamnesis, and are related in most cases with active replicated papilloma viruses. A surplus of autoantibodies against choriogonadotropin may be the reason for deficiency in this hormone, which is important for placenta development and maturation, as well as for cases of premature ovarian failure [Tuohy & Altuntas, 2007]. Excess of autoantibodies against Fc-fragments of IgG (Rheumatoid factor) is indicator of inflammatory processes of any localization. Elevated peak of autoantibodies against Spr-0.6 may be indication of declining fertility and in most cases is sensitive marker sign of endometritis and/or inflammatory processes in other pelvic organs. Abnormal rise of autoantibodies against insulin, thyroglobulin, ANCA, TrM-03, and KiM-05 in detected profiles may be markers of diabetic fetopathy, thyroidal abnormalities, vasculopathy and kidney-related disorders in pregnant women [Poletaev, 2010]. An early detection (especially before planned pregnancy) of relative deviations in serum content some of measured autoantibodies is especially important for revealing of individuals with elevated risk of abnormalities expected at pregnancy and implementation of necessary prophylactic measures.

10. Clinical illustrations

The main field for using of ELI-P-Complex method is screening of women planning their pregnancy, IVF including. Immune deviations revealed by this method are related to or reflect some individual health problems, and characteristic changes of autoantibodies profiles, that should be considered as prompting message for obstetrician about peculiar changes in woman' organism, which may be additionally investigated and effectively treated before pregnancy.

10.1 Some examples

In accordance to observations by Zhegulina [2002] 94% of women suffering from thyroid pathology were characterized by changes in serum content of embryotropic autoantibodies. Adequate preventive treatment under control of ELI-P-Complex method leads to 2,5-fold decreasing of unsatisfactory result frequency of the following pregnancy compared to pregnancy of women without immune control.

In accordance to observations by Nukhnin [2007] normal serum content of embryotropic autoantibodies has been found only in 7,4% of pregnant women with obstetrician complications in anamnesis, and deviations were typical in 93,6% of such women. Abnormal decreasing of numerous embryotropic autoantibodies was directly associated with miscarriages, placental insufficiency, and preeclampsia. Abnormal serum rise of them was typical for miscarriages, stillbirth, preeclampsia, and inborn anomalies.

In accordance to observations by Cherepanova [2008] there are direct relations between changes in serum content of some of embryotropic autoantibodies in early pregnancy and cases of pre-term abruption of placenta, preeclampsia at late pregnancy, and abnormal uterine bleedings at delivery. Special algorithm for evaluation of risk level of the noted complications was proposed. Abnormal decreasing of some of embryotropic autoantibodies as well as abnormal elevation was associated with deviations in the blood coagulation.

In accordance to observations by Makarov [2009] decreasing in serum content of some of embryotropic autoantibodies in early pregnancy gives possibility to screen women of the high risk for the future preeclampsia developing. Some changes in embryotropic autoantibodies serum levels provide possibility to differentiate between group of women with preeclampsia and chronic hypertension.

In accordance to Serova [2000] very different factors (infection agents, endocrine disfunction, environmental pollutions, drugs, chronic stresses, etc.) can be ground for steady changes in production and blood serum content of embryotropic autoantibodies. Characteristic of individual serum profiles of embryotropic autoantibodies may indicate to the main cause of revealing changes, and effective individualized correction (etiologic treatment) of women under control of embryotropic autoantibodies provides 5 to 8-fold rise of satisfactory result of pregnancy following.

In accordance to observations by Kluchnikov et al., [2001]., if children were born by women with the normal parameters of ELI-P-Complex method, at least 70% of them was evaluated as practically healthy persons at ages 4-6 years old. In opposite, no more then 15% children were evaluated as practically healthy if were born from women with steady deviated parameters of serum' autoantibodies.

Described examples represent only a small part of the general massive data obtained during the last twenty years and indicate clear necessity of wide using of preliminary evaluation of different embryotropic autoantibodies in women serum before planned pregnancy, especially in women belonging to a group of obstetrician risk.

Antigen	Possible clinical consequences of abnormal changes in relative serum content of according natural autoantibodies
Chorionic Gonadotropin	Excess of autoantibodies against this AG usually is indication of endocrine dysfunction and may be the cause of the functional insufficiency of choriogonadotropin. The last may lead to infertility, placental malformation, and placental insufficiency. Most cases of prolonged (months and years) abnormally elevated production of such autoantibodies is related to recent treatment by Pregnyl or Choragon during preparation for IVF. Besides excess of autoantibodies against this AG can be a marker sign of premature ovarian insufficiency. Rarely it may be indication for malignancy (tumor of pituary gland mostly).
DNA	Rise of autoantibodies against this AG may indicate for activation of apoptosis (virus-induced mainly). Rarely it may be indication for systemic autoimmune disease or malignancy. Excess of such autoantibodies may reveal embryotoxic effects.
B2-Glycoprotein I	Excess of autoantibodies against this AG is marker sign of anti-phospholipid syndrome which may be the cause of a small vessels thrombosis in placenta and other organs and leads to placental insufficiency. Rarely it may be indication for systemic autoimmune disease or malignancy. Excess of such autoantibodies may reveal embryotoxic effects.
Collagen II	Excess of such autoantibodies usually is indication for adhesions and scars formation. Besides excess of autoantibodies against this AG may be sign of pathological changes in a connective tissue. Excess of such autoantibodies may reveal embryotoxic effect.
Fc-fragment of IgG	Excess of autoantibodies against this AG (Rheumatoid factor) is indicator of inflammatory processes of any localization as well as of elevated production of proinflammatory cytokines. Excess of such autoantibodies may reveal embryotoxic effects.
Insulin	Excess of autoantibodies against this AG may be pathogenic factor for diabetic fetopathy. Besides elevated autoantibodies against insulin can be sign of the endothelial disfunction and vasculopathy, and may indicate initiated or forming gestational diabetes or insulin-dependent diabetes type I
Thyroglobulin	Excess of autoantibodies against this AG may be marker sign of the existing or forming disturbances in the thyroid gland. Excess of such autoantibodies may reveal embryotoxic effects.
S100	The most often reason for long-term elevated production of such autoantibodies is human papilloma virus infection (by mechanism of molecular mimicry). Excess of autoantibodies against S100 proteins may lead to deviations of general morphogenesis and cellular differentiation in embryo, and be cause for stillbirth at the beginning, in the middle, or at the end of pregnancy. Besides it may be reason of malformation of the nervous system because S100 is involved in differentiation and migration of neuroblasts of primordial nervous system.
Spr-06	Excess of such autoantibodies usually is marker sign of endometritis (in the most cases) and/or inflammatory processes in other pelvic organs (rarely). Excess of autoantibodies against Spr-06 may be cause of declining fertility in women and men.
ANCA	Excess of ANCA-specific autoantibodies is typical sign of different forms of small vessel vasculitis and vasculopathy. The last may be reason for deterioration of placental blood flow, as well as other organ malfunction related to the problems with blood circulation.
TrM-03	Excess of autoantibodies against TrM-03 is sign of trombocytopathy and may lead to the following deviations: 1) Elevated lysis of platelets which leads to pathological bleeding; 2) excessive aggregation of platelets (without their lysis) and trombotic events
KiM-05	Excess of autoantibodies against KiM-05 should be considered as marker sign of active inflammatory process in the renal tissue

Table 1. List of antigens used for detection and analysis of changes in relative serum contents of according autoantibodies by ELI-P-Complex method.

11. Acknowledgement

Author especially wish to thank *Dr. Sergey Skurydin and Dr. Sergey Humanov* for excellent help in preparation and translation of the text.

12. References

Backes C, Ludwig N, Leidinger P, Harz C, Homann J, Keller A, Meese E, Lenho H-P. Immunogenicity of autoantigens. BMC Genomics 2011; 12:340 doi:10.1186/1471-2164-12-340.

Balakhonov AV (2001). *Developmental errors*. ELBI-St.Pb Publishing, St. Petersburg, Russia.

Borisenko KK, Dolya OV, Loseva OK, Tumanova EL. Early inborn syphilis. Russian Med J 1998;15:12-16.

Budykina TS (1998). Meaning of autoantibodies against insulin, insulin receptors and NGF for diabetic fetopathy. *Dissertation PhD*, Moscow, Russia.

Cherepanova NA (2008). Analysis of the serum levels of some natural autoantibodies for evaluation of risk of pre-eclampsia. *Dissertation PhD*, Kazan, Russia,

Cohen IR, Young DB. Autoimmunity, microbial immunity and the immunological homunculus. Immunol Today 1991;12:105-110.

Cronise K, Kelly SJ. Does a maternal urinary tract infection during gestation produce a teratogenic effects in the Long-Evans rats? Soc Neurosci 1999;25 pt.2:2019.

De Baets S, Vandedrinck S, Vandamme EJ. (2000). "Vitamins and Related Biofactors, Microbial Production". *In: Lederberg J. Encyclopedia of Microbiology*. 4 (2 ed), pp. 837–853, Academic Press, New York, USA.

Dréau D, Culberson C, Wyatt S, Holder WD. Human Papilloma Virus in Melanoma Biopsy Specimens and Its Relation to Melanoma Progression. Ann Surg 2000;231:664–671.

Entrican G. Immune regulation during pregnancy and host-pathogen interactions in infectious abortion. J Comp Pathol 2002;126:79–94.

Finkenzeller D, Fischer B, McLaughlin J, Schrewe H, Ledermann B, Zimmermann W. Trophoblast cell-specific carcinoembryonic antigen cell adhesion molecule 9 is not required for placental development or a positive outcome of allotypic pregnancies. Mol Cell Biol 2000;20:7140-7145.

Gleicher N, Pratt D, Dudkiewicz A. What do we really know about autoantibody abnormalities and reproductive infertility? Contracept Fertil Sex 1995;23:239-254.

Grabar P (1968). About autoantibodies. In: *Problems of reactivity in pathology* (AD Ado, ed.), pp. 35-52. Meditsina, Moscow, Russia.

Grubb R, Midtvedt T, Norin E (eds). (1989). *The Regulatory and Protective Role of the Normal Microflora*. Macmillan, New York, USA.

Howes M. (2007). Maternal agency and the immunological paradox of pregnancy. *In: H. Kincaid and J. McKitrick (eds.), Establishing Medical Reality*, 179–198, Springer, Heidelberg, Germany.

O'Donoghue K. Fetal microchimerism and maternal health during and after pregnancy. Obstetric Medicine 2008;1:56-64.

Kaštelan S, Tomić M, Pavan J, Orešković S. Maternal immune system adaptation to pregnancy – a potential influence on the course of diabetic retinopathy. Reprod Biol Endocrinol 2010;8:124 doi:10.1186/1477-7827-8-124
http://www.rbej.com/content/8/1/124

Khaitov RM, Ignatyeva GA, Sidorovich IG. (2002). *Immunology*. Meditsina Publishing, Moscow, Russia.

Khlystova ZS (1987). *Immunogenesys in human fetus*. Meditsina Publishing, Moscow, Russia.

Kluchnikov SO, Poletaev AB, Budykina TS, Generalova GA (2001). Mew methods of immunobiotechnology in perinathology and pediatrics. In: *Lectures in Pediatrics* (VF Demin, SO Kluchnikov, eds.). RGMU Publishers, 243-267, Moscow, Russia.

Lacroix-Desmazes S, Kaveri SV, Mouthon L, Ayouba A, Malanchere E, Coutinho A, Kazatchkine MD. Self-reactive natural autoantibodies in healthy individuals. J Immunol Methods1998;216:117-137.

Kovaliov IE, Polevaya OY (1985). *Biochemical grounds for immunity against low-molecular chemical compounds*. Nauka Publishers, Moscow, Russia.

Landor M. Maternal-fetal transfer of immunoglibulins. Ann Allergy Asthma and Immunology 1995;74:279-283.

Landsteiner K van der Scher J. On cross reactions of immune sera to azoproteins. J Exp Med1936;63:325–339.

Lemke H, Lange H. Is there a maternally induced immunological imprinting phase a la Konrad Lorenz? Scand. J. Immunol 1999;50:348-354.

Levinson W, Jawetz E (2000). *Medical Microbiology & Immunology* 3rd ed., Appleton & Lange, Philadelphia, USA.

Lieberman M. A., & Marks A. (2008). *Basic Medical Biochemistry: a Clinical Approach*, 3rd edition, Lippincott Williams and Wilkins, Baltimore, USA.

Litvak OG (2001). Laparoscopy for treatment of tubulo-peritoneal infertility. *Dissertation PhD*, Moscow, Russia.

Makarov OV, Osipova NA, Poletaev AB. Autoantibodies and diagnosis of pre-eclampsy. Medicine – XXI Century 2009;14:28-32.

Matzinger P. The danger model: a renewed sense of self. Science 2002;296:301-305.

Mayanskiy AN (1999). *Microbiology for physicians*. NMGA Publishing, Nizhny Novgorod, Russia.

Medawar PB. Some immunological and endocrinological problems raised by the evolution of viviparity in vertebrates. Symposia-Society for Experimental Biology 1953;44:320-338.

Meroni PL, De Angelis V, Tedesco F (2007). Future Trends. In: *Autoantibodies*, (Y Shoenfeld, ME Gershwin, PL Meroni, Eds.), 823-826, Elsevier, B.V., Nederland.

Metchnokoff E. (1968). *Immunity in infective diseases*. Johnsom Reprint, New York, USA. (Original published 1901).

Niukhnin M.A. (2007). Autoantibodies analysis and the problem of optimization of the tactics of the pregnant women treatment. *Dissertation PhD*, Kazan, Russia.

Parnes O. From interception to incorporation: degeneration and promiscuous recognition as precursors of a paradigm shift in immunology. Molec Immunol 2004;40:985-991.

Poletaev AB. (2008). *Immunophysiology and immunopathology*. Medical Information Agency. Moscow, Russia.

Poletaev AB. (2010). *Physiological immunology*. Micklosh Publishing, Moscow, Russia.

Poletaev AB, Morozov SG. Changes of maternal serum natural antibodies of IgG class to proteins MBP, S100, ACBP14/18 and MP65 and embryonic misdevelopments in humans. Human Antibody 2000;9:215-221.

Poletaev AB, Morozov SV, Kovaliov IE. (2002). *The regulatory metasystem (united neuro-immuno-endocryne system in regulation of the physiologic functions)*. Meditsina Publishing, Moscow, Russia.

Poletaev A, Osipenko L. general network of natural autoantibodies as Immunological Homunculus (Immunculus). Autoimmunity Rev 2003;2:264-271.

Poletaev AB, Churilov LP. Immunophysiology, natural autoimmunity and human health. Anosia 2010;6:11-18.

Poletaev AB, Maltseva LI, Zamaleeva RS, Nukhnin MA, Osipenko LG. Application of ELI-P-Complex method in clinical obstetrics. Amer J Reprod Immunol 2007;57:294–301.

Pradeu T, Carosella ED. On the definition of a criterion of immunogenicity. Proc Nat Acad Sci 2006;103:17858–17861.

Radhupathy R. Th1-type immunity is incompatible with successful pregnancy. Immunol Today 1997;18:478-451.

Roberts RM, Xie S, Mathialagan N. Maternal recognition of pregnancy. Biol Reprod 1996;54:294–302.

Roubey RAS (2006). Antiphospholipid Syndrome. In: *The Autoimmune Diseases, (eds. Noel R. Rose and Ian R. Mackay)*, 4th Edition, pp. 381-392, Elsevier, Amsterdam, The Netherlands.

Sacks G, Sargent I, Redman C. An innate view of human pregnancy. Immunol Today 1999;20:114–118.

Sherer Y, Shoenfeld Y (2004). *The antiphospholipid syndrome*. Published by Bio-Rad Lautoantibodies, USA.

Serova OF (2000). Pre-gestational treatment of the women with habitual miscarriages. *Dissertation MD*, Moscow, Russia.

Shatavi SV, Llanes B, Luborsky JL. Association of unexplained infertility with gonadotropin and ovarian antibodies. Amer J Reprod Immunol 2006;56:286–291.

Spandorfer S, Bongiovanni A, Fasioulotis S, Rosenwaks Z, Ledger W, Witkin S. Prevalence of cervical human papillomavirus in women undergoing in vitro fertilization and association with outcome. Fertility a. Sterility 2006;86:765-767.

Sukhih GT, Van'ko LV (2003). *Immunology of pregnancy*. Russ. Acad. Med. Sci. Publishing, Moscow, Russia.

Talwar GP. Fertility regulating and immunotherapeutic vaccines reaching human trials stage. Human Reproduction Update1997;3:301–310.

Tong ZB, Gold L, De Pol A, Vanevski K, Dorward H, Sena P, Palumbo C, Bondy CA, Nelson LM. Developmental expression and subcellular localization of mouse MATER, an oocyte-specific protein essential for early development. Endocrinology 2004;145:1427-1434.

Tuohy VK, Altuntas CZ. Autoimmunity and premature ovarian failure. Reprod Endocrinol Curr Opinion in Obstetrics Gynecol 2007;9:366-369.

Zaichik AS, Churilov LP (2008). Basics of pathochemistry. OLBY-Press, St. Petersburg, Russia.

Zhegulina SG (2002). Perinatal problems in children from women with thyroid dysfunction; Immunology aspects. *Dissertation PhD*, Moscow, Russia.

3

Environmental Electromagnetic Field and Female Fertility

Leila Roshangar and Jafar Soleimani Rad

Tabriz University of Medical Sciences, Tabriz,
Iran

1. Introduction

Human beings are unavoidably exposed to ambient electromagnetic fields (EMFs) generated by every instrument that uses electricity. Electromagnetic fields are made by the combination of an electric field and a magnetic field and is propagated in a wave like manner. Thus sometimes called electromagnetic waves and or electromagnetic radiation. Under such condition the indoor and outdoor environment we live are bombarded by electromagnetic waves/radiations produced by home appliances; such as computer, television , mobile phone, industrial instruments; such as power transmission lines railway stations, medical and diagnostic tools; such as MRI, physiotherapy equipments and so on. The EMF which we are encountered everywhere, have a non ionizing nature and has two distinct parts; electrical and magnetic. The electrical part is generated by a voltage gradient and measured in volts. The magnetic part is produced by current flow and is measured in tesla. Therefore in any field, we are exposed to an electrical voltage gradient and a magnetic field. The electrical field is due to the difference between the voltage of the electricity used by the device and earth. The magnetic field is proportional to the current flowing through the device. Both types of field would induce biological effects, but magnetic field is more damaging because it penetrates living tissue more easily. Magnetic fields as low as around one microtesla can produce biological effects (Goldsworthy 2007; Sage et al. 2007; Jokela et al. 2004). The effect of EMF on human health vary widely depending on the frequency and intensity of the fields. Extremely low frequencies (ELF) such as those from home appliances are more potent than higher frequencies of radio waves (Genuis 2007; Zymslony 2007; Torregrossa 2005). According to WHO, EMFs of all frequencies represent one of the most common and fastest growing environmental influences, about which anxiety and speculation are spreading. All populations are now exposed to varying degree of EMF, and the levels will continue to increase as technology advances. It is obvious that in almost all societies the ambient EMFs are encountered everywhere and cause unavoidable exposure. There are body of information regarding adverse effects of EMF, especially chronic exposure to EMF (Wu 2008; Marek 2004; Adey 1993). Thus the concern about the public health hazards of EMFs has highly increased.

Based on the functional and or structural disorders it is shown that in a biological system, EMF may harm any organ. Epidemiological studies suggest a possible link between EMF exposures and clinically recognized medical disorders such as leukemia, brain cancer, breast cancer, kidney cancer and or cardiovascular disease (Kovacic and Pozos 2006; NRC 1996; UNEP/WHO/IRPA 1987). An ultra-structural study on rats shows that long term exposure to EMF could result in lymphatic organ disturbances and consequently weakening of immune system (Mohammadnejad et al. 2010). Some authors have reviewed risks of EMF exposure on reproduction and demonstrated that experimental exposure to EMF in laboratory animals has several adverse effects (Djeridane et al. 2008; Ozguner et al. 2005; Chung et al. 2005; Ahmed et al. 2002; elbetieha et al. 2002; Cheronff et al. 1992). There are numerous studies showing that EMF exposure of male rat/mice affects testicular architecture , spermatogenesis, sperm motility, leydig cell reduction, increased apoptosis of germ cells and in general subfertility and or infertility (Khaki et al. 2006; Lee et al. 2004; Soleimani Rad and Katebi 1997; Devita et al. 1995; Lokmatova 1993). In human and animal studies, it has been reported that female exposure to EMF cause some adverse effects and reviewed the potential effect of EMFs on infertility, implantation rate, number of living fetuses, sex ratio, miscarriages, premature births, growth retardation, low birth weight, congenital malformations and prenatal deaths (Roshangar and Soleimani Rad 2007; Lahijani et al. 2007; Feychting et al. 2005; Chiang et al. 1995; Huuskonen et al. 1993; Juutilainen et al. 1993; Mc Govern et al. 1990).

Although the epidemiological studies on the effect of EMF exposure in human, are not conclusive but the experimental findings on the effect of EMF on different organs would act as a corner stone for exploring the complicated topic of EMF effect on reproduction. As several organs are involved in the fertility of females and their well being are necessary for fertility, the present chapter will deal with the effect of EMF on three major female reproductive organs i.e. ovary, fallopian tubes and uterus.

2. Methods

In these series of experiments the Wistar rats are used as an experimental model and the studies were approved by the ethical committee of Tabriz University of Medical Sciences. For producing EMF, an EMF generating apparatus was designed in the Department of the Histology and Emberyology. The apparatus uses 220 V and 50 HZ alternative current and could generate up to 5 milli tesla EMF. In the presented studies, the adult female rats were exposed to 3 milli tesla, 4 hours/day for 2 months. After the experimental period the rats were sacrificed and their reproductive organs including; ovaries, uteri, and uterine tubes were dissected apart. Half of the samples were fixed in 10% formalin and paraffin-embedded sections were used for light microscopy and immunohistochemical studies. TUNEL techniques were used for detection of apoptosis and Ki-67 technique for proliferation assay. In both cases toluidine blue was used for counterstaining.

The other half of the samples were fixed in 2% glutaraldehyde and resin embedded ultra thin sections were used for electron microscopy.

3. Results

3.1 Ovarian effect of EMF exposure

Ovary is an organ involved in follicular development and germ cell production. In other word, the ovary provides a proper environment for oogenesis. Any disturbances in ovarian function may lead to the folliculogenesis disorder and or ceasing of ovulation. Several factors including hormonal disturbances, changes in ovarian stroma and or any factor that affect oocyte maturation would affect oogenesis.

3.1.1 Light microscopic studies

Light microscopy showed that, in control group, oocyte had a euchromatic nucleus and was encompassed with a homogenous zona pellucida, and well organized corona radiate and granulosa cells (Figure 1-A). In experimental group, the oocyte had a condensed nucleus so that it appeared small and darkly stained (Figure 1B). The cytoplasm of the oocytes were condensed and surrounding zona pellucida had changed and appeared narrower than that in control group (Figure 1B). The cells in granulosa and corona radiata layers were disorganized and contained dense nuclei (Figure 1B).

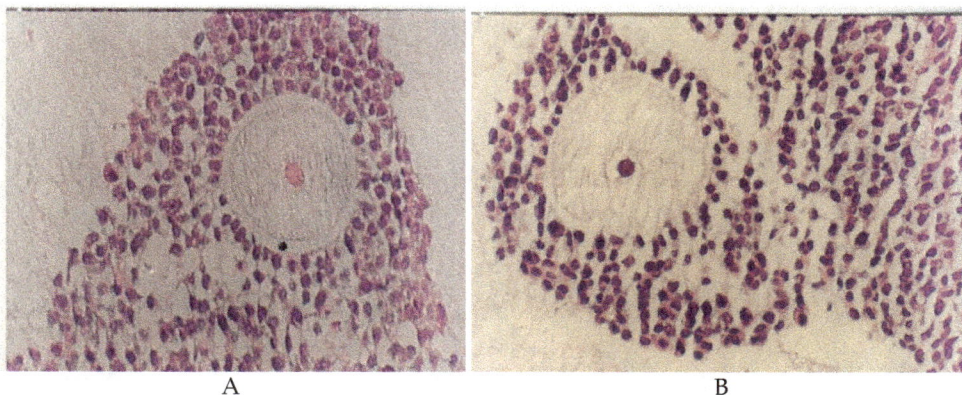

A   B

Fig. 1. Photomicrographs of ovarian sections from rat ovaries. A-from control group, showing part of a graffian follicle with oocyte and cumulus. B-from EMF-exposed group, showing an oocyte with condensed nucleus, surrounded with a faint zona pellucida and an irregularly arranged cumulus and corona radiata. H&E staining. 300X.

Ovarian stroma both in cortex and medulla contained several macrophages wich was rarely seen in control group and their number was higher in cortex than the medulla (Figure 2). Morphometric studies revealed that the number of ovarian follicles, in different stages of development, were higher in EMF-exposed group, but the number of corpora lutea were fewer than the control group. Atretic follicles in the EMF-exposed group were numerous than the control group.

3.1.2 Electron microscopic studies

Ultra structural studies revealed that granulosa cells in control group, were regularly arranged and the corona radiate layer was composed of columnar cells that were attached to eachother by intercellular junctions. Their microvilli were penetrated into zona pellucid and could be recognized in it. The cytoplasm of coronal cells contained different organels including spherical or ovoid mitochondria with limited cristae (Figure 3).

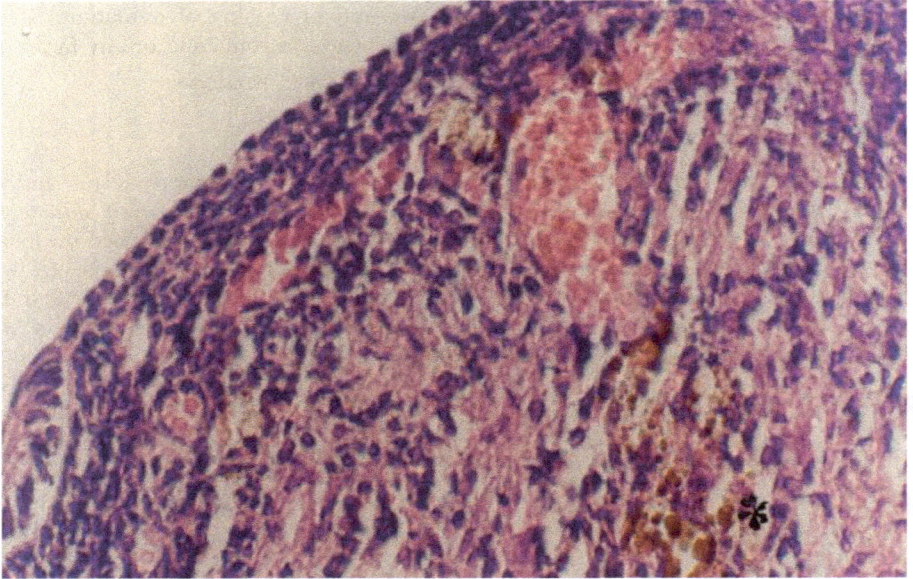

Fig. 2. Photomicrograph of a section of an ovary from EMF-exposed rat. Showing several macrophages with brownish residual bodies (*). H&E staining. 200X.

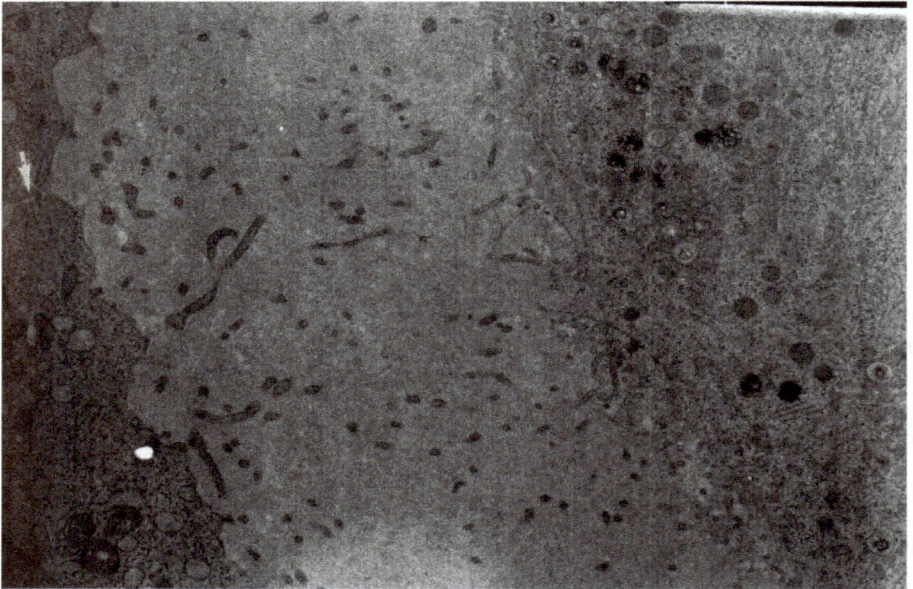

Fig. 3. Electron micrograph of developing follicle from a control rat ovary. Note the thickness of zona pellucida and sections of microvilli from oocyte and granulosa cells in it. cellular junction between granulosa cells is obvious (arrow). 15000X.

Cytoplasm of oocytes in this group contained numerous lamellae, scattered organells including round or ovoid mitochondriae with short and limited crista. The endoplasmic reticulum were poorly developed (Figure 4). The nuclei of oocytes were euchromatic and contained an obvious nucleolus. In the vicinity of granulosa cell layer the capillary-rich theca interna and outer to it the collagen-rich theca externa were present.

Ovary also contained several corpora lutei composed of large and round cells with a prominent nuclei and nucleoli. The luteal cells were pale and contained numerous mitochondria, an extensive rough endoplasmic reticulum, smooth endoplasmic reticulum and Golgi apparatus. The cells also contained numerous free ribosomes, lipid droplets and a few number of lysosomes and multivesicular bodies (Figure 5).

In EMF-exposed group, the zona pellucida was narrower than in control, 3.24 ± 0.25 µm VS 4.47 ± 0.42 µm, and the difference was significant ($p<0.001$). The number of microvilli profiles per unit area in this group was fewer than in control, 4.13 ± 0.83 VS 9.8 ± 0.56, which was statistically significant ($p<0.001$) and (Figure 7).The coronal cells were shrunken, separated from zona pellucid and lost contact from eachother (Figure 6).

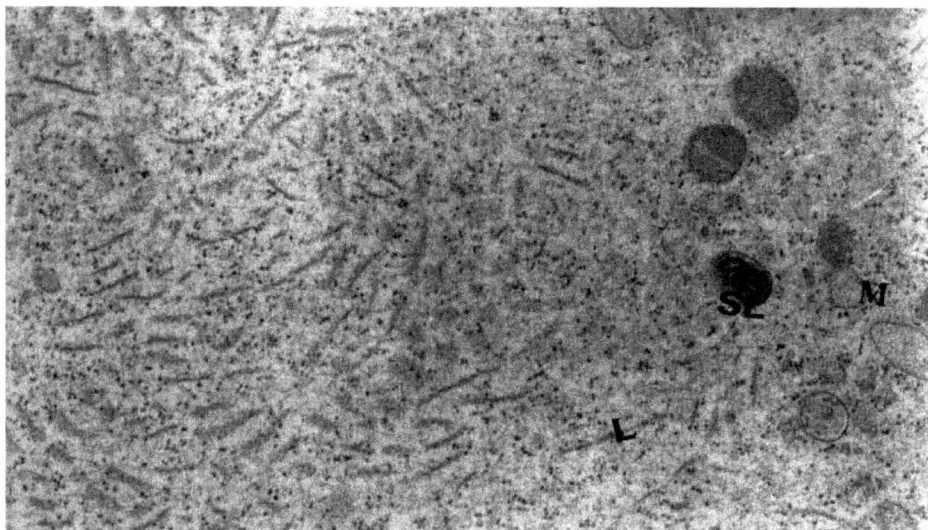

Fig. 4. Electron micrograph of cytoplasm of oocyte from a control rat ovary. Note mitochondria (M), lamellae (L), and secondry lysosome (SL). 15000 X.

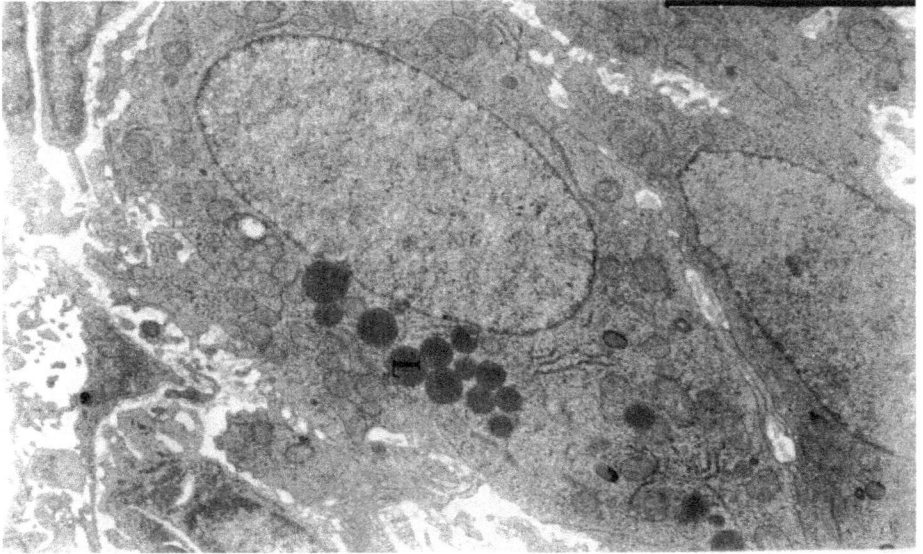

Fig. 5. Electron micrograph of corpus luteum from a control rat ovary. Note normal organels and some lipid droplets (L). 5000X.

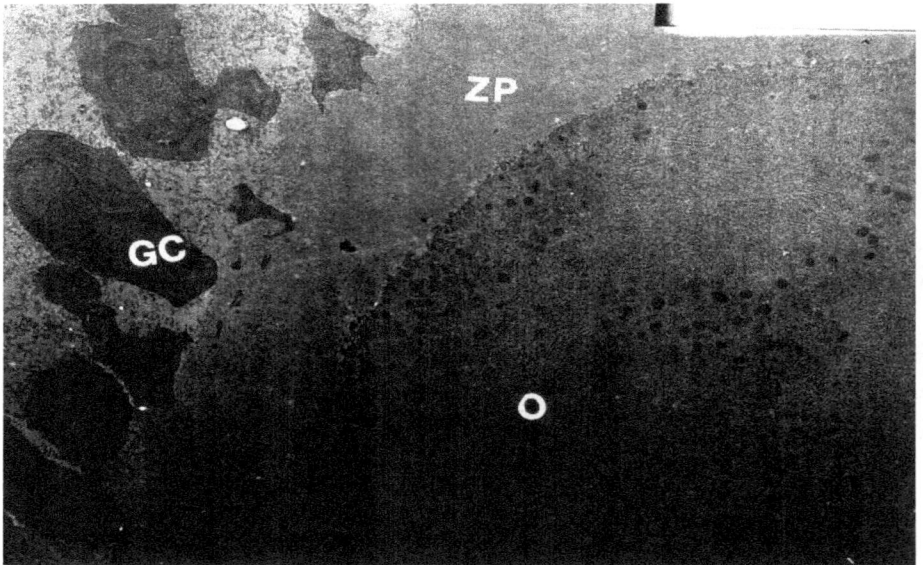

Fig. 6. Electron micrograph of an oocyte with zona pellucida and granulosa cells from EMF-exposed rat. Note condensed granulosa cells that lost contact from zona pellucida and neighboring cells (GC). Zona pellucid (ZP), and oocyte (O). 3000X.

The cytoplasm of oocytes showed fewer organell clusters and contained higher number of lamellae. The rough endoplasmic reticulum were poorly developed, mitochondria were smaller and numerous fat droplets were present in comparison to control group (Figure 7). The nuclei had irregular counter and nucleolus were condensed (Figures 8).

Numerous granulosa cells near the antrum had typical characteristics of apoptotic cells. They had condensed and cresent like nuclei and were separated from neighboring cells (Figure 9). The granulosa cells had also irregular basal lamina and in some follicles were broken. The thecal cells, in comparison to control group, had more condensed nuclei and contained; several lipid droplets, autophagic granules, apoptotic bodies, ruptured mitochondria, dilated nuclear membrane and cytoplasmic vesiculation (Figure 9). Similar changes were observed in the stromal cells from EMF-exposed group. In addition, several macrophages containing apoptotic bodies and multivesicular bodies were also present (Figure 10). These cells were mainly located near the blood vessels. The cells with cresent like nuclei, which is the characteristics of apoptotic cells, were present among stromal cells.

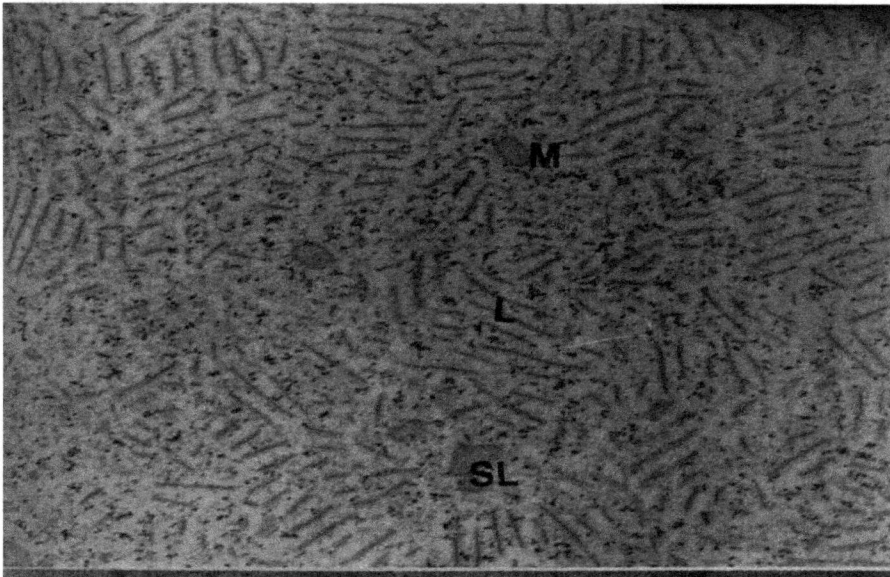

Fig. 7. Electron micrograph of cytoplasm of oocyte from EMF-exposed rat. Secondary lysosome (SL), lamellae (L), and mitochondria (M). 15000 X.

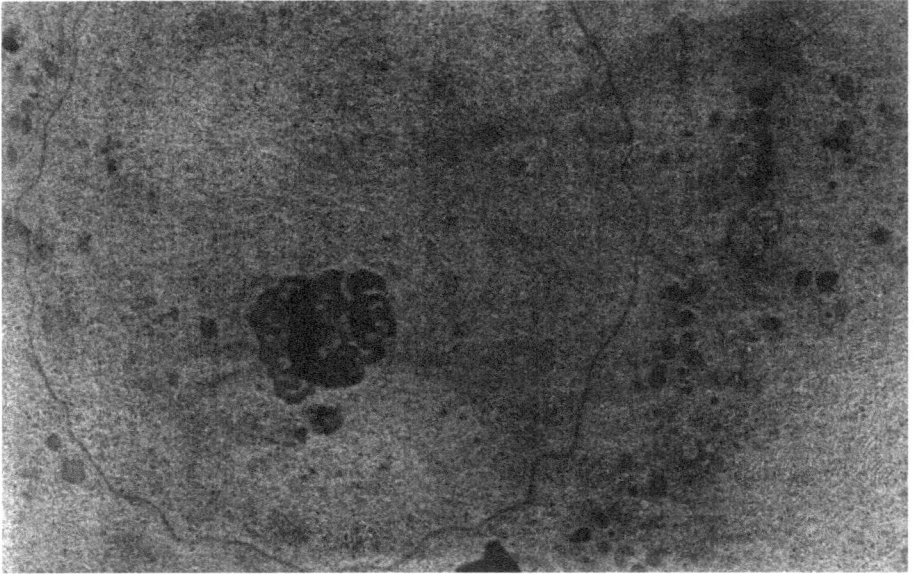

Fig. 8. Electron micrograph of oocyte nucleus and cytoplasm from an EMF-exposed rat. Note nucleus and nucleoulus. 10000 X.

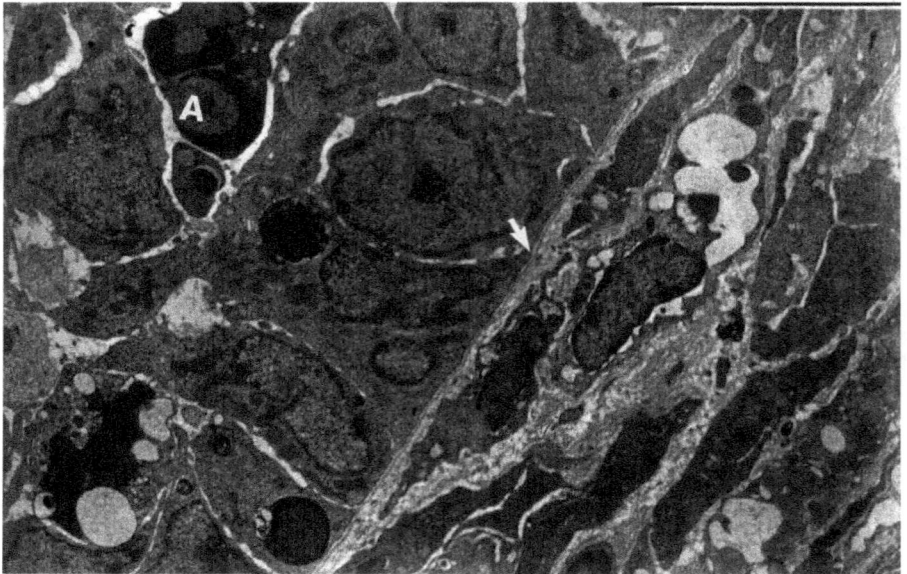

Fig. 9. Electron micrograph of a developing follicle from EMF-exposed rat. Apoptotic cell (A), basal lamina (arrow). 3000X.

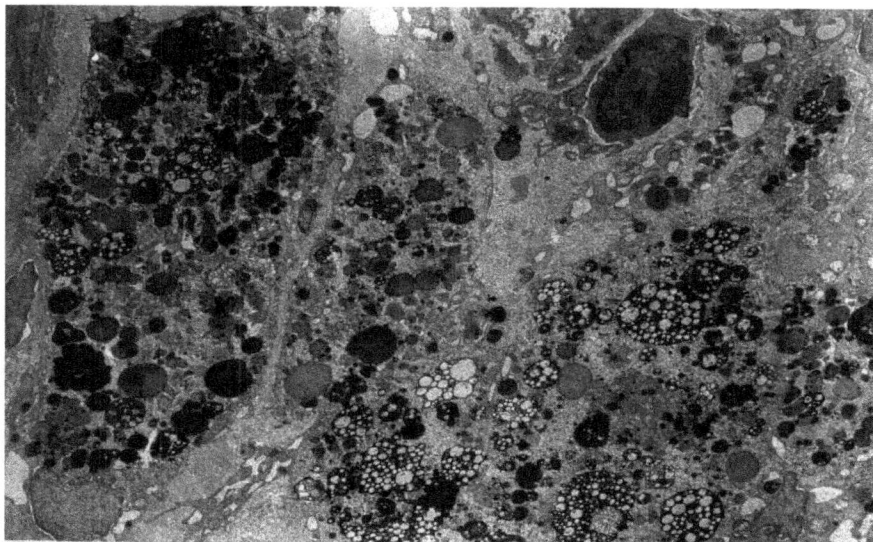

Fig. 10. Electron micrograph of ovarian stroma from an EMF-exposed rat. Note necrotic cells, and macrophages containing multivesicular and apoptotic bodies. 3700X.

3.1.3 Immunohistochemical studies

Immunohistochemical studies was performed on paraffin sections using TUNEL technique for detection of apoptosis and Ki-67 technique for proliferation assay. Both TUNEL positive and Ki-67 positive cells were distinct from nonpositive cells by their brownish color. In control group TUNEL positive cells were fewer and was limited to granulosa cells near the antrum of atretic follicles (Figure 11). Proliferative cells (Ki-67 positive cells), in this group, were observed in granulose layer close to the basement membrane.

In experimental group, exposed to EMF, apoptotic cells were mainly found near the antrum but also were present among cells close to basement membrane (Figure 12). TUNEL positive cells were not observed in thecal layers but were observed in ovarian stroma. The corpora lutea in the EMF-exposed group also contained numerous TUNEL positive cells. The result from apoptotic cells indicate that EMF exposure induces apoptosis not only in granulose cells but also in other parts of the ovary. Regarding Ki-67 assay, the number of Ki-67 positive cells in granulosa layer from EMF-exposed group were obviously fewer than that in control group meaning that EMF exposure inhibits proliferation.

In experimental group, exposed to EMF, apoptotic cells were mainly found near the antrum but also were present among cells close to basement membrane (Figure 12). TUNEL positive cells were not observed in thecal layers but were observed in ovarian stroma. The corpora lutea in the EMF-exposed group also contained numerous TUNEL positive cells. The result from apoptotic cells indicate that EMF exposure induces apoptosis not only in granulose cells but also in other parts of the ovary. Regarding Ki-67 assay, the number of Ki-67 positive cells in granulosa layer from EMF-exposed group were obviously fewer than that in control group meaning that EMF exposure inhibits proliferation.

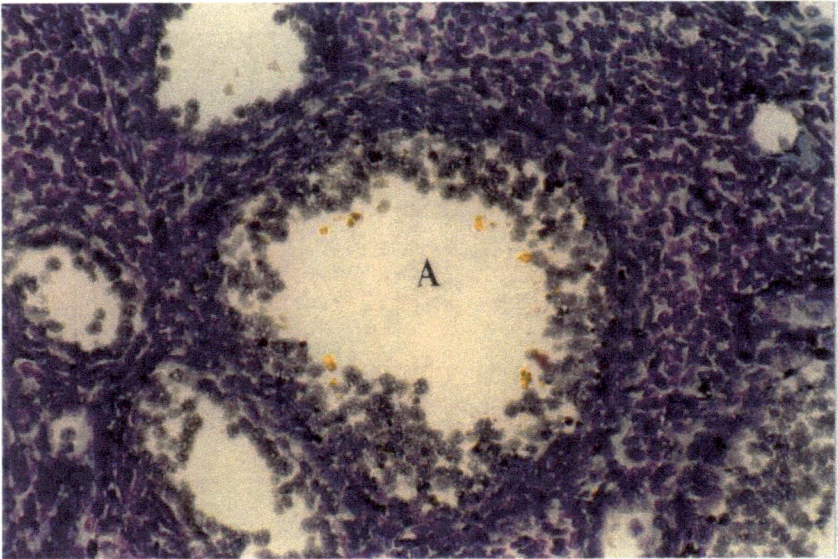

Fig. 11. Photomicrograph of a section from control rat ovary. An antral follicle (A), containing apoptotic cells with golden brown color at luminal surface. TUNEL method, counterstained with toluidine blue. 300X.

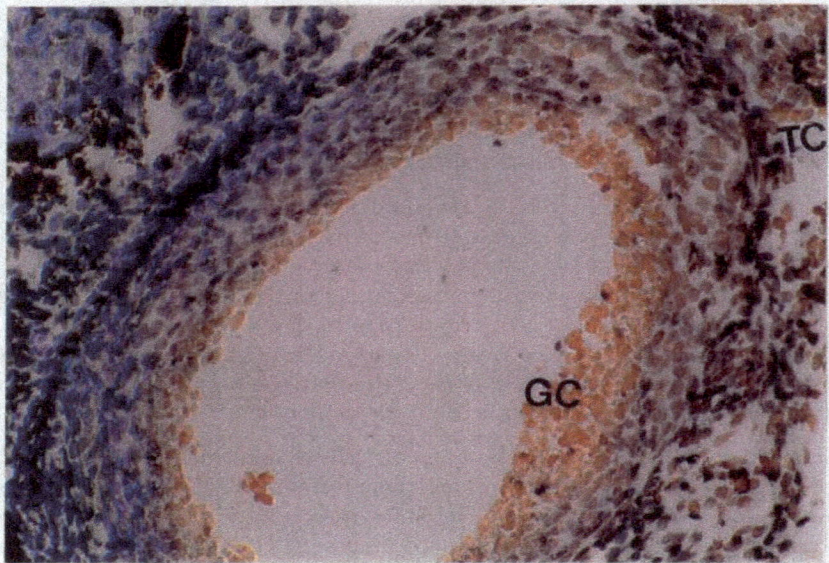

Fig. 12. Photomicrograph of an antral follicle from EMF-exposed rat ovary. Note numerous apoptotic cells with golden brown color among granulosa cells (GC), at luminal surface. Techa interna (TC). TUNEL method, counterstained with toluidine blue. 700X.

3.2 Effect of EMF on uterus

Different phases of the uterus is recognized according to the morphological characteristics of endometrium. The study was carried out in the proliferative phase. The phase was primarily selected based on estrous cycle and after sacrificing of the animals the morphological characteristics of the endometrium was used as the second criterion, otherwise the case was excluded from the study.

3.2.1 Light microscopic studies

In the control group, the endometrium is lined with simple columnar epithelium with nucleus located basally and contained limited uterine glands (Figure 13). In EMF-exposed group, the endometrial thickness was reduced and epithelial cells were smaller, shorter and had condensed nuclei (Figure 14). The difference between two groups was statistically significant (p<0.01). In experimental group, the cells in the stroma of the endometrium were smaller, contained condensed nuclei and blood vessels were less extensive. However, myometrium and perimetrium were similar in both groups.

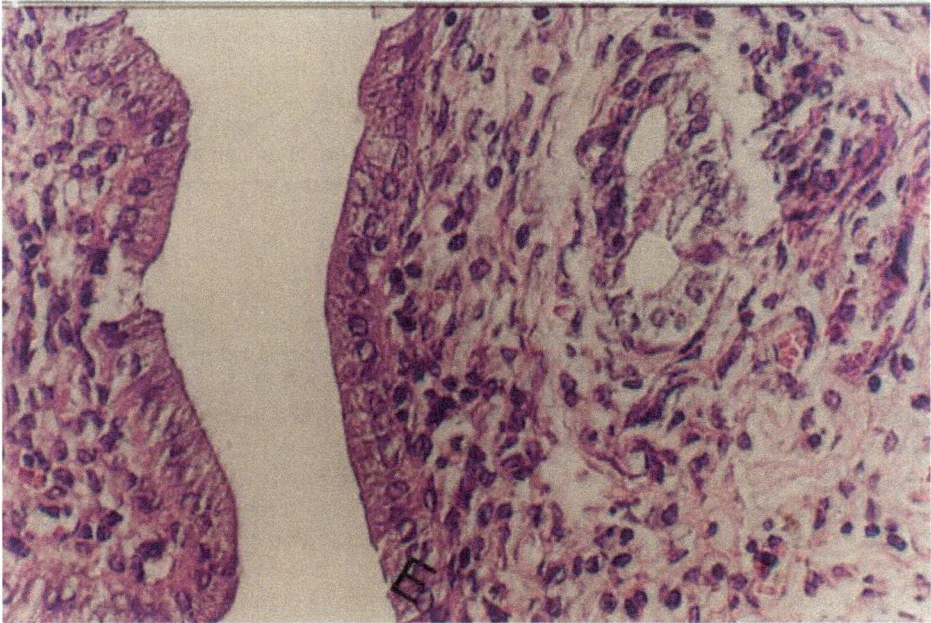

Fig. 13. Photomicrograph of uterine endometrium from a control rat. Note, columnar cells of endometrial lining (E). H &E staining, 200X.

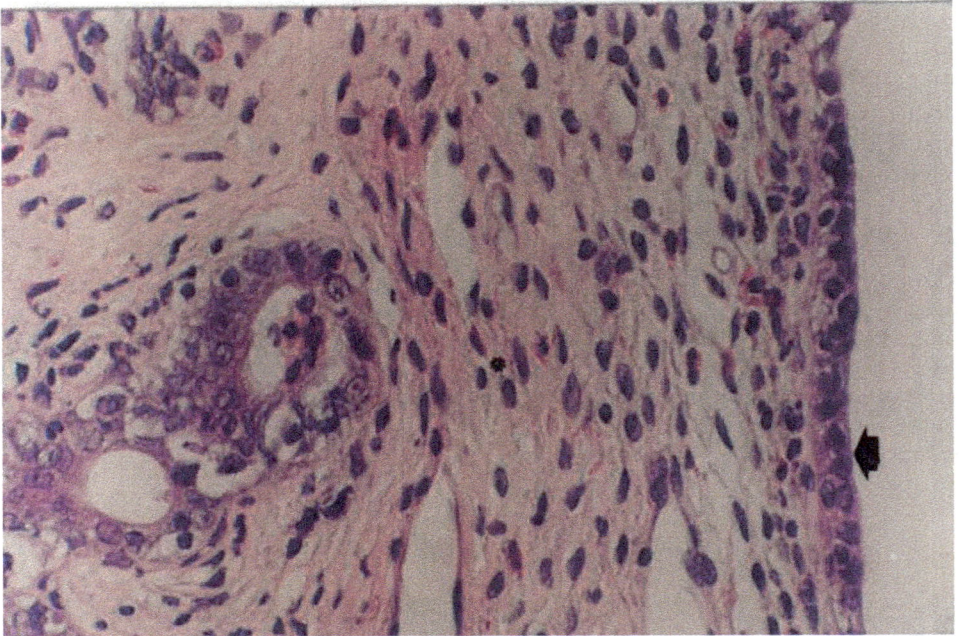

Fig. 14. Photomicrograph of uterine endometrium from an EMF-exposed rat. Note flattened endometrial epithelium (arrow head). H&E staining, 200X.

Stereological studies showed that the V/v of the nucleus to cytoplasm and axial ratio of the nuclei in the epithelial cells from experimental group was significantly lower than the control group (p<0.01).

3.2.2 Electron microscopic studies

Ultrastructural studies revealed that epithelial lining of the endometrium consist of two types of cell; ciliated and nonciliated cells. The ciliated cells are randomly scattered among the nonciliated cells. The nonciliated cells undergo morphological changes during different uterine phases. Both cell types contain euchromatic nuclei, a relatively well developed rough endoplasmic reticulum and Golgi apparatus, some apical secretory granules and some fat droplets. The cells prosses small and slender mitochondria. The cells at their lateral interface close to the apex show junctional complex, desmosomes and in some cases an interdigitation attaches the neighbor cells together. In addition to changes that observed with light microscope the electron microscopy showed that in experimental group the nuclear heterochromatin was increased and their mitochondria were condenser and sometimes ruptured in comparison to control group. Furthermore, the secretory granules were dispersed in the cytoplasm while in the control group they were localized to apical area. The rouph endoplasmic epithelium in experimental group was dilated and had a cystic appearance. The number of microvilli in experimental group was reduced in comparison to control group (Figures 15 and 16).

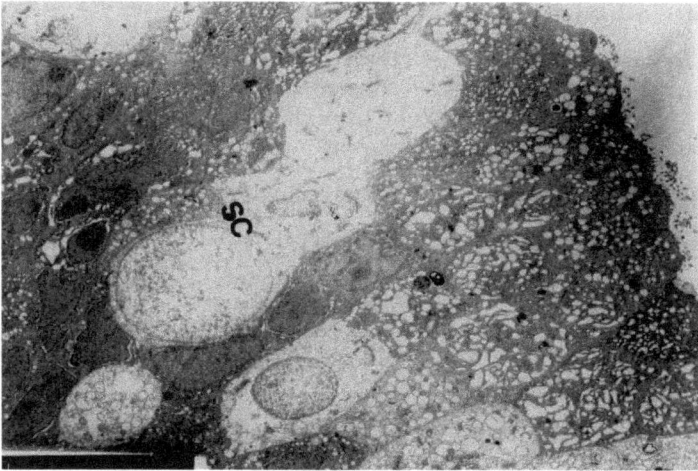

Fig. 15. Electron micrograph of uterine endometrial epithelium from control rat. Secretory cell (SC), ciliated cell (CC). 3500X.

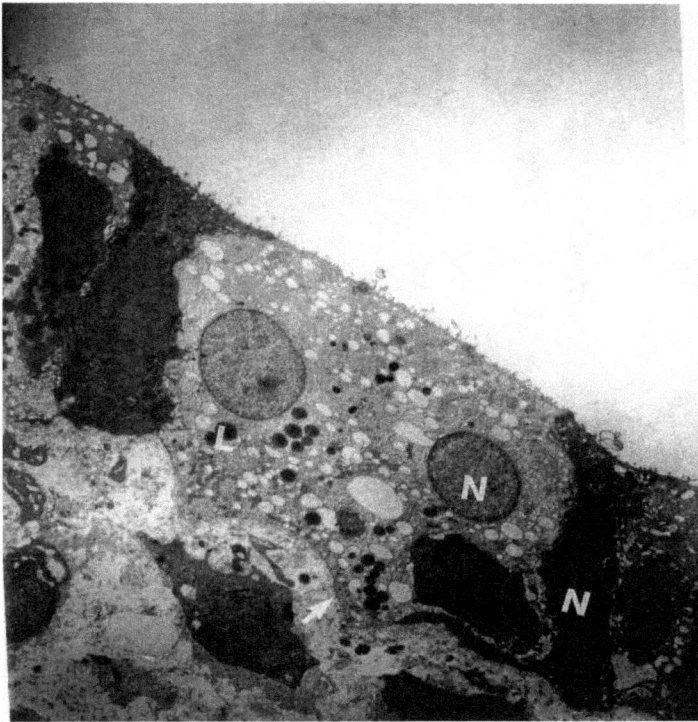

Fig. 16. Electron micrograph of uterine endometrial epithelium from EMF-exposed rat. Nucleus (N), lipid droplet (L), and irregular basal lamina (arrow). 3500X.

3.2.3 Immunohistochemical studies

Detection of apoptotic cells using TUNEL reaction technique showed that in control group the luminal epithelium appeared regular with some glycogen deposition but had almost no sign of apoptosis (Figure 17). In experimental group, the epithelium appeared irregular and there were several apoptotic cells in the luminal and glandular epithelium (Figure 18).

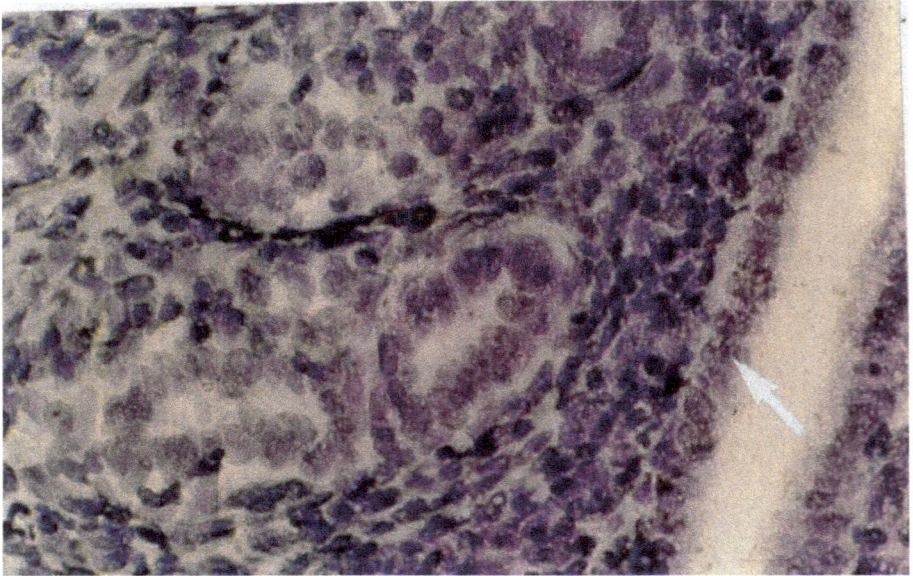

Fig. 17. Photomicrograph of a uterine section from control rat. Luminal epithelium (arrow), the uterine glands are seen. TUNEL method, counterstained with toluidine blue. 700X.

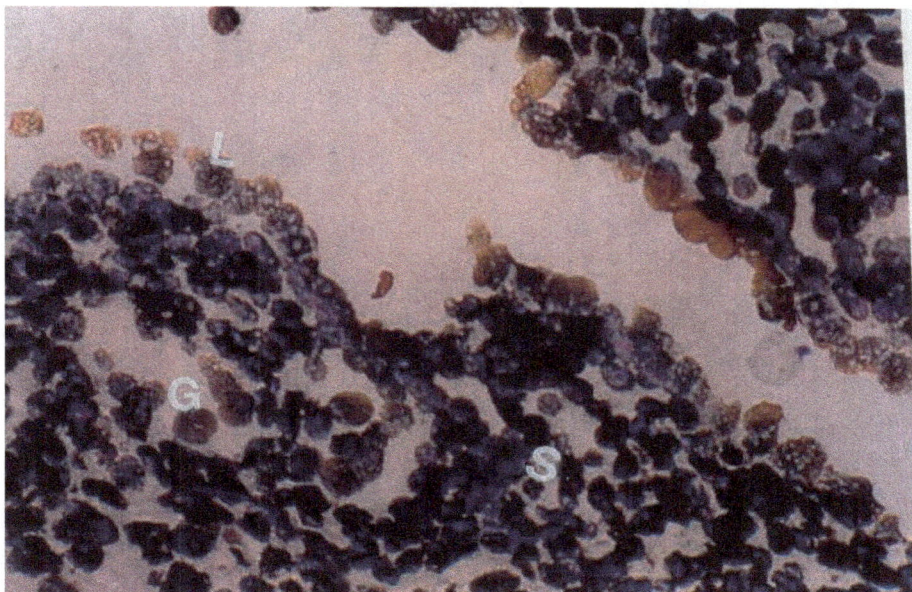

Fig. 18. Photomicrograph of uterine luminal epithelium from EMF-exposed rat. Note numerous TUNEL positive cells stained as golden brown. Luminal face (L), uterine gland (G), and uterine stroma (S). TUNEL method, counterstained with toluidine blue. 700X.

3.3 Effect of EMF on uterine tubes

The uterine tubes act as the site of fertilization and have a critical role in the conduction of zygote to the uterine cavity. Any changes in the structure and or function of uterine tubes would result in tubal pregnancies. The aim of the present study is evaluating the effect of EMF on uterine tubes by examining histological and morphological features using light and electron microscopy and immunohistochemical techniques.

3.3.1 Light microscopic studies

Light microscopic studies of uterine tubes from control group showed that: uterine tubes are lined with ciliated simple columnar epithelium and their cilia formed a smooth and orderly arranged ribbon at luminal face. The nuclei of epithelial cells were light and euchromatic. The epithelium was rested on a highly vascularized loose connective tissue (Figure 19). In the EMF-exposed group, epithelial cells were low columnar and mostly had lost their cilia. The nuclei of the epithelial cells were condensed and heterochromatic (Figure 20). Morphometric studies, based on final magnification, showed that the height of epithelial cells were decreased after EMF exposure, it was 2.77±0.19 mm VS 2.83±0.46 mm (Figure 21), the difference between two groups is significant (p<0.05).

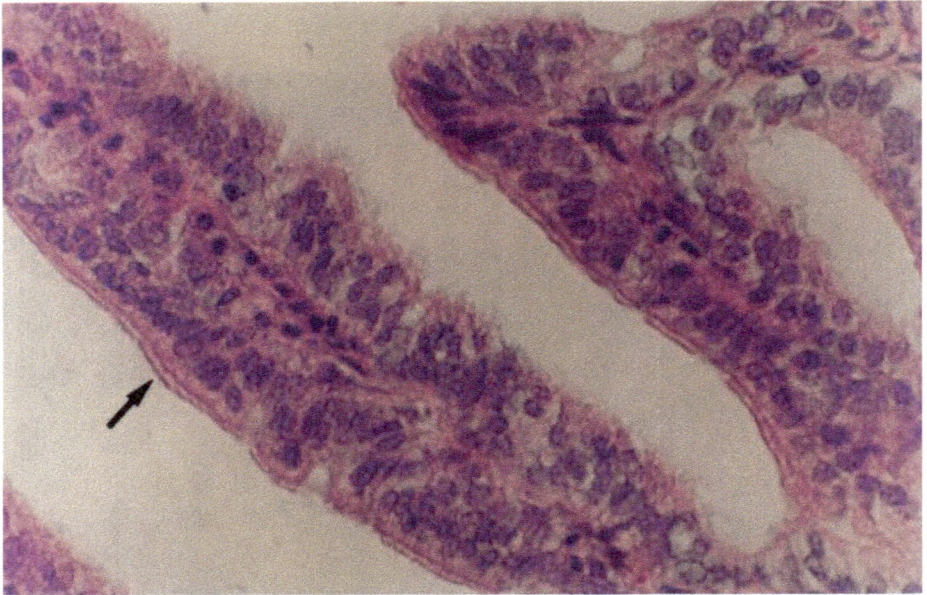

Fig. 19. Photomicrograph of uterine tube from control rat. Note epithelium with a ribbon-like cilia at luminal face (arrow). H&E staining. 600X.

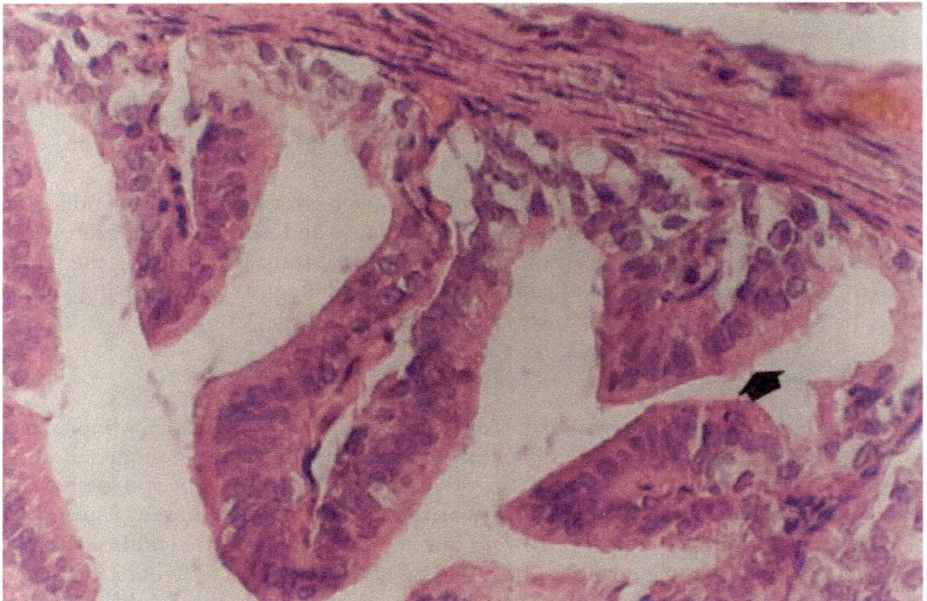

Fig. 20. Photomicrograph of a section of uterine tube from EMF-exposed rat. Note loss of cilia in epithelial cells, scattered cilia are left (arrow head). H&E staining. 600X.

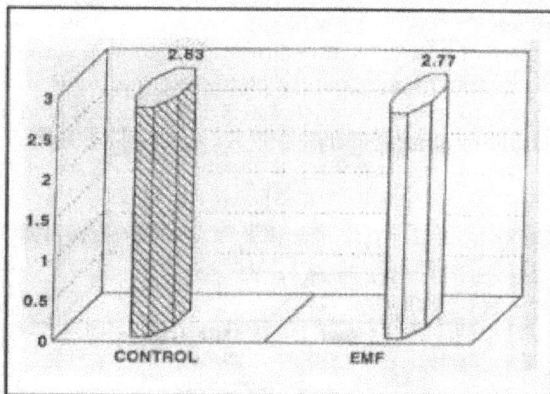

Fig. 21. A diagram showing the height of epithelial cells in uterine tubes (as mm) in control and EMF-exposed groups.

3.3.2 Electron microscopic studies

Electron microscopy showed clearly the ciliated and secretory cells in the epithelial lining of the uterine tubes. In the control group, the ciliated cells had a basal or central ellipsoid nuclei with a prominent nucleolus. The cytoplasm contained poorly developed organells. The apical cell surface bears numerous cilia. The secretory or non ciliated cells had a central elongated nuclei with a prominent nucleolus. The organells were well developed. Membrane bound granules were located at apical cytoplasm. The epithelial cells were held together by junctional complex and rested on a basal lamia (Figure 22).

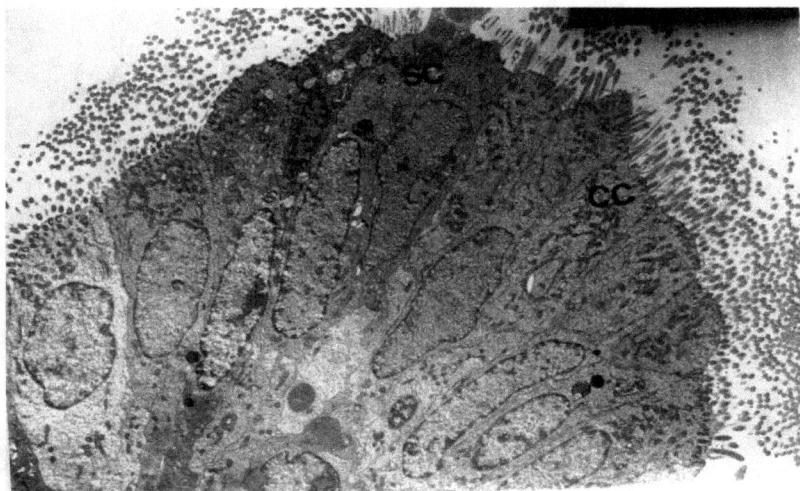

Fig. 22. Electron micrograph from uterine tube epithelium in control rat. Secretory cell (SC), ciliated cell(CC). 3000X.

In the EMF-exposed group, the nuclei were condensed, the apical cilia were apparently reduced and organells were sparsely distributed through the cytoplasm. Slight pyknosis, increased peripheral chromatin condensation and some degree of cytoplasmic condensation was observable. The most remarkable feature of the uterine tubes in this group was the presence of cells with preapoptotic characteristics i.e. flattened and cystic endoplasmic reticulum and nuclear condensation (Figure 23).

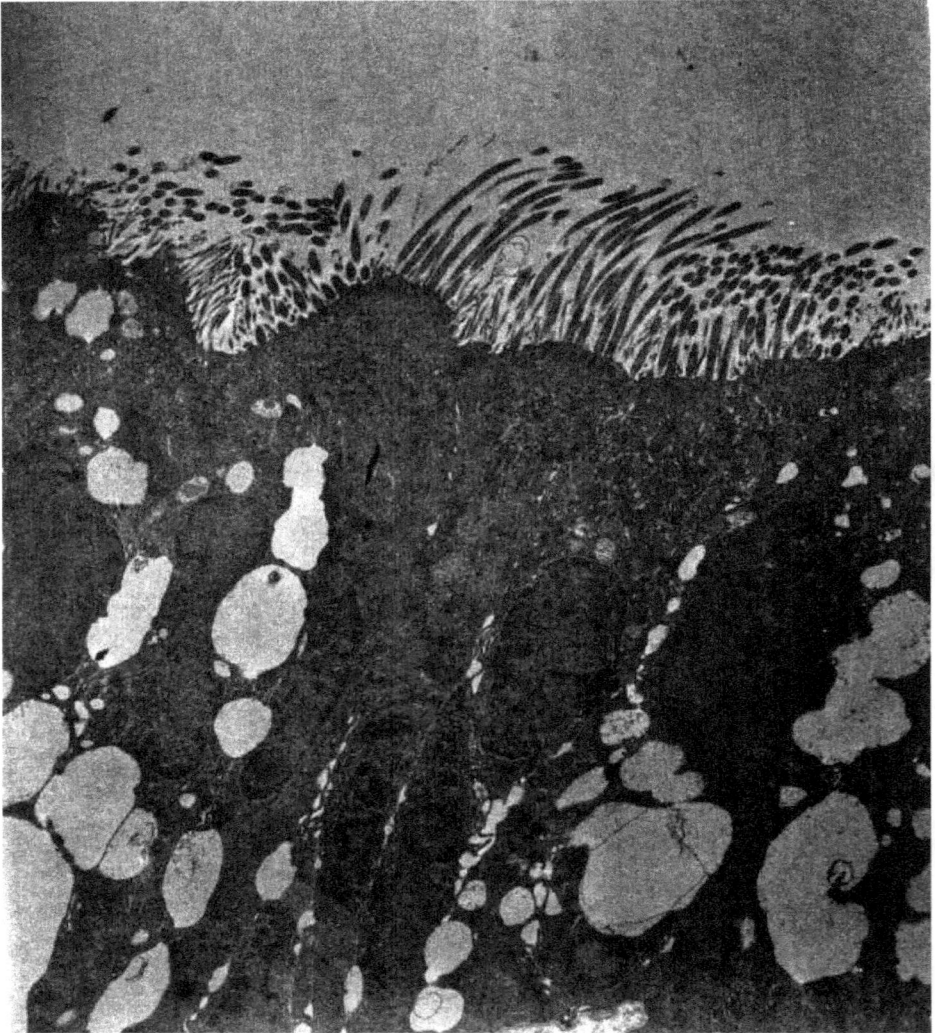

Fig. 23. Electron micrograph from uterine tube in EMF-exposed rat. Note decreased ciliar number and presence of intercellular spaces and cystic rER. 3500X.

3.3.3 Immunohistochemical studies

Immunohistochemical studies were restricted to TUNEL technique for detection of apoptotic cells. In the control group, with TUNEL assay, apoptotic cells was neither observed in the lining epithelium nor in the subepithelial layer (Figure 24). In the EMF-exposed group, there were numerous apoptotic cells in the lining epithelium. Apoptosis was observed both in secretory and ciliated cell types. Very few apoptotic cells was also present in the subepithelial layer (Figure 25).

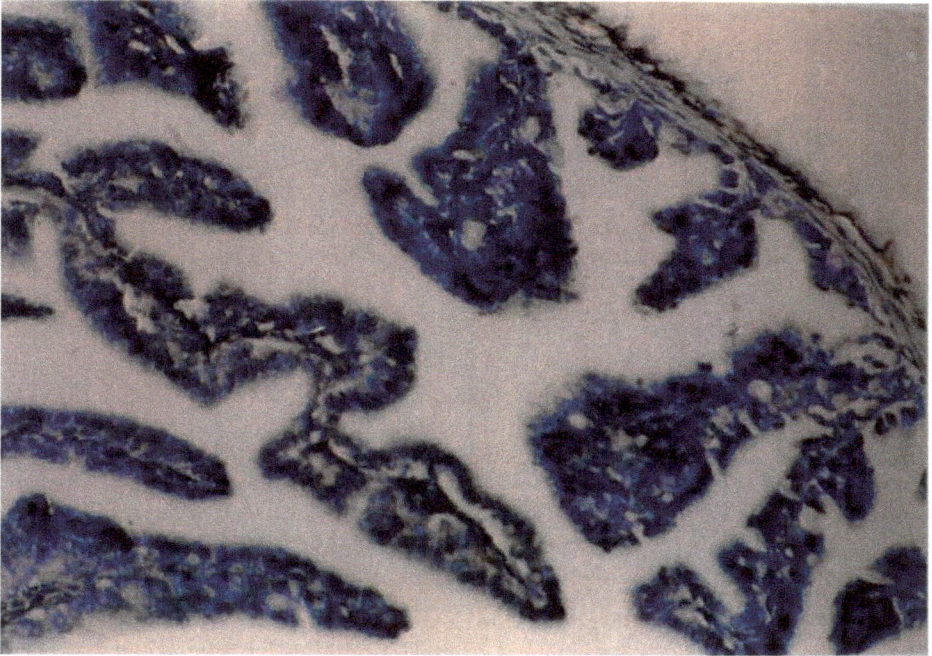

Fig. 24. Photomicrograph of a section from uterine tube in control rat. TUNEL method, counterstained with toluidine blue. 360X.

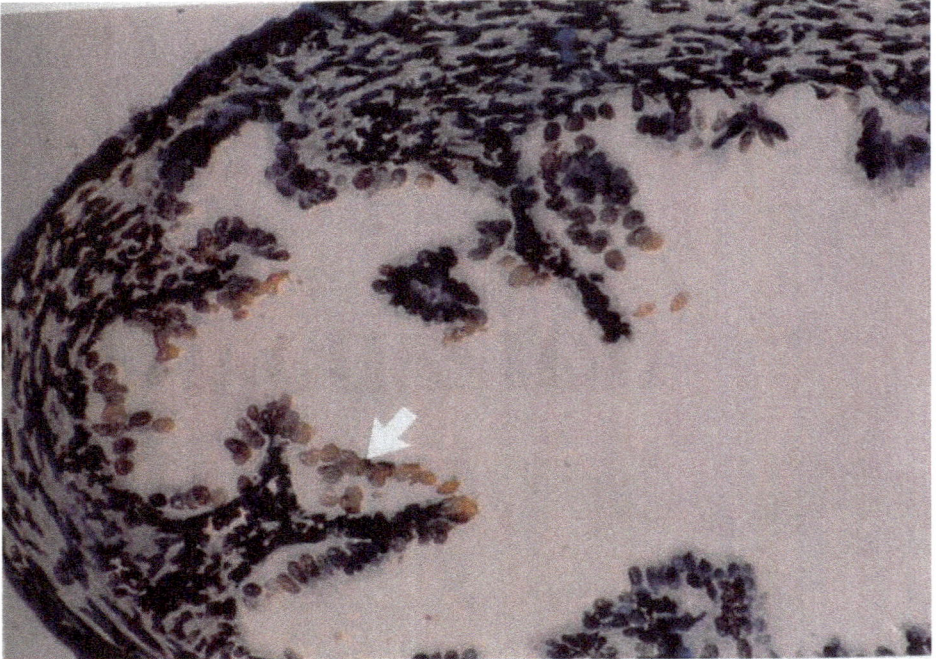

Fig. 25. Photomicrograph from uterine tube in EMF-exposed rat. Note apoptotic cells with golden brown color at luminal face (arrow). TUNEL method, counterstained with toluidine blue. 360X.

4. Discussion

This section is going to deal : 1) The morphological effects of EMF exposure on the genital organs including ovary, uterus, and Fallopian tubes using light and electron microscopy. 2) A possible role of apoptosis in the mediation of EMF-induced alterations using immunohistochemical techniques. To make it easier to explain, each organ is discussed separately, following the above theme, and made a general conclusion at the end.

4.1 EMF-induced morphological changes and apoptosis in ovary

The result of present study showed that EMF-exposure increased degenerative changes in the ovarian follicles. The results obtained from TEM studies have revealed that oocytes became shrunken, and the zona pellucida appeared narrower in the EMF exposed group in comparison to control group (Figs 1, 3, 4, 7). It was also shown that the number of microvilli in oocytes and coronal cells were decreased in experimental group. It is known that the microvilli of oocytes and granulosa cells are in contact, within the zona pellucida, by gap junction and are involved in oocyte nutrition (Martin et al. 2001; Takeo and Hokano 1995; Gondos 1982; Vazquez and Sotello 1967). The alterations produced by EMF could either be the result of initiation of apoptosis in the follicular cells or as a result of apoptosis in the oocytes themselves.

Comparison of oocyte degeneration with apoptosis since Wyllie et al. (Wyllie 1980) first described the morphological characteristics of physiological cell death (apoptosis) few studies have described the ultrastructure of the atretic oocyte and none have examined this in pubertal or adult animals. Most reviews of ovarian follicular atresia focused on changes in granulosa cells or equate the entire process with apoptosis (Tilly 1998; Kaipia and Hsueh 1996). Biochemical analysis of atretic follicles that have measured DNA integrity (188-189)or increases in cell death – related mRNA levels, including bax and Fas, fasL (Hsuhe et al. 1994; Mori et al. 1997), have confirmed that apoptosis is occurring in antral ovarian follicles. Because the oocyts is a very small component of these large follicles, such measurements most probably reflect the status of granulosa cells. Due to these restrictions, microscopic examination is required to study the process of atresia in oocytes in situ. Because ultrastructural characterization is a reliable method for the classification of cell death as apoptosis (Payne et al. 1995).

Alterations in oocytes from EMF-exposed ovaries mainly in rat atretic f'ollicles included: loss of both granulosa cell and oocyte microvilli from the zona pellucida, changes in cytoplasmic organelles such as lamellar condensation and shirinkage of oocytes. Loss of microvilli and cytoplasmic condensation do resemble apoptosis, but other events differed from those associated with traditional apoptosis. For example, the mitochondria do not maintain their characteristic appearance during, early stages of atresia, as normally occur in apoptosis. While, cytoplasmic condensation, which is reflected by an increase in electron density at the ultrastructural level, observed in degenerating oocytes. In support of the findings of the present study, condensed chromatin was never observed in oocytes of atretic follicles by other investigators (Devine 2000). These comparisons suggest that there are more differences than similarities between physiological oocyte cell death and apoptosis. Other reports attempting to identify the mechanism of oocyte death have not discussed the possibility of alternative, nonapoptotic, types of physiological death (Perez et al. 1999). Early ultrastructural studies occurred before apoptosis was characterized (Vazquez and Sotello 1967; Franchi and Mandl 1962). More recent studies using ovulated oocytes failed to prove definitively that apoptosis was the mechanism of oocyte death (Perez et al. 1999; Van et al. 1998; Phillips et al. 1992). Therefore, it seems likely that oocytes in postnatal rats have unique cell-death triggers, signal transduction pathways, and clearance mechanisms as compared with other cell types. Such flexibility has not been described for traditional apoptosis.

4.2 The unique aspects of oocytes

The unique nature of the oocyte relative to other cell types may be the cause for its unusual manner of cell death. Oocytes can remain arrested in meiosis for years, are surrounded by an acellular zona pellucida, are nonproliferating, and are known to rely on surrounding granulosa cells for survival (Hirshfield 1991). Apoptosis is an active process thought to protect the rest of an organism from an aberrant cell. Meiotic oocyte may not be required to undergo apoptosis, because they pose no threat of excessive proliferation and tumor formation.   Overall, the results presented here support that oocyte loss in atretic follicles of postnatal rats can be morphologically distinguished from the two more widely described mechanisms of cell death, necrosis, and apoptosis. While it is generally accepted that granulosa cells are lost by apoptosis, the ability of the oocyte to undergo apoptosis is still in question. Based on ultrastructural criteria traditionally associated with apoptosis (Wyllie et al. 1972), oocyte death should be assigned to a different class of physiological cell death. Such variations in the mechanisms of cell death are becoming more widely accepted (Chernoff et al. 1992) and will be the subject of future investigations.

In the present study, we characterized the degeneration of rat ovarian tissue after the exposure to EMF, cell death of the interstitial tissue in ovary was shown to be apoptotic by morphological criteria with TEM. Taken together, our results suggest that apoptosis play a critical role in the degeneration of in situ ovarian cortical and interstitial tissue, after the exposure to EMF.

Some follicles with intact oocytes contain several layer of granulosa cells and fail to form follicles consisting of multiple layers of granulosa cells. We hypothesized that this lack of increase in granulosa cell number is due to either a lack of granulosa cell proliferation or to an increase in granulosa cell apoptosis. In contrast, ovary demonstrated large number of TUNEL-positive granulosa cells (Fig. 12), suggesting that most of the granulosa cells especially near the lumen are apoptotic cells. It appears that soon after oocyte degeneration, granulosa cell begins to undergo apoptosis in the follicles of the EMF-exposed ovary.

In summary, EMF-induced changes in ovary may interfere with oogenesis, fertility, and is an indication of the cytotoxic effect of EMF on maturation of oocytes.

In EMF-exposed rats, granulosa cells have a nucleus with condensed chromatin, apoptotic bodies and several autophagic vacuoles. The presence of granulosa cells with condensed nuclei and their separation from zona pellucida and neighbouring cells, corresponds with the characteristic of apoptotic cells and constitutes the classical land mark of follicular atresia (Hardwick 2004; Tilly et al. 1992; Hurwitz and Adashi 1991). While the proportion of granulosa cells with condensed nuclei was low in control group, this was evidenced by few number of apoptotic cells. This study demonstrates induction of programmed cell death by EMF and suggest a role for EMF in increasing of follicular atresia in rat ovary.

Based on the sequential ultrastructural observations of this study as well as previous works, the following model is proposed to explain the initiation of apoptosis in ovaries. Alterations occur in the granulosa cells include; nuclear condensation, apoptotic body formation and blebbing of the cytoplasm (present study and Peluso et al. 1977). As the follicle enters into the apoptotic changes, pyknotic nuclei, apoptotic bodies and numerous autophagic vacuoles develop. The autophagic vacuoles are associated with the granulosa cells close to the basal lamina. The fact that these vacuoles contain acid phosphatase activity indicates that they are lysosomal in origin (Elfont et al. 1977) and in part responsible for the deterioration of the granulosa cell layer. Autophagic vacuoles are also observed in the thecal layers, and interstitial tissue particulary associated with the thecal cells and interstitial cells near the blood vessels. The deterioration of both granulosa and thecal cell layers is also enhanced by invasion of macrophages which occurs after many of the granulosa cells have undergone apoptosis. From all morphological standpoints cytoplasmic bodies apparently corresponding to phagolysosomes, these large cells have been identified as macrophages. It has been proposed that such cells induce the invasion of macrophages (Byskov 1974) possibly by releasing a chemotactic factor (Gaytan et al. 1998). Regarding the mechanism whereby macrophages promote granulosa cell change it is postulated that macrophages have the capacity to produce oxidative products such as nitric oxide (Bredt et al. 1994), superoxide radicals, and hydrogen peroxide (Sugino et al. 1996); and in addition, macrophage-derived cytokines such as transforming growth factor and have been found to induce apoptosis in ovarian cells (Foghi et al. 1996). The present study describe not only the ultrastracture of follicle in rat ovaries but also the increased degenerative changes within follicle committed to undergo apoptosis after EMF-exposure (Roshangar and Soleimani Rad, 2007). In support of this idea several studies reported (Roshangar and Soleimani Rad 2001; Kaipia et al. 1997; Hughes and Gorospe 1991; Zamboni 1972) increased of macrophages after the EMF exposure. It is believed that the cell fragments produced by apoptosis are phagocytosed by macrophages. These macrophages do not release cytokines that would initiate an inflammatory response (Andrew et al. 1998).Thus the granulosa and thecal cells would be destroyed, leaving only fibroblasts and other connective tissue elements to represent the follicular wall, thereby transforming the follicle into a cystic follicle. It has been reported that macrophages were involved in the apoptotic process (Leonardo and Skeel 1980). This clearly indicates that increased number of macrophages in experimental group (Soleimani Rad and Roshangar 2000) potentially increases cell damages. Using rat ovaries, the present study confirms that the follicular granulosa cells undergo apoptosis after the EMF exposure on the basis of their microscopic features, i.e., condensation of nuclear chromatin to the margin of the nucleus, and presence of apoptotic bodies, both changes being characteristic of apoptosis (Ker et al. 1972), even more evidence is occurring in parallel with the above- mentioned morphological changes. As far as we aware, the fate of the dying granulosa cells in the ovarian follicles is unclear.

In the present study in rats, we demonstrated that large amount apoptotic and internalized granulosa cells and their fragments. The factors responsible for this basic difference are as yet unknown. In summary, this model is proposed to foster and more clearly focus future research on the mechanisms of follicular apoptosis after the EMF exposure.

Our results demonstrate that a remarkable proportion of oocytes in the rat ovary degenerate during the EMF exposure by the mechanism of apoptosis. This is already evident at experimental period, with a high number of apoptotic oocytes and increasing of macrophages and autophagic vacuoles in some occasional granulosa cells, and several lipid droplets in thecal and luteal cells. Previous TEM studies (Takeo and Hokano 1995) suggested that the process of apoptosis of the ingested cells was assumed to progress through the following steps. The nuclei of ingested cells underdog degenerative changes of successive karyopyknosis, karyorrhexis and karyolysis. The nuclear envelope and the two layers of cell membranes separating the ingested cell from the phagocytic cell were destroyed, and finally, a phagocytic vacuole was formed within the phagocytic cell.

The molecular mechanisms underlying apoptosis are poorly understood at this time. However, there are several models of apoptotic initiation that are now accepted. Apoptosis has been found to be induced via the stimulation of several different cell surface receptors in association with caspase activation. For example, the CD95(APO-Ifas) receptor ligand system is a critical mediator of several physiological and pathophysiological processes, including homeostasis of the peripheral lymphoid compartment and CTL - mediated target cell killing . Upon cross-linking by ligand or agonist antibody, the fas receptor initiates a signal transduction cascade which leads to caspase-dependent programmed cell death. The simplest way to observe this phenomenon in vitro is to use a cell permeant DNA-staining fluorescent dye such as Hoechst 33342, which allows a striking visualization of the chromatin condensation (Gartner and Hiatt 2001).

Apoptosis is over 20 times faster than mitosis. Seeing of dying cells in vivo are therefore rare. Apoptotic cells are engulfed and degraded by neighboring cells without a trace. For cell homeostasis to be maintained, a balance between the increase (by differentiation from precursors and by proliferation) and decrease (by further differentiation and cell death) in the number of a cell population has to be neatly balanced. If mitosis proceed without cell death, an 80-year-old person would have 2 tons of bone marrow and lymph nodes, and a gut 16 Km long.

Apoptotic death can be triggered by a wide variety of stimuli, and not all cells necessarily will die in response to the same stimulus. Among the more studied death stimuli is DNA damage (by irradiation or drugs used for cancer chemotherapy), which in many cells leads to apoptotic death via a pathway dependent on p53. Some hormones such as corticosteroids lead to death in particular cells (e.g., thymocytes), although other cell types may be stimulated. Some cell types express Fas, a surface protein which initiates an intracellular death signal in response to cross-linking. In other cases cells appear to have a default death pathway which must be actively blocked by a survival factor in order to allow cell survival, a survival factor normally binds to its cell surface receptor. When the survival factor is removed, the default apoptotic death program is triggered (Andrew et al. 1998).

Biochemical correlates of these morphological features have emerged during the subsequent years of study of this phenomenon. The first and most dramatic is DNA fragmentation, which was described by Brocklehurst 1996; McLauchlan 1981; and Wyllie 1980. When DNA from apoptotically dying cells was subjected to agarose gel electrophoresis, ladders with – 200 bp repeats were observed, corresponding histone protection in the nucleosomes of native chromatin. Subsequent pulsed field gel techniques have revealed earlier DNA cleavage patterns into larger fragments. Since even a few double stranded DNA breaks will render the cell unable to undergo mitosis successfully, such DNA fragmentation can be regarded as a biochemical definition of death. However, in some apoptotic systems (e.g., Fas killing of tumor cells) artificially enucleated cells lacking a nucleus still die, showing that the nucleus is not always necessary for apoptotic cell death.

The changes in the apoptotic cell which trigger phagocytosis by non-activated macrophages have been investigated by several groups. Macrophages appear to recognize apoptotic cells via several different recognition systems, which seem to recognize recognition used preferentially by different macrophage subpopulations. There is good evidence that apoptotic cells lose the normal phospholipid asymmetry in their plasma membrane, as manifested by the exposure of normally inward-facing phosphatidyl serine on the external face of the bilayer. Macrophages can recognize this exposed lipid head group via an unknown receptor, triggering phagocytosis.

Another biochemical landmark of apoptotic death which increasingly appears general is the activation of caspases, which are cysteine proteases related to ced-3, the "death gene" of the nematode Caenorhabditis elegans. caspases seem to be widely expressed in an inactive proenzyme form in most cells. Their proteolytic activity is characterized by their unusual ability to cleave proteins at aspartic acid residues, although different caspases have different fine specificities involving recognition of neighboring amino acids. Active caspases can often activate other pro-caspases, allowing initiation of a protease cascade. While several protein substrates have been shown to be cleaved by caspases during apoptotic death, the functionally important substrates are not yet clearly defined. Persuasive evidence that these proteases are involved in most examples of apoptotic cell death has come from the ability of specific caspase inhibitors to block cell death, as well as the demonstration that knockout mice lacking caspase 3, 8 and 9 fail to complete normal embryonic development. A critical issue is how caspases become initially activated, which seems to be an irreversible commitment towards death. It seems that aggregation of some pro-caspases (those with large pro- domains) allows them to become autoactivated. Recent experiments make it clear that mitochondria are involved in one major pathway involving activation of pro- caspase-9. Other experiments show that ligands crosslinking death receptors such as Fas trigger formation of a cytoplasmic complex in which pro-caspase-8 is aggregated and activated. In both cases these initiator caspases in turn activate a cascade of other pro-caspases leading to death (Andrew et al. 1998).

While there is much to be learned about the molecular pathways leading to apoptotic cell death, it is increasingly clear that cell death is a normal part of normal biological processes. This had not been appreciated until relatively recently, and our understanding of such death, and our ability to manipulate it, could allow therapeutic intervention in major diseases such as cancer, heart disease, stroke, AIDS, autoimmunity, degenerative diseases, and others.

We can only speculate how our EMF would fit into one of these models for induction of apoptosis. One such model is apoptotic initiation by intracellular perturbation. Examples of this model are ionizing radiation and chemotherapeutic ionizing agents, which cause DNA damage and initiation of apoptosis. An electromagnetic field could have a similar effect (Norman et al. 1997).

Additionally, it has been shown that the overexpression of c-myc portion leads to apoptosis. It is interesting that EMFs have been shown to increase specifically transcription of c-myc in several cell lines (Lin et al 1998). This is just one of the numerous possible mechanisms that could be inducing apoptosis. Another possibility is EMF-inducing apoptosis is mediated through the production of free radicals. It is shown that EMF exposure may result in production of free radicals (Lucia et al. 2004; Brocklehurst and McLauchlan 1996; Grundler et al. 1992; Alexander 1954). It is also shown that addition of antioxidants, such as vitamine E reduces EMF-induced changes *in vivo* and *in vitro* (Mohammadnejad and Soleimani Rad 2010). On the other hand free radicals as an inducer of apoptosis is also established (Formica and Silvestri 2004).

The findings with TEM about apoptosis-induced by EMF is confirmed using TUNEL assay. TUNEL positive cells are localized in granulosa layer, thecal cells, luteal cells and interstitial cells. The localization of apoptotic cells are well correlate with TEM studies. It is proposed that combining other methods such as microscopic evaluation of morphological changes with TUNEL POD test can substantiate the specificity of results.

Although the mechanisms underlying follicular atresia are not well known at this time, DNA damage, which can be initiated by oxidative free radicals, has been proposed as a possible mechanism that leads to the activation of the apoptotic cascade in atretic follicles (Gougeon 1996). Macrophages have the capacity to produce oxidative products such as nitric oxide (Bredt and Synder 1994), superoxide radicals, and hydrogen peroxide (Sugino et al. 1996). Macrophage-derived cytokines such as transforming growth factor α induce apoptosis in ovarian cells (Foghi et al. 1997).

In addition to the ovarian follicles the apoptotic status and nuclear condensation is observed in corpora lutea and ovarian stroma. These findings was also confirmed with the presence of TUNEL positive cells. Ultrastractural characteristics of apoptotic cells in the corpora lutea in this study is similar to those reported by Shikone et. al. 1996. Another finding in the present study was the presence of numerous macrophages in the stroma and granulosa layer in EMF exposed rats. Since the presence of macrophages in the granulosa layer of atretic follicles and the degenerating corpora lutea of rats was demonstrated by Bulmer (Bulmer 1964), macrophages have been thought to scavenge degenerated cells in the ovary (Lauber et al 2004; Anderson et al. 2003).

In addition to apoptotic changes induced by EMF exposure the other ultrastructural changes include mitochondrial disruption, condensation and or their cristae disappearance, rER dilatation and in some occasion, cytoplasmic membrane dissolution. All these alterations are the sign of cell damage and necrosis rather than apoptosis. The rational explanation would be that: EMF induces both apoptosis and necrosis depending on its strength and cell types. For example typical degenerative changes were never observed in oocytes, while it occurred in many granulosa cells. The cytotoxic effect of EMF could be attributed to its production of local heat and free radicals. This hypothesis is evidenced by the studies have shown that EMF could produce heat and free radicals (Dandrea et al. 2003; Grundler et al. 1992; Alexander and Charlesby 1954).

In this regards, it has been shown that electromagnetic fields from power lines, household currents and video display terminals, microwaves, and ultrasound have also been studied with regard to their reproductive risks. Biological plausibility plays an even more important role in their evaluation than with ionizing radiation. EMF has the capacity to produce hyperthermia, which is a proven reproductive toxin. Numerous animal experiments have demonstrated that intrauterine exposures to hypertheimia from microwaves and ultrasound and EMFs can produce malformations, growth retardation, and embryonic loss. But the usual population exposures to EMFs are below the exposures that result in hyperthermia. Furthermore, those mechanisms that are involved in reproductive toxicity, such as cytotoxicity and abnormal differentiation and cell migration do not occur at the population exposures to these agents. Evaluations of pregnancy loss from intrauterine exposures to environmental toxicants presents special problems, especially if it is the only reproductive effect being evaluated. Many studies have ignored the basic concepts of reproductive toxicology and the biological plausibility of their findings. Investigators should be cautious about biological Investigator epidemiological studies dealing with pregnancy loss without concurrent collecting other reproductive endpoints. Studies evaluating multiple reproductive endpoints have markers to assist them in determining the validity of the fertility loss data (Byene 1999).

In summary, the present data suggest that the currently applied EMF levels under certain circumstances might induce biological effects. Results indicate that the genetic constitution of cells determined by loss of P53 function can influence EMF related cellular responses. Whereas wild-type cells were insensitive. It remains to be elucidated, whether EMF induced changes of expression levels of regulatory genes may be compensated or normalized, or would result in sustained biological effects in vivo. Further studies are needed to analyze the whole transcription of EMF exposed cells by genomics technologies, such as cDNA microchips or serial analysis of gene expression (SAGE), because of conflicting epidemiological data on human EMF exposure (Repacholi 1998).

For biological effects of EMF, non thermal mechanisms are also proposed. These include: 1) Free radical formation. 2) Removal of Ca ions from membranes and and making them more likely to tear and keak. 3) DNAase leaking through the lysosomal membrane and DNA damage. 4) Leakage of Ca ions into the cytosol and acting as metabolic stimulant (Goldsworthy 2007). With regard to the effect of free radicals, it has been proposed that free radical could affect membrane integrity, produce DNA damage, and protein structures (Alexander and Charlesby 1954). This type of changes, would result in cell damage and induction of apoptosis (Formica and Silvestri 2004).

No conclusion can be drawn for electromagnetic fields and radiofrequencies because of lack of data, but there is no convincing evidence today that EMFs of the sort pregnant women or potential fathers meet in occupational or daily life exposures do any harm to the human reproductive process (Cheronff et al. 1992).

Additionally, it has been hypothesized that electromagnetic fields initially affect cells at their surface, since these low energy fields cannot directly access the cell interior because of the high resistance of the cell plasma membrane (Luben et al. 1982). The proteins that span the width of the plasma membrane therefore, have been hypothesized to act as potential sensors of ELF electromagnetic so that their actions may be transmitted to intracellular enzymes and organelles (Adey 1990).

Moreover, transformed cells and normal ones show different electrical characteristics as extensively documented by several scientists (Capko et al. 1996; Shulyakovskaya et al. 1993; Goller et al. 1986). These results led to the hypothesis that EMF of more than 1 mT, may through their effect on motion of charged matter, have a selective action on cell signaling which influences cell survival mechanisms in transformed cell, inhibiting their growth and differentiation (Tofani 1999). Also EMF have been shown to affect different aspects of biomolecular synthesis in cell, including the kinetics of DNA, RNA, and protein production (Libof 1985). Increased DNA and proteoglycan synthesis have been observed in chondrocytes (Rodan et al. 1978). In fibroblasts, low – intensity electric and magnetic fields altered collagen and proteoglycan synthesis (Farndale and Murray 1985). A complex range of effects was observed depending on the exact magnetic field configurations.

Gap junctions are specialized areas of the plasma membranes between two contiguous cells where a" pore" is formed that allows for the passage of small molecules between cells (Dean et al. 2002; Loewenstein 1979). These gap junctions are composed of proteins called connexins which have extracellular regions that attach to other connexin proteins of a contiguous cell as well as having intramembranous and cytoplasmic domains. Thus connexin proteins could also be targets of electromagnetic fields. Gap junctions have been ultrastructurally described in bone (Doty 1981). They occur among osteoblasts and osteocytes (Takahashi 2002; Boone and Tsang 1997). It has been noted that gap junctions can be regulated by change in cellular Ca^{2+} concentration. Micromolar concentration of Ca^{2+} have been demonstrated to decrease gap junction intercellular communication in a variety of tissues including cardiac muscle and liver (Li et al. 1999; Hertzberg et al. 1981). Thus it would be important to understand if changes in intracellular Ca^{2+} metabolism that may occur with exposure to ELF magnetic fields would be related to alterations in gap junction dependent intercellular communication (Luben 1991).

Research on the effects of electromagnetic fields on cells has known to alter some important physiological pathways. Of note are ionic conductances with such species as calcium ion (Ca^{2+}) which is a known interacellular messenger in cell functions such as proliferation and intercellular communication. Specifically, with respect to extremely low-frequency (EMF) (<300 Hz) magnetic fields, Ca^{2+}, uptake into lymphocytes was shown to increase (Lednev 1991). Walleczek (1992), summarized the effect of ELF magnetic fields, showing that such fields could either increase or decrease Ca^{2+} uptake into lymphocytes, depending on the time of exposure, the frequency and shape of the signal, and concomitant induced electric field intensity.

Mechanisms of interaction of ELF fields have been reviewed by Blank (1995), NRC (1996), Tenforde et al. (1996), and Valberg et al. (1997). A well-known mechanism of interaction of exposure of biological tissues to ELF fields is the induction of time- varying electric currents and fields. At sufficiently high levels, these can produce direct stimulation of excitable cells such as nerve and muscle cells. At the cellular level, the interaction induces voltages across the membranes of cells sufficient to stimulate nerves to conduct or muscles to contract. This mechanism accounts for the ability of humans and animals to perceive electric currents in their bodies and to experience electric shocks.

Our results have also been demonstrated the junctional changes that occur after EMF-exposure (Figs. 7, 9). Moreover, it is postulated that developmental exposure to EMF may reduce oocyte differentiation and diminish folliculogenesis at earlier stages of oocyte and follicular nest formation. Both of which could result in decreasing of ovarian reservoir and thus the individual will be prone to subfertility in adulthood.

4.3 EMF-Induced ultrastractural changes and apoptosis in uterus and fallopian tubes

Other findings in the present study are the effects of EMF on the lining epithelium of endometrium, uterine glands and Fallopian tubes. Ultrastractural results from EMF exposed rats revealed that the height of epithelial and glandular cells both in uterus and Fallopian tubes were reduced, indicating metabolic activity of cells were decreased. On the other hand, there were condensation and cilliary loss, which could be considered as pre apoptotic changes.

This postulation was confirmed by apoptosis assay, using TUNEL reaction technique which was revealed apoptotic cells (TUNEL positive cells) in both endometrial surface and glandular epithelium of uterus and covering epithelium of Fallopian tubes. Ultrastractural changes corresponding to cytotoxic effect of EMF were also observed. These changes include; accumulation of numerous fat droplets in the secretory cells, presence of secondary lysosomes and morphological changes of mitochondria.

As we know, endometrial surface epithelium plays a key role in blastocyst implantation and an implantation window is required for the process of implantation to begin (Marti et al. 2001; Otasuki 2001). Additionally, increasing of secretion is usually occurs in preimplantation stage (Marti et al. 2001). Any changes in the amount and or nature of secretory substance would obviously affect implantation process. Similarly, the activity of ciliated and nonciliated cells in the covering of Fallopian tubes are very important factor for transport and early development of preimplant embryo. The structural changes produced by EMF could affect both development and transport of early embryo.

There is no doubt that cell damages are the basis of all disorders occurs after EMF exposure. In support of our findings Sandra et. al. (Sandra et al. 2000) suggested that EMF-exposure might impair mammalian female reproductive potentiality by reducing the capacity of the follicles to reach a developmental stage that is an essential pre requisite for reproductive success.

The acceleration of cell damage with EMF-exposure in reproductive organs in rathas previously been reported (Roshangar and Soleimani Rad 2002; Soleimani Rad and Roshangar 2000; Byskov 1974). To elucidate the mechanisms underlying the acceleration of cell damage (Armstrong et al. 2001; Chun et al. 1996), in the present study, the earlier step of cell damage on the cellular membrane integrity, mitochondrial features, appearance of apoptotic bodies, nucleus condensation, and lipid droplet accumulation is investigated with EM and TUNEL assay. Each of these end points showed a parallel correlation with apoptosis when the animals exposed to EMF for long time.

These findings may explain the acceleration and increasing of apoptotic process by the conditioning dose. Contrary to the acceleration of apoptosis shown in the present study, in some types of cells, such as malignant cells (Ohnishi et al. 2002) and mouse spleen cells (Takahashi et al. 2002). As a possible mechanism, the attenuation of P53 response has been postulated (Dean et al. 2002; Doty 1981). In cellular responses to ionizing radiation, P53 plays very important roles. It regulates DNA repair, which leads cells to die. The partial involvement of P53 in the regulation of apoptosis is also suggested (Perez et al. 1999; Vousden 2005).

The recent evidence pointing to the role of caspases in activating DNA degradation (Green and Reed 1998; Liu et al 1997) suggest that in order for ovarian cells to complete the apoptotic program they must contain caspase-3, and an endogenous nuclear DNAase. Boone et.al. (Boone and Yan 1995) demonstrated that granulosa and luteal cells contain endogenous nuclear DNAase, and they hypothesized that these cells would therefore only require a signal to activate this enzyme in order to degrade their DNA in an apoptotic fashion (Laun et al. 2000; Boone and Tsang 1997).

4.4 Conclusion

In conclusion, we have shown that EMF-exposure causes a large proportion of oocytes in the rat ovary to degenerate by a mechanism similar to apoptosis. This is evident in the EMF-exposed group with a large number of degenerative oocytes. Other findings of the study are: an increased number of macrophages; autophagic vacuoles in some granulosa cells; and appearance of several lipid droplets in thecal and luteal cells. The present study has also shown the increased number of macrophages not only in the corpora lutea but also in the growing follicles in the EMF-exposed group. Based on our TEM, we have proposed a model that can explain the initiation of apoptosis by EMF-exposure in ovaries.

The aim of this work was to monitor the reproductive effect of exposure to a magnetic field in rat. Taken together, our results suggest that apoptosis plays a critical role in the degeneration of ovarian cortical tissue, luminal epithelium, glandular epithelium and stromal cells in uterus and luminal epithelium in fallopian tube. The present EMF- exposure model can be used when striving to find ways to improve the viability of ovarian tissue in order to grow follicles for subsequent IVF treatment, and or to protect reproductive organs from EMF effect. Regarding the human effect of EMF, the public concern about EMFs is motivated mainly by the fact that they are ubiquitous and nobody can totally avoid this type of exposure. The available epidemiologic studies all have limitations that prevent to draw clear-cut conclusions on the effects of EMFs on human reproduction.

5. References

Adey WR. (1990). Electromagnetic fields, cell membrane amplification, and cancer promotion'. In: Wilson BW, Stevens RG, Anderson LE (eds) *Extremely Low Frequency Electromagnetic Fields: the Question of Cancer.* Battelle Press, Columbus, Ohio, pp 211-249.

Ahmed E. Mohd Ali A. Homa D. (2002). Long-term exposure of male and female mice to 50 HZ magnetic field: Effect on fertility. *Bioelectromagnetics,* 23: 168-172.

Alexander D. Charlesby A. (1954). Energy transfer in macromolecules exposed to ionizing radiation. *Nature,* 113: 578-579.

Anderson HA. Maylock CA, Williams JA, Pawelez CP, Shu H, Shactor E, (2003). Serum-derived protein S binds to phosphatidylserine and stimulates the pliaoocytosis of apoptotic cells. *Nat. Immunol,* 4: 87-91.

Andrew W. Vicki D. Bertram F. Hill D. Mansow S. (1998). *Apoptosis and cell proliferation.* 2nd ed, Boehringer Mannheim. pp 112-122.

Armstrong BG. Deadman J. McBride ML. (2001). The determinants of, Canadian children's personal exposure to magnetic Fields. *Bioelectromagneticsm,* 22: 161-169.

Blank M, (1995). Electric stimulation of protein synthesis in muscle. *Adv Chem,* 250: 143-153.

Boone DL, Yan 1y. (1995). : Identification of a deoxy ribon LIC lease I-like endonuclease in rat granulosa and luteal cell nuclei. *Biol Reprod,* 53: 1057-1067.

Boone DL, Tsang BK. (1997). Identification and localization of Dnase I in rat ovary. *Biol Reprod,* 57: 813-821.

Bredt DS, Snyder SH. (1994). Nitric oxyde: a physiologic messenger molecule. *Anna Rev biochem,* 63:175-195.

Brocklehurst B, McLauchlan KA. (1996). Free radical mechanism foi- the effects of' environmental electromagnetic fields on biological systems. *Int J Radiat Biol,* 69: 3-24.

Bulmer D. (1964). The histochernistry of ovarian macrophages in the rat. *Journal of Anatomy,* 98: 313-319.

Byene J. (1999). Long-term genetic and reproductive effects of ionizing radiation. *Teratology,* 58: 210-215.

Byskov AGS. (1974). Cell kinetic studies of follicular atresia in the mouse ovary. *J Reprod Fertil,* 37: 277-285.

Capko D. Zhuravko A. Davis RJ. (1996). Transepithelial depolarization in brest cancer. *Breast Res Treat,* 41: 230-235.

Chernoff N. Rogers JM. Kavet R. (1992). A review of the literature on potential reproductive and developmental toxicity of electric and mangnetic fields. *Toxicology,* 74: 91-126.

Chiang H. Wu RY. Shao BJ. Fu YD. Yao GD. And Lu DJ. (1995). Pulsed magnetic field from video display terminals enhances teratogenic effects of cytosine arabinoside in mice. *Bioelectromagnetics,* 16: 70-74.

Chung MK. Lee SJ. Kim YB. Park SC. Shin DH. Kim SH. Kim JC. (2005). Evaluation of spermatogenesis and fertility in F1 male rats after in utero and neonatal exposure to extremely low frequency electromagnetic fields. *Asian J Androl*, 7: 189-194.

Chun SY. Eisenhauer KM, Minami S, Billig H, Perlas E, Hsueh AJ. (1996). Hormonal regulation of apoptosis in early antral follicles. *Endocrinology*, 137: 1447- 1456.

Dandrea JA, Elenor R, Lorge OD. (2003). Behavioral and cognitive effects of Microwave exposure. *Bioelectromagnetic*, 6:39-62.

Dean T. Huaeng J, Ma D, Wane KC. (2002). Inhibition of gap junction intercellular communication by extremely low-frequency electromagnetic fields in osteoblastlike models is dependent on cell differentiation. *J. Cell Physiology*, 180: 180-188.

Devine P.J. Payne CM, McCuskey MK. (2000). Ultrastructural Evaluation of Oocytes During Atresia in Rat Ovarian Follicles. *Biology of Reprod*, 63: 1245- 1252.

Devita R. Cavallo D. Raganella L. Eleuteri P. Grollino MG. Calugi A. (1995). Effect of 50 HZ magnetic fields on mouse spermatogenesis monitored by flow cytometric analysis. *Bioelectromagnetics*, 16: 330-334.

Djeridane Y. Touiyou Y. De Seze R. (2008). Influence of electromagnetic fields emitted by GSM-900 cellular telephones on the circadian patterns of gonadal, adrenal and pituitary hormones in men. *Radiate Res*, 169: 337-343.

Doty SB. (1981). Morphological evidence of gap junctions between bone cells. *Calcif Tissue Int*, 33: 509-512.

Elbetieha A. Al-Akhras MA. Darmani H. (2002). Long term exposure of male and female mice to 50 HZ magneticfield: effects on fertility. *Bioelectromagnetics*, 23: 168-172.

Elfont EA, Roszka JP, Dimino MJ. (1977). Cytochemical studies of acids phosphatase in ovarian follicles: a suggested role for lysosomes in steroldogenesis. *Biol Reprod*, 17: 787-795.

Farndale RW. Murray JC. (1985). pulsed electromagnetic fields promote collagen production in bone marrow fibroblasts via athermal mechanisms. *Calcif Tissue Int*, 37: 178-182.

Feychting M. Ahlbom A. Kheifets L. (2005). EMF and health. *Ann Rev Public Health*, 26: 89-165.

Foghi A. Teeds Kj. Van der Donk H. Dorrington J. (1997). Induction of apoptosis in rat thecal/interstitial cells by transforming growth factor a plus transforming growth factorβ in vitro. *J Endocrinol*, 153: 169-170.

Formica D. Silvestri S. (2004). Biological effects of exposure to magnetic resonance imaging. *Bio Medical Engineering*, 3: 111-112.

Franchi LL, Mandl AM. (1962). The ultrastructure of oogonia and oocytes in the foetal and neonatal rat. *Proc R Soc Lond*, 157: 99-114.

Gartner LP, Hiatt JL. (2001). Color Textbook of Histology, Second edition, W.B Saunders company. New York, pp 125-175.

Gaytan F. Morales C. Bellido C. Aguilar E. (1998). Ovarian follicle macrophages: Is follicular atresia in the immature rat a macrophage-mediated event. *Biol Reprod*, 58: 52-59.

Genuis SJ. (2007). Fielding a current idea: Exploring the public health impact of electromagnetic radiation. *Public Health*, 18.

Goller DA, Weidema WF. Davies RJ. (1986). Transmural electrical potential as an early marker in colon cancer. *Arch Surg*, 121: 345-350.

Goldsworthy A. (2007). The Biological Effects of Weak Electromagnetic Fields. *http://www.scribd.com/doc/19203269/The*-Biological-effects-of-weak-Electromagnetic-Fields.

Gondos B. (1982). Ultrastructure of follicular atresia. *Gamete Res*, 5: 199-206.

Gougeon A. (1996). Regulation of ovarian follicular development in primates: Facts and hypotheses. *Endo Rev*, 17: 121-155.

Green DR, Reed JC. (1998). Mitochondria and apoptosis. *Science*, 281: 1309-1312.

Grundler W. Kaiser F. Keilmann F, Walleczek J. (1992). Mechanisms of electromagnetic interaction with cellular systems. *Naturwissenschaften*, 79: 551- 559.

Hardwick M. (2004). The role of apoptosis in the female uterine and ovarian cycles. *WWW. Intellectual.corn*.

Hertzberg EL, Lawrence TS, GIILila NB. (1981). Gap junctional communication. *And Rev Physiol*, 43: 479-491.

Hirshfield AN. (1991). Development of follicles in the mammalian ovary: *Int Rev Cytol*, 124: 43-101.

Hsueh AJW. Elsenhatier K, Chun SY, Hsu SY, Billig H. (1996). Gonadal cell apoptosis. *Recent Prog Horm Res*, 51: 433-455.

Hsueh AJW. Billig H, Tsafriri A. (1994). Ovarian follicle atresia: a hormonally controlled apoptotic process. *Endocr Rev*, 15: 707-724.

Hurwitz A, Adashi EY. (1991). Ovarian follicular atresia as an apoptotic process. *Mol Cell Endocrinol*, 84: 19-23.

Hughes FM, Gorospe WC. (1991). Biochemical identification of apoptosis (programmed cell death) in granulosa cells: evidence for a potential mechanism underlying follicular atresia. *Endocrinology*, 129: 2415-2422.

Huuskonen H. Juutilainen J. and Komulainen H. (1993). Effects of low frequency magnetic fields on fetal development in rats. *Bioelectromagnetics*, 14: 205-213.

Jokela K. Puranen L. Sihvonen A-P. (2004). Assessment of the magnetic field exposure due to the battery current of digital mobile phones. *Health Physics* 86: 56-66.

Juutilainen J. Matilainen P. Saarikoski S. Laara E. Suonio S. (1993). Early pregnancy loss and exposure to 50 HZ magnetic fields. *Bioelectromagnetics*, 14: 229-236.

Kaipia A, Hsueh AJW. (1997). Regulation of ovarian follicle atresia. *Annu Rev Physiol*, 59: 349-363.

Kerr JFR. Wyllie AH, Currie AR. (1972). Apoptosis: a basic biological phenomenon with wide-ranging implications in tissue kinetics. *Brit. J. Cancer*, 26: 239-257.

Khaki AA. Tubbs RS. Shoja MM. Rad JS. Khaki A. Farahani RM. Zarrintan S. Nag TC. (2006). The effects of an electromagnetic field on the boundary tissue of the seminiferous tubules of the rat: a light and transmission electron microscope study. *Folia Morphol*, 65: 105-110.

Lahijani MS. Nojooshi SE. and Siadat SF. (2007). Light and electron microscopic studies of effect of 50 HZ electromagnetic fields on preincubated chick embryo. *Electromag Biol Med*, 26: 83-89.

Lauber K. Sibylle G, Waibel M, Wesselborg S. (2004). Clearance of apoptotic cells: Getting rid of the corpses. *Molecular Cell*, 14: 277-286.

Laun P. Pichova A. Madco F. Fuchs J. Ellinger A. Kohlwein S. Dewes I. Frohlich KU. Breitenbach M. (2000). Aged mother cells of Saccharomyces cervisdiae show markers of oxidative stress and apoptosis. *Mol Microbial*, 39: 1166-1173.

Lednev VV. (1991). Possible mechanism for the influence of weak magnetic fields on biological systems. *Bioelectromagnetics,* 12: 71-75.

Lee JS. Ahn SS. Jung KC. Et al. (2004). Effects of 60 HZ electromagnetic field exposure on testicular germ cell apoptosis in mice. *Asian J Androl,* 6: 29-34.

Leonard EJ, Skeel AH. (1980). Enhancement of spreading, phagocytosis and cliernotaxis by macrophage stimulating protein (MSP). *Adv Exp Med Biol,* 121B: 181-194.

Li CM, Chiang H, Fu YD, Shao BJ, Shi JR, Yao GD. (1999). Effects of 50 Hzmagnetic fields on gap junctional intercellular communication *Bioelectromagnetics,* 20: 290-294.

Libof AR. (1985). Cyclotron resonance in membrane transport. In Chiabrera A. Nicolini C. Schwan HP: "Interaction electromagnetic fields and cells.'" London : Plenurn, P 281, 1985.

Lin H. Head M. Blank M, Han L. Jin M. Goodman R.(1998). Myc-mediated transactivation of HSP70 expression following exposure to magnetic fields. *J Cell Biochem,* 69: 181-188.

Liu X, Zou H, Wang X. (1997). Dff a heterodimeric protein that functions downstream of caspase-3 to trigger DNA fragmentation during apoptosis. *Cell,* 89: 175-184.

Loewenstein WR. (1979). Junctional intercellular communication and the control of -rowth. *Biochim Biophys Acta,* 1: 560-565.

Lokmatova A. (1993). Ultrastructural analysis of testes in mice subjected to long-term exposure to a 17-KHZ electric field. *Radiobiology,* 33: 342-346.

Luben RA, Cain CD, Chen MC-Y, Rosen DM, Adey WR. (1982). Effects of electromagnetic stimuli on bone and bone cells in vitro: inhibition of responses to parathyroid hormone by low-energy low-frequency fields. *Proc Natl Acad Sci USA,* 79: 4180-4184.

Luben RA. (1991). Effects of low-energy electromagnetic fields (pulsed and DC) on membrane signal transduction processes in biological systems. *Health Phys,* 61: 15-28.

Lucia P. Luigi C, Piatti E, Umberta A. (2004). Effect of static magnetic field exposure on different DNA. *Bioelectromagnetics,* 25: 352-355.

Marek Z. Elzabieta R. Pawel M. Piotr P. Jolata J. (2004). The effect of weak 50 HZ fields on the umber of free oxygen radicals in rat lymphocytes in vitro. *Bioelectromagnetics,* 25: 607-612.

Martin H, Johnson E, Barry E. (2001). Essential reproduction. Fifth edition, *Iowa state university press A Blackwell science company,* Chapter 5.

Mc Givern RF. Sokol RZ. Adey WR. (1990). Prenatal exposure to a low frequency electromagnetic field demasculinizes adult scent marking behavior and increases accessory sex organ weights in rats. *Teratology,* 41: 1-8.

McLauchlan KA. (1981). The effects of magnetic fields on chemical reactions. *Sci Prog,* 67: 509- 529.

Mohammadnejad D. Soleimani Rad J. Azami A. et al. (2010). Protective effect of vitamin E supplement in electromagnetic field induced damages in spleen: An ultrastructural and light microscopic studies. *Global Veterinaria,* 4. 4: 416-421.

Mori T, Xu JP, Mori E, Sato E, Saito S, Guo MW. (1997). Expression of Fas- Fas ligand system associated with atresia through apoptosis in marine ovary. *Horm Res,* 48: 11-19.

Norman CB, Ricci J, Breger L, Zychlinsky A. (1997). Effect of Low-intercity AC and /or DC electromagnetic fields on cell attachment and induction of apoptosis. *Bioelectromagnetics,* 18: 264-272.

NRC (1996). Possible health effects of exposure to residential electric and magnetic fields. *National Research Council, Washington: National Academy Press.*

Ohnishi T. Wang X, Takahashi A. (2002). Low-dose-rate radiation attenuates the response of the tumor suppressor TP53. *Radiat Res,* 151: 369-372.

Otasuki Y. (2001). Apoptosis in human elIC1011ICtl-ILIIII. *Health & Disease,* 12: 211- 222.

Ozguner M. Koyu A. Cesur G. et al. (2005). Biological and morphological effects on the reproductive organ of rats after exposure to electromagnetic field. *Saudi Med J,* 26: 405 410.

Payne CM, Bernstein C, Bernstein H. (1995). Apoptosis overview emphasizing the role of oxidative stress, DNA damage and signal-transduction pathways. *Leak Lymphoma,* 19: 43-93.

Peluso JJ, Steger RW, Hafez E. (1977). Surface ultrastructural changes in granulosa cells of atretic follicles. *Biol Reprod,* 16: 600-605.

Perez GI, Tao XJ, Tilly JL. (1999). Fragmentation and death (a.k.a. apoptosis) of ovulated oocytes. *Mol Hum Reprod,* 5: 414-420.

Phillips PL, Haggren W, Thomas WJ, Ishida-Jones T, Adey WR. (1992). Magnetic field – induced changes in specific gene transcription. *Biochim Biophys Acta,* 1132: 140- 144.

Repacholi MH. (1998). Low-level exposure to radiofrequency electromagnetic fields. *Bioelectromagnetics,* 19: 1-19.

Rodan GA, Bourrett LA, Norton LA. (1978). DNA-synthesis in cartilage cells is stimulated by oscillating electric fields. *Science,* 199: 690-692.

Roshangar L. and Soleimani Rad J. (2007). Ultrastructural alterations and occurrence of apoptosis in developing follicles exposed to low frequency electromagnetic field in rat ovary. *Pakistan Journal of Biological Sciences,* 10. 24: 4413-4419.

Roshangar L, Soleimani Rad J. (2001). The effect of electromagnetic field on follicular maturation. *5th international congress on Anatomical sciences. Tehran Iran.*

Roshangar L, Soleimani Rad J. (2002). Electron microscopic study of folliculogenesis after exposure to electromagnetic field. *Anatomical science J,* 1: 47-51.

Roshangar L. Soleimani Rad J, Khaki A. (2003). Light and electron microscopic evaluation of the effect of electromagnetic field on oocyte maturation. Twin- Meeting Alpha-andrology, Antwerp Belgium.

Sage C, Johansson O, Sage SA. (2007). Personal digital assistant (PDA) cell phone units produce elevated extremely low frequency electromagnetic field emissions. *Bioelectromagnetics.* DOI 10.1002/bem.20315 Published online in Wiley InterScience (www.interscience.wiley.com).

Sandra M, Cecconi S, Gualtieri G, Bartolome AD, Troiani G. (2000). Evaluation of the effects of extremely low frequency electromagnetic fields on mammalian follicle development. *Hum Reorod,* 15 (11): 2319-2325.

Shikone T, Yamoto M, Kokawa K, Yamashita K. Nishimori K, Nakano R. (1996). Apoptosis of human corpora lutea during cyclic luteal regression and early pregnancy. *J Clin Endocrinol Metab,* 81: 2376-2380.

Shulyakovskaya T, Sumegi L, Gal D. (1993). In vivo experimental studies on the role of free radicals in photodynamic therapy. *Biochem Biophys Res Commun,* 195(2): 581-587.

Soleimani Rad J. and Katebi M. (1997). Studying the effect of electromagnetic field on spermatogenesis. *Med J University of Tabriz,* 31: 36-41.

Soleimani Rad J, Roshangar L, Karimi K. (2001). The effect of electromagnetic field on Fallopian tubes. IFFS, Selected Free Comunications, Monduzzi Editor, International Proceedings Division, Melbourne Australia, November 25-30.

Soleiniani Rad J, Roushangar L. (2000). Inhibitory effect of electromagnetic field on folliculogensis: with and without hMG-induced ovulation. 7`" Annual meeting of Middle East fertility society (MEFS), 2000; Lebanon. MEFS journal, Vol 5, Suppl 2:7.

Sugino N. Shimamura K, Tamura H, Ono M, Nakamura Y, Ogino K. (1996). Progesterone inhibits superoxide radical production by mononuclear phagocytes in pseudopregnant rats. *Endocrinol,* 137: 749-754.

Takahashi A. Asakawa I. Yuki K. (2002). Radiation-induced apoptosis in the scid mouse spleen after low dose-rate irradiation. *Int J Radiat Biol,* 78: 689-693.

Takeo Y, Hokano M. (1995). An electron microscopic study of apoptosis in the granulose layer of ovarian follicles in rats. *Med Electron Microsc,* 28(1): 38-44.

Tenforde TS, Polk C, Postow E. (1996). Interaction of ELF magnetic fields with living systems and Biological effects of electromagnetic fields. *Boca Raton: CRC Press,* p 185-230.

Tilly JL. Kawalski KI, schomberg, DW, Hsueh AJ. (1992). Apoptosis in atretic ovarian follicles is associated with selective decreases in messenger ribonucleic acid transcripts for gonadotropin receptors and cytochrome P450 aromatase. *Endocrinol,* 131:1670-1676.

Tilly JL. (1998). Molecular and genetic basis of normal and toxicant-induced apoptosis in female germ cells. *Toxicol Lett,* 102 (31): 497-501.

Tofani S. (1999). Physics may help chemistry to improve medicine: a possible mechanism for anticancer activity of static and ELF magnetic fields. *Phys Media,* 15(4): 291-294.

Torregrossa MV. (2005). Biological and health effects of electric and magnetic fields at extremely low frequencies. *Ann Ig,* 17: 441-530.

UNEP/WHO/IRPA (1987). United Nations Environment Programme/ International Radiation Protection Association/ World health Organization. *Environmental Health Criteria,* 69: Magnetic Fields. WHO. Geneva.

Valberg PA. PA. Kavet R. Rafferty CN. (1997). Can low-level 50/60 Hz electric and magnetic fields cause biological effects? *Radiat Res,* 148: 2-21.

Van Blerkom J, Davis PW. (1998). DNA strand breaks and phosphatidylserine redistribution in newly ovulated and cultured mouse and human oocytes: occurrence and relationship to apoptosis. *Hum Reprod,* 13:1317-1324.

Vazquez-Niri GH. Sotello JR. (1967). Electron microscope study of the atretic oocytes of the rat. *ZZellforsch Mikrosk Anat,* 80: 518-533.

Vousden KH. (2005). Apoptosis. P53 and PUMA: a deadly duo. *Science,* 309: 1685-1686.

Walleczek J. (1992). Electromagnetic field effects on cells of the immune system: The role of calcium signalling. *FASEB J,* 6: 3177-3185.

Wu W. Yao K. Wang KJ. Lu DQ. He JL. Et al. (2008). Blocking 1800 MHZ mobile phone radiation-induced reactive oxygen species production and DNA damage in lens epithelial cells by noise magnetic fields. *Zhejiang Da Xue Xue Bao Yi Xue Ban,* 37: 34-38.

Wyllie AH. Kerr JFR. Currie AR. (1972). Cell death: the significance of apoptosis. *Int Rev Cytol,* 68: 251-307.

Wyllie AH. (1980). Glucocorticoid-induced thymocyte apoptosis is associated with endogenous endogenous activation. *Nature,* 284: 555-556.

Zamboni L. (1972). Comparative studies on the ultrastructure of mammalian oocytes. In: Biggers ED, Schuetz AW (eds.), Oogenesis. *Baltimore: University Press,* pp. 5-46.

Zymslony M. (2007). Biological mechanisms and health effects of EMF in view of requirements of reports on the impact of various installations on the environment. *Med Pr,* 58: 27-36.

4

Role of Tumor Marker CA-125 in the Detection of Spontaneous Abortion

Batool Mutar Mahdi
Al-Kindy College of Medicine - Baghdad University,
Iraq

1. Introduction

Spontaneous abortion represents a common pregnancy adverse outcome and is a serious emotional burden for women. Loss of pregnancy is a distressing problem for both the patient and physician.

The clinical diagnosis of threatened abortion is presumed when any bloody vaginal discharge or bleeding appears during the first trimester of pregnancy. A prospective study on women with threatened abortion reported that women older than 34 years had an odds ratio of 2.3 for miscarriage (Falco et al., 1996). Some women who bleed in early pregnancy, approximately half of them, will abort (Weiss et al., 2004). Occasionally, bleeding may persist for weeks, and then it becomes essential to decide whether there is any possibility of continuation of the pregnancy or not. The diagnosis of spontaneous abortion currently depends on a combination of ultrasonography and nine hormonal methods including serum human chorionic gonadotropin (HCG), estradiol (E2), estrone, estriol, progesterone, human placental lactogen, cortisol, urine HCG and urine estrogen (Gerhavd and Runnebaum 1984; Zeimet et al., 1998; Osmanagaoglu et al., 2010). Another parameter that could be used as a predictive marker for a spontaneous abortion or subsequent outcome of pregnancy is Cancer Antigen-125 (CA-125). This antigen is a cell surface high molecular weight glycoprotein. It is a mucin like coelomic antigen, which is detected in 80% of non-mucus epithelial carcinomas of ovary. This antigen is secreted from normal tissues, such as coelomic epithelium, amnion and their derivatives including respiratory system, mesenteric organs and epithelium of female genital system (Berek 2002). An increased CA-125 level is due to genital or non-genital origins. Non-genital causes include hepatic diseases, peritonitis, renal failure, breast, colon and lung cancer, and tuberculosis. Genital causes include: pelvic inflammatory diseases, endometriosis, adenomyosis, leiomioma, ectopic pregnancy, endometrial and ovarian cancer.

Serum CA-125 levels are increased in early pregnancy and immediately after birth (Cunningham 2005; Speroff and Fritz 2005), implicating the disintegration of the maternal decidua (i.e., blastocyst implantation and placental separation) as a possible source of the tumor marker elevation (Ayaty et al., 2007). There is a cyclic change in the serum concentration of CA-125 in normal menstruating women. It indicates that CA-125 was produced from normal endometrium (Zeimet et al., 1993). Generation of potential immunogenic peptide (YTLDrDSLYV) derived from CA-125 that bind to human leukocyte antigen (HLA A2,1) leading to elicit peptide – specific human cytotoxic T lymphocytes that effectively kill ovarian tumors expressing CA-125 antigen (Kabawat et al., 1983; Bellon et al., 2009) .

Regarding the level of CA-125 in pregnancy, conflicting results have been reported. There is a positive correlation between CA-125 levels elevated 18-22 days after conception and spontaneous abortion, while repeated measurements at 6 weeks of gestation did not correlate with the outcome (Check et al., 1990). The distribution of CA-125 during pregnancy was highest in first trimester than second and third trimester (Brumsted et al., 1988). This may be due to the secretion of CA-125 and placenta protein 14 (PP14) by the glandular epithelium of the endometrium (Julkunen et al., 1986a; Julkunen et al., 1986b; Dalton et al.,1995; Dalton et al.,1998). Serum concentration of these parameters may increase during the first trimester of pregnancy as the concentration of progesterone rise to a maximum in the first trimester. These observations suggest that CA-125 is synthesized by normal endometrium in non pregnant female and by deciduas in pregnant women (Jacobs et al., 1988). Quirk et al. (1988) hypothesized that decidual CA-125 gains access to the maternal compartment via a "tubal reflux" resulting in subsequent absorption via the peritoneal lymphatics. They speculated further that the drop in maternal serum CA-125 might well be related to a functional obstruction of the tubes that occurs as pregnancy advances, with fusion of the decidua capsularis and the decidua parietalis.

The serum CA-125 level is higher in normal pregnancy compared to ectopic pregnancy 2-4 weeks after a missed menses due to impaired interaction between the fetal trophoblast and tubal mucosa (Niloff et al., 1984; Sadovsky et al., 1991; Predanic 2000). Increase in serum CA-125 levels was found in patients with vaginal bleeding and impending spontaneous abortion due to extensive decidual destruction and trophoblast separation from decidual cells (Kobayashi et al., 1993). Sequential determinations of maternal CA-125 measurements appear to be a highly sensitive prognostic marker in the patients with viable pregnancy at an abortion risk (Schmidt et al., 2001). Transient elevation of the CA-125 level occurs in maternal serum during early pregnancy and just after delivery because of the destruction of decidual tissues may cause this transient elevation of CA-125 (Shin et al., 2003). Therefore the elevated serum CA-125 levels in women with normal intrauterine pregnancies may be clinically useful in early pregnancy monitoring. This test is rather sensitive to differentiate the normal pregnancy and threatened abortion. There was not a significant correlation between CA-125 levels and gestational weeks (Yamane et al., 1989). Consequently, an increase in serial CA-125 measurements in the follow-up of pregnancies with vaginal bleeding could be an early signal in determining the progression to the pregnancy loss. It had been found that women with symptoms of imminent abortion, who have a CA-125 level of ≥43.IU/ml, should be considered at a greater risk of miscarriage (Fiegler et al., 2003; Sotiriadis et al., 2004) (Table-1).

Patients who eventually aborted had values of CA-125 more than 125 IU/ml while the control had a value not more than 93 IU/ml (Check et al., 1990; Ocer et al., 1992). In addition to that, an extremely high CA-125 level (over 2000 IU/mL) indicates a karyotype associated with fetal anomalies and CA-125 levels returned to normal after spontaneous abortion eliminated the possibility that some other condition caused the marked increase (Munné et al., 1995). Although elevated CA-125 levels have been found previously in patients suffering from ovarian hyperstimulation syndrome and this merely reflect an increase in number of follicles (Bischof et al., 1989). Mordel et al. (1992) reported that CA-125 existed in significant amounts in the follicular fluid of periovulatory follicles of IVF and embryo transfer patients, but that there was no correlation between CA-125 concentrations and follicular fluid oestradiol, progesterone, testosterone, oocyte fertilization, embryo quality or pregnancy rates. It was stated that a possible ovarian tissue–blood barrier might preclude the passage of CA-125 from the follicular fluid to the serum (Fleuren et al., 1987). Endometrial receptivity is an important factor in IVF pregnancy success, and may be the origin of the changes in serum CA-125 that occur mostly from the endometrium. Bersinger et al. (1993) have investigated the considerable contribution of the endometrium to serum CA-125 concentrations and found that it reflects a favourable endometrium. The ability to predict the chances of pregnancy before embryo transfer might assist clinicians in deciding whether embryos have a greater chance of implantation if they are transferred in a subsequent cycle. It was noted that CA-125 concentrations on the day of oocyte retrieval were the best predictors of pregnancy, with concentrations >10 IU/ml having an accuracy of 86.6% for pregnancy. Thus, in intracytoplasmic sperm injection cycles, women with high serum CA-125 concentrations (>10 IU/ml) on the day of oocyte retrieval had very high pregnancy rates (Tavmergen et al., 2001) (Table 2).

Favorable prognostic factors	Adverse prognostic factors
History	
Advancing gestational age	Maternal age >34 years
	Increasing number of previous miscarriages
Sonography	
Fetal heart activity at presentation	Fetal bradycardia
	Discrepancy between gestational age and crown to rump length
	Empty gestational sac >15-17 mm
Maternal serum biochemistry	
Normal levels of these markers	Free β-hCG value of 20 ng/ml
	hCG increase <66% in 48 hrs
	Bioactive/immunoreactive ratio hCG <0.5
	Progesterone <45 nmol/l in 1st trimester
	Inhibin A <0.553 multiples of median
	CA-125 level ≥43.1 U/mL in 1st trimester

Table 1. Prognostic factors in cases of threatened abortion

Characteristic	Non-pregnant mean ± SEM	Pregnant mean ± SEM	P Values
No. of oocytes retrieved	7.58 ± 1.02	9.54 ± 0.92	NS
No. of mature oocytes	4.98 ± 0.58	6.43 ± 0.54	NS
Grade I embryo rates (%)	47.5	54.3	NS
No. of embryos transferred	3.0 ± 0.3	4.66 ± 0.3	<0.001
Peak oestradiol conc. (pg/ml)	1483.17 ± 129.9	2002.3 ± 114.8	0.004
Endometrial thickness (mm)	12.6 ± 0.38	13.45 ± 0.42	NS

NS: not significant (t test and x^2 test; P > 0.05).

Table 2. Value of serum CA-125 concentrations as predictors of pregnancy in assisted reproduction cycles

An observation suggests CA-125 correlates less well with endometrial development in women suffering from recurrent miscarriage (Scrapellini et al., 1995). The concentration of CA-125 in the pregnant women who subsequently aborted were higher than those who did not, thus suggesting that serum CA-125 are not so important in maintaining successful pregnancy (Azogui et al., 1996). CA-125 may be useful in the assessment of endometrial development in recurrent miscarriage patients and this suggested the importance in preparing the endometrium for embryo implantation (Yu et al., 2008). High level of serum CA-125 with high lactate dehydrogenase indicates more extensive trophoblastic tissue damage (Madendag et al., 2008). Some found that single serum CA-125 level determinations is valuable in women with imminent abortion presenting with abdominal pain, vaginal bleeding or both while others are in disagreement with this result (Fiegler et al., 2003). Possibly it may be attributed to the method of CA-125 measurement like the radioimmunoassay or the enzyme immune sorbent assay method.

The prognostic predictive value of maternal serum CA-125 measurement in threatened abortion can be useful to determine the extent of decidual destruction which is directly related to the outcome of pregnancy. So one can conclude a hypothesis of a tropho-decidual origin of this marker suggesting its possible usefulness in the prognostic evaluation of first trimester threatened abortion. To predict the outcome of patients with threatened abortion at an early stage of gestation is clinically important. CA-125 and hormones associated with pregnancy serum human chorionic gonadotropin beta-subunit, serum progesterone, serum cortisol, serum human placental lactogen, serum estrone, serum estradiol, serum estriol, urine human chorionic gonadotropin progesterone, inhibin A, and urine estrogen. Serum CA-125 concentrations may be helpful as predictors and serve as a judge of good prognosis in threatened abortion indicators in association with other tests like ultrasonography because others found that serum CA-125 levels are not predictive of spontaneous abortion in the first trimester and failed to discriminate among missed abortions, threatened abortions, and normal pregnancies (Mahdi 2010) (Table 3).

Test	Group I End with abortion n=42	Group II Normal pregnancy n=20
Serum Ca-125 Cut-off value up to 30 IU/ml	39.9±15.4	28.03±4.5
p-value	NS	NS

Table 3. Level of CA-125 in the serum of pregnant women expressed as mean ± standard error mean

The single measurement of free beta-hCG or progesterone levels can be useful in the prediction of first trimester spontaneous abortions, but using progesterone may be recommended since it has high availability and low cost.

As a conclusion, the measurement of serum CA-125 is not of value to predict the outcome of threatened abortion because it is secreted from different origins. There is no correlation between CA-125 level and outcome of pregnancy. CA-125 may have a predictive role in the successful outcome in ICSI cycles, but it has to be further investigated

2. References

Ayaty S, Roudsari FV, Tavassoly F. CA-125 in normal pregnancy and threatened abortion. Iranian J Reprod Med 2007;5:57-60.

Azogui G, Yaronovski A, Zohar S, Ben-Shlomo I. CA-125 are elevated in viable pregnancies destined to be miscarried, a prospective longitudinal study. Fertil Steril 1996;65:1059-1061.

Bellon S, Anfossi S, O'Brien TJ, Cannon MJ, Silasi DA, Azodi M, Schwartz PE, Rutherford TJ, Pecorelli S, Santin AD. Generation of CA-125 specific cytotoxic T lymphocytes in human leukocytes antigen –A2, 1 positive healthy donors and patients with advanced ovarian cancer. Am.J.Obstet.Gynecol 2009;200:75e1-e10.

Berek S.J "Novak's Gynecology", 13th Ed. Lippincott William & Wilkins; 2002:518.

Bersinger, N.A., Sinosich, M.J., Baber, R. et al. Development of an endometrial explant model for the investigation of uterine readiness for implantation in the human. In Gianaroli, L., Campana, A. and Trounson, A.O. (eds), Implantation in Mammals. Serono Symposia 91. Raven Press, New York.1993. pp. 301–308.

Bischof P, Therese MM, Cedard L. Are pregnancy-associated plasma protein-A (PAPP-A) and CA-125 measurements after IVFET possible predictors of early pregnancy wastage? Hum Reprod 1989;4:84-87.

Brumsted JR, Nakajima ST, Badger G, Riddick DH, Grudzinskas JG. The distribution of CA-125 in the reproductive tract of pregnant and non-pregnant women. Br J Obstet Gynecol 1988; 95:1190 -1194.

Check JH, Nowroozi K, Winkel CA. Serum CA-125 levels in early pregnancy and subsequent spontaneous abortion. Obstet Gynecol 1990; 75:742-744.

Cunningham F.G, "Williams's obstetrics", 22nd ed.USA, Appleton & Lange, 2005.

Dalton CF, Laird SM, Serle E etal. The measurement of CA-125 and placental protein 14 in uterine flushing in women with recurrent miscarriage relation to endometrial morphology .Hum.Reprod 1995; 10:2680-2684.

Dalton CF,Laird SM, Estdale SE,Saravelos HG and Li TC.Endometrial protein PP14 and CA-125 in recurrent miscarriage patients ,correlation with pregnancy outcome. Human Reprod 1998;13:3197-3202.

Falco P, Milano V, Pilu G, David C, Grisolia G, Rizzo N, Bovicelli L. Sonography of pregnancies with first-trimester bleeding and a viable embryo: a study of prognostic indicators by logistic regression analysis. Ultrasound Obstet Gynecol 1996;7:165-9.

Fiegler P, Katz M, Kaminski K, Rudol G. Clinical value of a single serum CA-125 level in women with symptoms of imminent abortion during the first trimester of pregnancy.J Reprod Med 2003 ;48:982-988.

Fleuren, G.J., Nap, M., Aalders, J.G. *et al.* Explanation of the limited correlation between tumor CA-125 content and serum CA-125 antigen levels in patients with ovarian tumors. Cancer 1987; 60:2437–2442.

Gerhavd I and Runnebaum B. Predictive value of hormone determinations in the first half of the pregnancy. Eur. J. Obstet. Gyne. Reprod. Biol 1984; 17:1-17.

Jacobs IJ, fay TN, Stabile I, Bridges JE, Oram JE and Grudzinskas JG. The distribution of CA-125 in the reproductive tract of pregnant and non pregnant women. Br.J.Obst.Gyne.1988.95:1190-1194.

Julkunen M, Rutanen EM, Koskimies A etal. Distribution of placental protein 14 in tissues and body fluids during pregnancy. Br.J.Obstet. Gynaecol.1986a.92:1145-1151.

Julkunen M, Koistinen R, Sjoberg.J. etal. Secretory endometrium synthesis placental protein 14 Endocrinology.1986b.118:1782-1786.

Kabawat SE, Bast RC, Welch WR et al .Immunopatholgic characterizations of a monoclonal antibody that recognizes common surface antigen of human ovarian tumors of serous , endometeriod and clear cell types. Am.J .Clin.Pathol.1983.79:98-104.

Kobayashi F, Takashima E, Sagawa N, Mori T, Fujii S. Maternal serum CA-125 levels in early intrauterine and tubal pregnancies. Arch Gynecol Obstet 1993; 252: 185-189.

Madendag Y, Col-Madendag I, Kanat-Pektas M and Danisman N.Predictive power of serum CA-125 and LDH in the outcome of first trimester pregnancies with human chorionic gonadotropin levels below discriminatory zone. Arch. Gynecology .Obstet 2009 ; 279:661-666.

Mahdi BM. Estimation of Ca-125 in first trimester threatened abortion. Int J Gyn Obs. 2010;12:1.

Mordel, N., Anteby, S.O., Zajicek, G. *et al.* CA-125 is present in significant concentrations in periovulatory follicles of *in vitro* fertilization patients. Fertil Steril 1992 ; 57:377–380.

Munné, S., Alikani, M., Tomkin, G. *et al.* (1995) Embryo morphology, developmental rates, and maternal age are correlated with chromosome abnormalities. Fertil. Steril 1995;64 :382–391.

Niloff JM, Knapp RC, Schaetzl E. CA-125 antigen levels in obstetric and gynecologic patients. Obstet Gynecology 1984; 64:703-707.

Ocer F, Bese T, Saridoqan E, Aydinli K and Astasu T. The prognostic significance of maternal serum Ca-125 measurement in threatened abortion. Eur J Obs Gyn Rep Biolo 1992; 46: 137-142.

Osmanagaoglu MA, Erdogan I, Eminagaoglu S, Karahan SC, Ozgun S, Can G and Bozkaya H. The diagnostic value of beta-human chorionic gonadotropin, progesterone, CA-125 in the prediction of abortions. J Obs Gyn 2010; 30: 288-293.

Predanic M. Differentiating tubal abortion from viable ectopic pregnancy with serum CA-125 and beta human chorionic gonadotropin determinations. Fertile Steril 2000;73:522-525.

Quirk JG, Brunson GL, Long CA, Bannon GA, Sanders MM, O'Brien TJ. CA-125 in tissues and amniotic fluid during pregnancy. Am J Obstet Gynecol 1988; 159 :644-9.

Sadovsky Y, Pineda J , Collins JL. Serum CA-125 levels in women with ectopic and intrauterine pregnancies. J Reprod Med 1991; 36:875-878.

Schmidt T, Rein DT, Foth D. Prognostic value of repeated serum CA-125 measurements in first trimester pregnancy. Eur J Obstet Gynecol Reprod Biol 2001; 97:168-173.

Scrapellini F, Mastrone M, Sbracia M and Scarpellini L. Serum Ca-125 and first trimester abortion. Int J Obs Gyn 1995; 49: 259-264.

Shin JS, Kim TJ and Kim YM. Maternal Serum CA-125 Levels in Intrauterine Pregnancy and Abortion in the First Trimester. Korean J Perinatol 2003; 14:284-289 .

Sotiriadis A, Papatheodorou S and Makrydimas G. Threatened miscarriage: evaluation and management . BMJ 2004; 329 : 152-155.

Speroff L, Fritz M, A .Clinical Gynecology endocrinology and infertility. 7th ed., Lippincott Williams and Wilkins 2005; 11-12.

Tavmergan E, Sendag F, Coker E and Levi R. Value of serum CA-125 concentrations as predictors of pregnancy in assisted reproduction cycles. Human Repod 2001; 16:1129- 1134.

Weiss JL, Malone FD, Vidaver J, et al. Threatened abortion: A risk factor for poor pregnancy outcome, a population-based screening study. Am J Obstet Gynecol 2004; 190:745-50.

Yamane Y, Takahashi k and Kiotao M. Prognostic potential of serum CA-125 and pregnant markers in threatened abortion. Nippon Sanka Fujinka Gakkai Zasshi 1989 ; 41:1999-2004.

Yu X, Cohen J, Deshmukh H, Zhang R, Shin JY,Osann K,Husain A, Kapp DS, Chen L and Chan JK. The association of serial ultrasounds and CA-125 prior to diagnosis of ovarian cancer –Do they improve early detection.Gynecol Oncol 2008; 111:385-386.

Zeimet AG, Offner FA, Muller-Holzner E. etal. Peritoneum and tissues of the female reproductive tract as physiological sources of Ca-125. Tumor boil 1998 ;19:275-282.

Zeimet AG, Muller-Holzner E. Marth C. etal. Tumor markers CA-125 in tissues of female reproductive tract and in serum during the normal menstrual cycle. Fert.Steril 1993; 59:1028-1035.

5

The Effect of Prepregnancy Body Mass Index and Gestational Weight Gain on Birth Weight

Hiroko Watanabe
Department of Clinical Nursing, Shiga University of Medical Science
Japan

1. Introduction

Birth weight is an important predictor in infant mortality and morbidity, growth, development and wellbeing in adult life (Goldfrey & Barker, 2000). Reduced-size-at-birth infants, which include low birth weight (LBW: birth weight <2,500 g) and small-for-gestational age (SGA: below the 10th percentile for gestational age) infants, are at greater risk of having reduced educational capacity, school performance, and intellectual development than are infants of normal birth weight (Lagerstrom et al., 1991).

Some adult health risks also have a clear negative correlation with infant birth weight. In 1980′, Barker & Osmond in the UK reported that differences around the UK in neonatal mortality as maker for LBW in 1921-1925 predicted death rates from stroke and heart disease in 1968-1978 (Barker & Osmond, 1986). They found that LBW and weight at one year were associated with an increased risk of death from cardiovascular disease. There was an approximate two times of the mortality rate from the highest to the lowest extremes of birth weight (Barker et al., 1989).

Over recent decades, accumulating evidence around the world has suggested that LBW may be associated with an increased risk of subsequent development of a variety of complications in adulthood including cardiovascular disease, non-insulin-dependent diabetes mellitus, hypertension, and dyslipidemia (Li et al., 1998; Rich-Edwards et al., 1999). These studies have led to discoveries of the developmental, fetal origins of adult health and disease; fetal programming theory states that fetal growth restriction, secondary to under nutrition, has long-lasting physiologic and structural effects that predispose the fetus to diseases later in life.

On the other hand, high birth weight relates to complications during delivery including shoulder dystocia and caesarean sections and to obesity during child- and adulthood (Stotland et al., 2004; Weiss et al., 2004). Increased numbers of high birth weight infants (>4,000 g) and large-for-gestational age infants (LGA; birth weight above the 90th percentile for gestational age) have been reported in North America and Europe (Kramer et al., 2002; Surkan et al., 2004). In the past three decades, there has been a 116 g increase in singleton birth weight (Catalano, 2007). Fetal growth is affected by maternal obesity and by mothers being overweight during pregnancy. Recent evidence suggests that LGA infants are also at increased risk for childhood and subsequent adult obesity as well as type two diabetes (Parsons et al., 2001). Thus, birth weight may be an important parameter of adult disease.

Numerous factors are associated with birth weight, such as parity and the sex of the child (Bonellie et al., 2008), maternal and gestational diabetes (Langer et al., 2005), maternal smoking during pregnancy (Ward et al., 2007), maternal overweight status (Larsen et al., 1990), and gestational weight gain (GWG) (Kiel et al., 2007). Of these factors, previous studies have suggested particularly that both prepregnancy body mass index (BMI; weight (kg)/ height (m)^2) and GWG are positively associated with birth weight in the offspring and are related to risks of both low and high offspring birth weight (Brown et al., 2002; Rode et al., 2007). Women with a normal prepregnancy BMI and those who meet the recommended weight gains are healthiest and have healthier children. Adequate GWG contributes to better pregnancy outcomes in both mothers and infants, for short- and long-term health. Prepregnancy BMI and GWG management may be a key factor influencing the health of women during pregnancy and the development of the fetus. This review focuses on the effect of prepregnancy BMI and adequate GWG on birth weight.

2. Optimal birth weight for low neonatal mortality rate

Birth weight is the single strongest predictor of infant survival. One determinant of birth weight is gestational age: as the fetus matures, it grows. The other determinant is gestational age, because birth weight is a summary of fetal growth. Susser et al. (1972) reported that when gestational age and weight are analyzed simultaneously, birth weight accounts for 90% of the variance of perinatal mortality, whereas gestational age accounts for barely 5%. On the other hand, Wilcox & Skjaerven (1992) stated that an infant benefits as much from an increase in gestational age as from an increase in its weight, relative to the weights of others at the same gestational age.

Birth weight between the 10th and 90th percentile has been generally accepted as appropriate fetal growth and classified as an appropriate gestational age (AGA) infant. However, what birth weight range in single term infants is optimal to reduce the neonatal mortality rate? National weight-for-gestational-age charts are created from the weight distributions of livebirths at each age using population-based data from each country. According to Japanese Vital Statistics, the lowest early neonatal mortality rate per 1000 live births in 2005 was 0.3 for infants weighing 3,000–3,999 g. The rate increased with decreasing birth weight: 0.4 for 2,500–2,999 g, 1.7 for 2,000–2,499 g and 10.9 for 1,500–1,999 g (Ministry of Health, Labour and Welfare, Japan, 2006).

The National Center for Health Statistics in the United States reported similar findings for the year 1995–2002, using singletons data (Joseph et al., 2009). For centuries, gestational maturity has been understood as important to infant survival. Research establishing an association between birth weight and neonatal morbidity/ mortality rates in term livebirth infants is limited. Joseph et al. (2009) show the birth weight-specific rates of serious neonatal morbidity and neonatal mortality in 17,554,934 livebirths from perinatal mortality data files of the National Center for Health Statistics for the years 1995-2002. All were singleton livebirths with a clinical estimate of gestation between 36 and 42 weeks born to white or black mothers in the United States (Figure 1). Based on empirical observation, birth weight-specific patterns of serious neonatal morbidity or neonatal death follow a specific pattern, that is, that neonatal morbidity/mortality rates decrease exponentially with increasing birth weight in the LBW range. This declining pattern changes to a flat, stable rate at "optimal" birth weight before serious neonatal morbidity/neonatal mortality rates increase with increasing birth weight. In the regression model, the low optimal birth weight at 40 weeks' gestation was 2,982 g (95% confidence interval (CI): 2,965-2,999 g) for females and 3,012 g (95% CI: 3,008-3,018 g) for males. Similarly, the high end of optimal birth weight range was 3,813 g (95% CI: 3,774-3,852 g) for females and 3,978 g (95% CI: 3,976-3,980 g) for males.

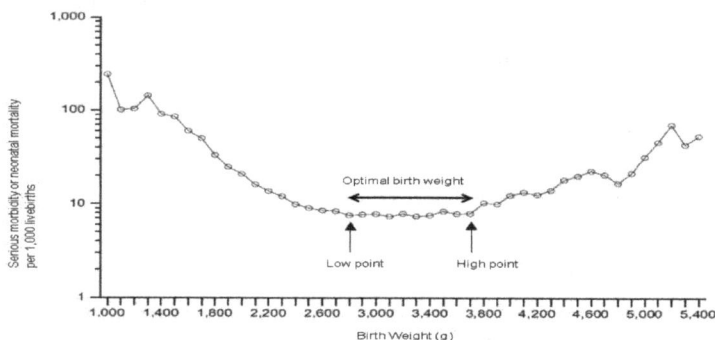

Source; Reference [Joseph KS., et al.,2009]

Fig. 1. Birth weight specific rates of serious neonatal morbidity and neonatal mortality at 37 weeks' gestational age among singletons

The optimal birth weight range may vary according to the age, race, ethnicity, and size of the mother, as maternal growth constraint may protect the health of the mother and baby. A study of 16.4 million women using the National Center for Health Statistics' 1983-1987 national lived birth/infant death data sets, examined the association between birth weight and neonatal mortality rate in adolescent (aged 15-18 years) and adult mothers (aged 19-34 years) of black and white race. Minimum neonatal mortality rates occurred at the same birth weight (3,500 to 4,499 g white and 3,000 to 3,999 g black) whether mothers of the infants were adolescents or adults. The most favorable range of birth weight, in which survival was greatest, commenced at 3,000 g for all mothers and terminated at 3,999 g for most black adolescents and black adults, at 4,499 g for most white adolescents, and at 4,999 g for white adults. Of infants born to mothers < or = 16 years old, 33% were lighter and 1.5% were heavier than the favorable birth weight range (Rees et al., 1996). Assisting mothers to bear infants with birth weight in the optimal weight range corresponding with low neonatal mortality in each country is an appropriate goal of clinical management.

3. Optimal weight gain recommendation

Adequate weight gain by prepregnancy BMI is important for optimal pregnancy outcomes. The Institute of Medicine (IOM) released new gestational weight guidelines (IOM, 2009) to reinforce those released in 1990 (IOM, 1990), because many key aspects of the health of women of childbearing age have changed, such as the increasingly high rates of overweight and obese women, increasing GWG, and the increasing age of women becoming pregnant. There are several salient differences. First, the new guidelines change the BMI categories to those commonly used for other adult health outcomes. Second, they provide a closed gestational weight gain range for obese women, based on data from women with BMI values of 30-34.9 kg/m².

According to the new guideline, underweight women (BMI<18.5 kg/m²) should gain 12.5-18.0 kg during pregnancy, normal weight women (BMI 18.5-24.9 kg/m²) should gain 11.5-16.0 kg, and overweight women (BMI 25.0-29.9 kg/m²) should gain 7.0-11.5 kg. This is the standard for weight gain worldwide (IOM, 2009) (Table 1). This guideline will be used in clinical practice as an effective weight management tool, and it will help to evaluate the association between these gestational weight ranges and pregnancy outcomes worldwide. Weight gain within the guidelines has been associated with healthy fetal and maternal outcomes.

Prepregnancy BMI (kg/m²)	Total Weight Gain		Rates of Weight Gains* 2nd and 3rd Trimester	
	Range in kg	Range in lbs	Mean (range) in kg/week	Mean (range) in lbs/week
Underweight	12.5-18	28-40	0.51	1
(<18.5)			(0.44-0.58)	(1-1.3)
Normal weight	11.5-16	25-35	0.42	1
(18.5-24.9)			(0.35-0.5)	(0.8-1)
Overweight	7-11.5	15-25	0.28	0.6
(25.0-29.9)			(0.23-0.33)	(0.5-0.7)
Obese	5-9	11-20	0.22	0.5
(≥30.0)			(0.17-0.27)	(0.4-0.6)

* Calculations assume a 0.5-2 kg (1.1-4.4 lbs) weight gain in the first trimester

Source; Reference [Institute of Medicine, 2009]

Table 1. 2009 IOM recommendations for total and rate of weight gain during pregnancy by prepregnancy BMI

In the 1990 IOM guideline, two thirds of women exceeded the recommended weight gain (Schieve et al., 1998). In a study of over 4,000 women from the University of California's San Francisco Perinatal Database, 23% of underweight women, 49% of normal-weight women, and 70% of overweight women exceeded the 1990 IOM recommendations (Carmichael et al., 1997). On the other hand, newly released, 2009 IOM recommendations were assessed by Park et al. (2011) in a population-based, retrospective cohort study of 570,672 women with singleton, full-term livebirths in Florida from 2004 to 2007. They found that 31.6% of underweight women, 42.8% of normal-weight women, and 65.0% of overweight women exceeded the 2009 IOM recommendations. These results suggest that interventions including nutritional education and behavioral strategies to promote healthy and appropriate weight gain during pregnancy should approach obese women in particular.

4. Trends of reproductive age-women's body composition

4.1 The prevalence of overweight or obese women

Maternal size before conception plays a key role in determining pregnancy outcomes. BMI is an appropriate indicator of prepregnancy nutrition when assessed in women who are well-nourished (Saldana et al., 2004). Overweight status and obesity have become serious global public health issues. Nearly two thirds of reproductive-aged women in the United States are currently overweight or obese (≥25 kg/m²). In the National Health and Nutrition Examination Survey (NHANES), the prevalence of obesity (BMI ≥30 kg/m²) in women aged 20-49 years continues to be high, exceeding 30% after 1999 (Flegal et al., 2010)(Fig. 2).

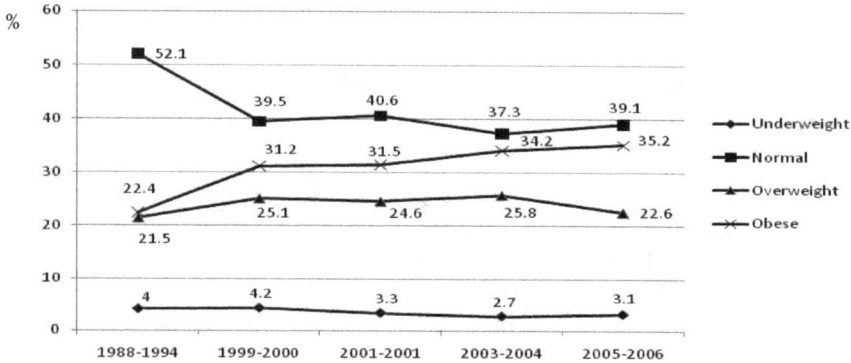

BMI categories (kg/m²); Underweight, <18.5; Normal, 18.5-24.9; Overweight, 25.0-29.9; Obese, ≥30.0.

Fig. 2. Trends of underweight, normal, overweight, and obese among U.S. women aged 20-40 y

In the latest NHANES data from 2007-2008 of 877 women aged 20-39 years, the prevalence of overweight status (BMI ≥25 kg/m²) and obesity were 59.5% and 34.0%, respectively. Trends are similar by age. The prevalence in all classes of obesity [(class I (30–34.9 kg/m²), class II (35–39.9 kg/m²), and class III (≥40 kg/m²))] is lowest in white, non-Hispanic women, and highest in non-Hispanic black women in the United States (Flegal et al., 2010). Other developed countries have observed similar trends. In Australia in 2007-2008, 44.5% women aged 25-34 years and 55.3% women aged 35-44 years were overweight or obese, which constituted a marked increase over the previous 20 years (Australian Institute of Health and Welfare, 2010). In the UK, more than 50% of women in the reproductive age category of 25-44 years are overweight or obese. There has been a 69% increase in maternal obesity from 1990 to 2004, a period of only 15 years (Heslehurst et al., 2007). Thus, the increased number of overweight and obese reproductive-aged women is a worldwide phenomenon.

4.2 The prevalence of underweight women

The prevalence of underweight status (BMI<18.5 kg/m²) was only 3.1 % of reproductive-aged women in 2005-2006 (Flegal et al., 2010). Underdeveloped regions, such as South Asia or Africa, where undernutrition is generally highest, or there are socio-economic characteristics or food poverty, report the highest prevalence of underweight women (Macro International Inc, 2007). However, even some developed countries such as Japan show high prevalence rates. Over the last two decades in Japan, the prevalence of underweight women has increased from 19.6% to 21.2% in those aged 20-29 years, and from 8.6% to 13.3% in those aged 30-39 (Hayashi et al., 2006). A low body mass index in highly industrialized countries is not, in all probability, a result of environmental factors such as periodic food shortages and malnutrition; therefore, one must consider it an expression of constitutional low weight or a result of cosmetically induced starvation. Excessive thinness has been glamorized among reproductive aged women, and unhealthy dieting to lose weight has become a popular practice in that age group. Body image in younger women is susceptible to societal influence through mass media, such as television, movies, and magazines.

5. Influence of prepregnant BMI and GWG on birth weight

5.1 SGA infant

Low prepregnancy BMI and low GWG have been associated with the delivery of smaller infants. There is strong evidence for an association between weight gains below the IOM guidelines and the risk of having an SGA infant (Nielsen et al., 2006; Park et al., 2011). In a study undertaken of 26,028 women in California, those with gestational weight gains below the IOM guidelines had a significantly higher risk of SGA infants when compared with women with a weight gain above IOM guidelines, adjusting for prepregnancy BMI (Park et al., 2011).

Similar results were also observed in a study among Swedish women with singleton full-term births. The risks for SGA were higher when gaining <8 kg (95% CI: 1.68-2.35) and lower when gaining >16 kg (95% CI: 0.50-0.61) (Cedergren, 2006). Merchant et al. (1999) reported lower mean birth weights of newborns among Pakistani women with prepregnancy BMI<19 kg/m2 who gained >12.5 kg compared to those who gained 12.5 kg. Women in the lowest quartile for both prepregnancy BMI and GWG were 5.6 times more likely to have intrauterine growth restriction (IUGR) infants, compared to women in the upper quartile (Naidu & Rao, 1994). The research among 3,071 Japanese women who gave birth to single-term infants found that underweight women were 1.7 times and 1.5 times more likely to give birth to a SGA or LBW infant, respectively (Watanabe et al., 2007). However, an increase in GWG eliminated or reduced the incidence of SGA.

Current evidence indicates that GWG, particularly during the second and third trimesters, is an important determinant of fetal growth (Althuizen et al., 2006; Kaiser et al., 2008). Inadequate weight gain during these trimesters is associated with an increased risk of LBW or IUGR. Health care providers should give women individual graphs of their weight gains at each antenatal check up, having viewed valuable sources of information on diet and nutrition.

5.2 LGA infant

The mean birth weight has continuously increased in United States, Canada, Europe, and Asia (Kramer et al., 2002). In Australia, LGA births have increased from 9.2% to 10.8% in male infants and from 9.1% to 11% in female infants from 1990 to 2005 (Hadfield et al., 2009). The 25% to 36% increase in maternal BMI over the past decade has translated to approximately a 25% increase in the incidence of newborns with high birth weight (Surkan et al., 2004). The possible reason may be increased maternal body weight and/or excess weight gain during pregnancy beyond the recommended IOM guideline. Strong evidence confirms the association between excessive GWG and increased birth weight in all BMI categories.

A population-based retrospective cohort study was reported of 570,672 women aged 18-40 years, examining the association between the 2009 IOM recommendations and adverse infant outcomes by prepregnancy BMI reported that fifty-one percent of women were above the IOM guidelines. Gains of greater than the recommended amount were associated with increased odds of LGA (95% CI: 1.27-5.99), and gains less than those recommended were associated with decreased odds of LGA (95% CI: 0.27-0.77) (Park et al., 2011). Similar findings observed that the proportions of LGA increased with high prepregnancy BMI, but the proportions of SGA decreased. Obese women with lower weight gain or weight loss during pregnancy had lower risk of LGA and higher risk of SGA (Nohr et al., 2008).

6. Long-term effects of fetal environment for offspring

Many animal models have demonstrated that altering the environment in utero leads to lifelong consequences, such as high blood pressure (Mamun et al, 2009), impaired glucose tolerance (Fraser et al., 2010), insulin resistance (Ozanne & Hales, 1999), and altered hepatic architecture and function (Ozanne et al., 2001). Population-based prospective cohort studies starting from different geographical regions in the preconception period or in early fetal life and following the offspring from early fetal life until young adulthood seem to be the most suitable epidemiological design (Geelhoed & Jaddoe, 2010; Jaddoe & Witteman, 2006) (Fig. 3).

There is now increasing evidence supporting the effect of the in utero environment on the development of obesity and risk factors for adult diseases (Ong, 2006; Pettitt & Jovanovic, 2007). Epidemiological studies confirm that the relationships between human birth weight and adult obesity, hypertension, or insulin resistance are U-shaped curves rather than inverse linear associations over a full range of birth weight distributions (Barker, 1998) (Fig. 4). That is, children born at both the lower - classified as SGA - and the upper – classified as LGA – ends of the birth weight spectrum are at risk of obesity and, subsequently, a range of adult diseases in later life.

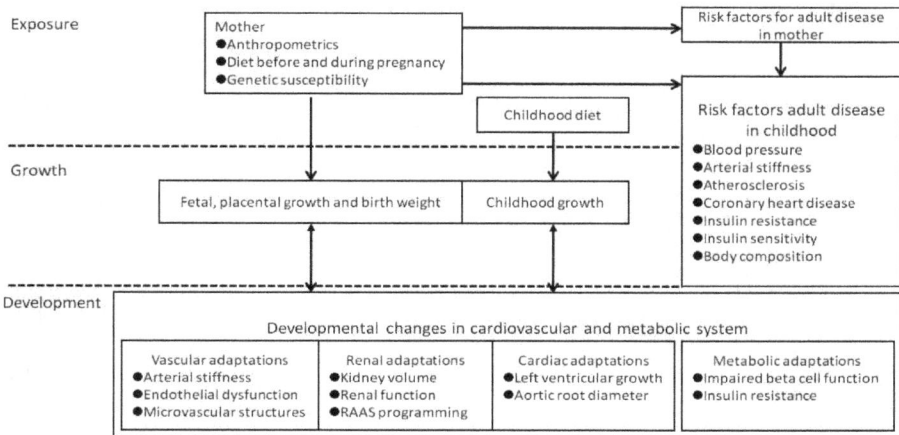

Source; Reference [Geelhoed & Jaddoe, 2010; Jaddoe & Witteman, 2006]

Fig. 3. Models for studying the fetal origins of adult diseases hypotheses in epidemiological studies.

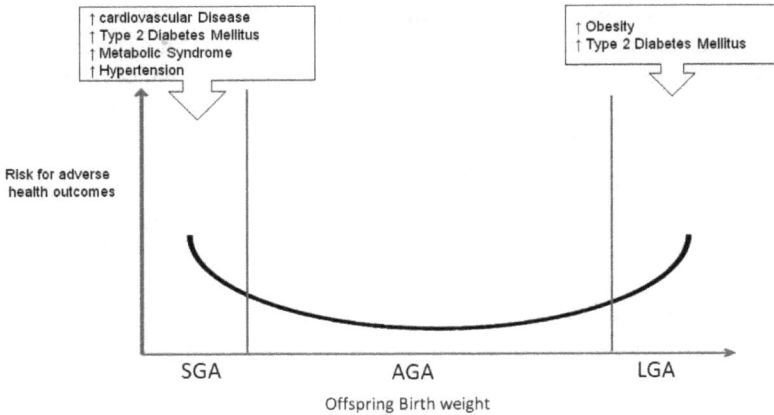

Source; Reference [Barker DJ, 1998]

Fig. 4. Hypothesized U-shaped relationship between offspring birth weight and risk for postnatal adverse health outcomes

6.1 The consequence of being SGA

LBW and SGA infants are at risk for hypertension, cardiovascular disease, insulin resistance, and diabetes mellitus type 2 in adult life (Saenger, 2007). A recent systematic review of the literature relating to the birth weight/type 2 diabetes relationship noted that for every one-kg increase in weight at birth, the risk of diabetes in adulthood decreased by 25% (OR 0.75, 95%CI: 0.70-0.81) (Whincup et al., 2008). In an Indian study of young adults, which followed up at birth and every six months until the age of 21 years, plasma glucose concentrations and insulin resistance were inversely related to birth weight, and impaired glucose tolerance and diabetes were associated with lower weight and BMI at the age of 1 year, after adjusting for adult BMI (Bhargava et al., 2004).

Studies linking birth weight to kidney disease and hypertension in adulthood have also been reported. LBW infants have lower kidney weight with a decreased number of nephrons, which indicates that hypertensive patients have lower nephron numbers (Hughson et al., 2003). A histomorphometric study observed a 13% decrease of nephron number in LBW infants (Manalich et al., 2000). Schmidt et al. (2005) investigated kidney length or volume in early life in SGA infants compared to AGA infants. They found that being SGA was associated with small kidneys at birth and impaired kidney growth in early childhood. Hotoura et al. (2005) compared SGA infants with a gestational age of 31 to 36 weeks with a control group of AGA infants. They reported that SGA infants had shorter kidney length at birth compared with AGA infants. Similar findings were observed in the SGA term infant, but the association disappeared in later childhood (Giapros et al., 2006).

In addition, a recent study reported that SGA was associated with adult psychological disorders. Children born full term but weighing 2,475 g had increased psychological distress in later life, and a 1SD decrease in birth weight for gestational age was associated with increased psychological distress in adulthood (Wiles et al., 2005).

6.2 The consequence of being LGA

High birth weight and LGA infants are prone to induce neonatal complications (Das & Sysyn, 2004) and to developing insulin resistance (Giapros et al., 2007), obesity, and diabetes in later life (Boney et al., 2005; Dietz, 2004). LGA infants have increased fat mass at birth compared with AGA infants (Armitage et al., 2008). McCance et al. (1994) examined birth weight and diabetes in later life among Pima Indians. Diabetes rates among persons with high birth weight (≥4500 g) were almost twice as high as among those with a birth weight between 2,500 and 4,500 g. Similar findings were observed in a meta-analysis where infants with high birth weight (>4,000 g) had 1.36 times higher (95%CI: 1.07-1.73) incidence of type 2 diabetes in later life than normal birth weight (2,500-4,000 g) infants did.

Furthermore, a recent study has shown that obese women have a high risk for gestational diabetes mellitus, providing a future risk for type 2 diabetes mellitus (Catalano et al., 2009). Diabetes in pregnancy that results in high birth weight and early onset of diabetes in the offspring represents a vicious cycle (Knowler et al, 1990), with the offspring of women who had diabetes during pregnancy being very likely to have already developed diabetes by the time they reach their childbearing years. Boney et al. (2005) conducted a longitudinal cohort study to determine whether children who were LGA at birth and offspring of mothers with or without gestational diabetes mellitus were at increased risk for developing the metabolic syndrome in childhood at age 6 to 11 years. They found that children who were LGA at birth and exposed to an intrauterine environment of either diabetes or maternal obesity were at increased risk of developing metabolic syndromes.

7. Conclusion

Birth weight is an important predictor in infant mortality and morbidity, growth, development, and wellbeing in adult life. Women with a normal prepregnancy BMI and within the adequate range of GWG associated with minimal risk for SGA and LGA have better pregnancy outcomes in both mothers and infants, for short- and long-term health. However, nearly two thirds of reproductive-aged women are currently overweight or obese. On the other hand, the number of women with BMI below 18.5 has increased in some countries. In addition, only 28% of women actually adhere to the guidelines for optimum birth weight; over half gain in excess of the recommended weight gain.

Prepregnancy BMI and pregnancy weight gain reflect maternal nutritional status before and during pregnancy; this status plays a crucial role in creating an optimal intrauterine environment. Understanding the relationship between maternal nutrition and birth outcomes may provide a basis for developing nutritional interventions that will improve birth outcomes and long-term quality of life. All women of reproductive age should be encouraged to follow the government recommendations and eat a well-balanced diet. A critical goal for women is to make behavior changes to achieve good nutritional status before, during, and after conception, which may lead to improved birth outcomes.

8. References

Althuizen, E.; van Poppel, M.N.; Seidell, J.C.; van der Wijden, C. & van Mechelen, W. (2006). Design of the New Life (style) study: a randomized controlled trial to optimize maternal weight development during pregnancy. *BMJ Public Health*, Vol. 6: 168.

Armitage, J.A.; Poston, L. & Taylor, P.D. (2008). Developmental origins of obesity and the metabolic syndrome: the role of maternal obesity. *Front Horm Res*, Vol. 36: 73-84.

Australian Institute of Health and Welfare (AIHW). (2010). *Australia's health 2010: The eighth biannual health report of the AIHW*. Australian Institute of Health and Welfare, Canberra.

Barker, D.J. & Osmond, C. (1986). Infant mortality childhood nutrition, and ischaemic heart disease in England and Wales. *Lancet*, Vol. 1(8489): 1077-81.

Barker, D.J.; Winter, P.D.; Osmond, C.; Margetts, B, & Simmonds SJ. (1989). Weight in infancy and death from ischaemic heart disease. *Lancet*, Vol. 2(8663): 577-80.

Barker, D.J. (1998). In utero programming of chronic disease. *Clin Sci*, Vol. 95(2): 115-28.

Bhargava, S.K.; Sachdev, H.S.; Fall, C.H.; Osmond, C.; Lakshmy, R.; Barker, D.J.; Biswas, S.K.; Ramji, S.; Prabhakaran, D. & Reddy, K.S. (2004) Relation of serial changes in childhood body mass index to impaired glucose tolerance in young adulthood. *N Eng J Med*, Vol. 350(9): 865-75.

Bonellie, S.; Chalmers, J.; Gray, R.; Greer, I.; Jarvis, S. & Williams, C. (2008). Centile charts for birthweight for gestational age for Scottish singleton births. *BMC Pregnancy Childbirth*, Vol. 8: 5.

Boney, C.M.; Verma, A.; Tucker, R. & Vohr, B.R. (2005). Metabolic syndrome in childhood: association with birth weight, maternal obesity, and gestational diabetes mellitus. *Pediatrics*, Vol. 115(3), pp. e290-6.

Brown, J.E.; Murtaugh, M.A.; Jacobs, D.R. Jr. & Margellos, H.C. (2002). Variation in newborn size according to pregnancy weight change by trimester. *Am J Clin Nutr*, Vol. 76(1): 205-9.

Carmichael, S., Abrams, B. & Selvin, S. (1997). The pattern of maternal weight gain in women with good pregnancy outcomes. *Am J Public Health*, Vol. 87(12): 1984-8.

Catalano, P.M. (2007). Management of obesity in pregnancy. *Obstet Gynecol*, Vol. 109(2 Pt 1): 419-33.

Catalano, P.M.; Presley, L.; Minium, J.; Hauguel-de Mouzon, S. (2009). Fetuses of obese Mothers develop insulin resistance in utero. *Diabetes Care*, Vol. 32(6): 1076-80.

Cedergren, M. (2006). Effects of gestational weight gain and body mass index on obstetrics outcome in Sweden. *Int J Gynaecol Obstet*, Vol. 93(3): 269-74.

Das, U.G. & Sysyn, G.D. (2004). Abnormal growth: intrauterine growth retardation, small for gestational age, large for gestational age. *Pediatr Clin N Am*, Vol. 51(3): 639-54.

Demographic and Health Surveys, Macro International Inc, Access on June 1, 2011, http://www.measuredhs.com/countries/

Dietz, W.H. (2004). Overweight in childhood and adolescence. *N Engl J Med*, Vol. 350(9): 855-7.

Flegal, K.M.; Carroll, M.D.; Ogden, C.L. & Curtin, L.R. (2010). Prevalence and trends in obesity among US adults, 1999-2008. *JAMA*, Vol. 303(3): 235-41.

Fraser, A.; Tilling, K.; Macdonald-Wallis, C.; Sattar, N.; Brion, M.J.; Benfield, L.; Ness, A.; Deanfield, J.; Hingorani, A.; Nelson, S.M.; Smith, G.D. & Lawlor, D.A. (2010). Association of maternal weight gain in pregnancy with offspring obesity and metabolic and vascular traits in childhood. *Circulation*, Vol. 121(23): 2557-64.

Geelhoed, J.J. & Jaddoe, V.W. (2010). Early influences on cardiovascular and renal development. *Eur J Epidemiol*, Vol. 25(10): 677-92.

Giapros, V.; Drougia, A.; hotoura, E.; Papadopoulou. F.; Argyropoulou, M. & Andronikou, S. (2006). Kidney growth in small-for-gestational-age infants: Evidence of early accelerated renal growth. *Nephrol Dial Transplant*, Vol. 21(12): 422-7.

Giapros, V.; Evagelidou, E.; Challa. A.; Kiortsis, D.; Drougia. A. & Andronikou, S. (2007). Serum adiponectin and leptin levels and insulin resistance in children born large for gestational age are affected by the degree of overweight. *Cli Endocrinology 2*, Vol. 66(3): 353-9.

Goldfrey, K.M. & Barker, D.J. (2000). Fetal nutrition and adult disease. *Am J Clin Nutr*, Vol. 71 (5 Suppl), pp.1344S-52S.

Hadfield, R.M.; Lain, S.J.; Simpson, J.M.; Ford, J.B.; Raynes-Greenow, C.H.; Morris, J.M. & Roberts, C.L. (2009). Are babies getting bigger? An analysis of birthweight trends in New South Wales, 1990-2005. *Med J Aust*, 190(6): 312-5.

Hayashi, F.; Takimoto, H.; Yoshita, K. & Yoshiike, N. (2006). Perceived body size and desire for thinness of young Japanese women: a population-based survey. *Br J Nutr*, Vol. 96(6): 1154-62.

Heslehurst, N.; Ells, L.J.; Simpson, H.; Batterham, A.; Wilkinson, J. & Summerbell, C.D. (2007). Trends in maternal obesity incidence rates, demographic predictors, and health inequalities in 36,821 women over a 15-year period. *BJOG*, Vol. 114(2): 187-94.

Hotoura, E.; Argyropoulou, M.; Papadopoulou, F.; Giapros, V.; Drougia, A.; Nikolopoulos, P. & Andronikou, S. (2005). Kidney development in the first year of life in small-for-gestational-age preterm infants. *Pediatr Radiol*, Vol. 35(10): 991-4.

Hughson, M.; Farris, A.B.; Douglas-Denton, R.; Hoy, W.E. & Bertram, J.F. (2003). Glomerular number and size in autopsy kidneys: the relationship to birth weight, *Kidney Int*, Vol. 63(6): 2113-22.

Institute of Medicine. (1990). *Nutrition during pregnancy: part I, weight gain; part α, nutrient supplements*. National Academies Press, Washington, DC.

Institute of Medicine. (2009). *Weight gain during pregnancy: reexamining the guidelines*. National Academies Press, Washington, DC.

Jaddoe, V.W. & Witteman, J.C. (2006). Hypotheses on the fetal origins of adult diseases: contributions of epidemiological studies. *Eur J Epidemiol*, Vol. 21(2): 91-102.

Joseph, K.S.; Fahey, J.; Platt, R.W.; Liston, R.M.; Lee, S.K.; Sauve, R.; Liu, S.; Allen, A.C. & Kramer, M.S. (2009). An outcome-based approach for the creation of fetal growth standards: do singletons and twins need separate standards? *Am J Epidemiol*, Vol. 169(5): 616-24.

Kaiser, L.; Allen, L.H. & American Diabetic Association. (2008). Position of the American Dietic Association: nutrition and lifestyle for a healthy pregnancy outcome. *J Am Diet Assoc*, Vol. 108(3): 553-61.

Kiel, D.W.; Dodson, E.A.; Artal, R.; Boehmer, T.K. & Leet, T.L. (2007). Gestational weight gain and pregnancy outcomes in obese women: how much is enough?. *Obstet Gynecol*, Vol. 110(4): 752-8.

Knowler, W.C.; Pettitt, D.J.; Saad, M.F. & Bennett, P.H. (1990). Diabetets mellitus in the Pima Indians: incidence, risk factors and pathogenesis. *Diabetes Metab Rev*, Vol. 6(1): 1-27.

Kramer, M.S.; Morin, I.; Yang, H.; Platt, R.W.; Usher, R.; McNamara, H.; Joseph, K.S. & Wen, S.W. (2002). Why are babies getting bigger? Temporal trends in fetal growth and its determinants. *J Pediatr*, Vol. 141(4): 538-542.

Lagerstrom, M.; Bremme, K,; Eneroth, P. & Magnusson, D. (1991). School performance and IQ-test scores at age 13 as related to birth weight and gestational age. *Scand J Psychol*, Vol. 32 (4): 316 – 24.

Langer, O.; Yogev, Y.; Most, O. & Xenakis, E.M. (2005). Gestational diabetes: the consequences of not treating. *Am J Obstet Gynecol*, Vol. 192(4): 989-97.

Larsen, C.E.; Serdula, M.K. & Sullivan, K.M. (1990). Macrosomia: influence of maternal overweight among a low-income population. *Am J Obstet Gynecol*, Vol.162(2), pp. 490-4.

Li, R.; Haas, J.D. & Habicht, J.P. (1998). Timing of the influence of maternal nutritional status during pregnancy on fetal growth. *Am J Hum Biol*. Vol. 10: 529-39.

McCance, D.R.; Pettitt, D.J.; Hanson, R.L.; Jacobsson, L.Y.; Knowler, W.C. & Bennett, P.H. (1994). Birth weight and non-insulin-dependent diabetes: thrifty fenotype, thrifty phenotype, or surviving small baby genotype? *BMJ*, Vol. 308(6934): 942-5.

Mamun, A.A.; O'Callaghan, M.; Callaway, Williams, G.; Najman, J. & Lawlor, D.A. (2009). Associations of gestational weight gain with offspring body mass index and blood pressure at 21 years of age: evidence from a birth cohort study. *Circulation*, Vol. 119(13): 1720-7.

Manalich, R.; Reyes, L.; Herrera, M.; Melendi, C. & Fundoral, I. (2000). Relationship between weight at birth and the number and size of renal glomeruli in humans; A histomorhometric study. *Kidney Int*, Vol. 58(2): 770-3.

Merchant, S.S.; Momin, I.A.; Sewani, A.A. & Zuberi, N.F. (1999). Effect of prepregnancy body mass index and gestational weight gain on birth weight. *J Pak Med Assoc*, Vol. 49(1): 23–5.

Ministry of Health, Labour and Welfare, Japan, Mothers' & Children's Health Division. (2006). *Maternal and Child Health Statistics of Japan*, Mothers' & Children's Health Organization, Tokyo (in Japanese).

Naidu, A.N. & Rao, N.P. (1994). Body mass index: a measure of the nutritional status in Indian populations. *Eur J Clin Nutr*, Vol. 48 (Suppl 3): S131-40.

Nielsen, J.N.; O'Brien, K.O.; Witter, F.R.; Chang, S.C.; Mancini, J.; Nathanson, M.S. & Caufield, L.E. (2006). High gestational weight gain does not improve birth weight in a cohort of African American adolescents. *Am J ClinNutr*, Vol. 84(1): 183-9.

Nohr, E.A.; Vaeth, M.; Barker, J.L.; Sorensen, T. & Olsen, J. (2008). Rasmussen KM. Combined associations of prepregnancy body mass index and gestational weight gain with the outcome of pregnancy. *Am J Clin Nutr*, Vol. 87(6): 1750-9.

Ong, K.K. (2006). Size at birth, postnatal growth and risk of obesity, Horm Res, Vol. 65 (Suppl 3): 65-9.

Ozanne, S.E. & Hales, C.N. (1999). The log-term consequences of intrauterine protein malnutrition for glucose metabolism. *Proc Nutr Soc*, Vol. 58: 615-9.

Ozanne, S.E.; Dorling, M.W.; Wang, C.L. & Nave, B.T. (2001). Impaired PI 3-Kinase activation in adipocytes from early growth-restricted rats. *Am J Physiol*, Vol. 280(3): E534-9.

Park, S.; Sappenfield, W.M.; Bish, C.; Salihu, H.; Goodman, D. & Bensyl, D. (2011). Assessment of the institute of medicine recommendations for weight gain during pregnancy: Florida, 2004-2007. *Matern Child Health J*, Vol. 15(3): 289-301.

Parsons, T.J.; Power, C. & Manor, O. (2001). Fetal and early life growth and body mass index from birth to early adulthood in 1958 British cohort: longitudinal study. BMJ, Vol. 323(7325): 1331-5.

Rees, J.M.; Lederman, S.A. & kiely, J.L. (1996). Birth weight associated with lowest neonatal mortality: infants of adolescent and adult mothers. *Pediatrics*, Vol. 98(6 Pt 1): 1161-6.

Pettitt, D.J. & Jovanovic, L. (2007). Low birth weight as a risk factor for gestational diabetes, diabetes, and impaired glucose tolerance during pregnancy. *Diabetes Care*, Vol. 30 (Suppl 2): S147-9.

Rich-Edwards, J.W,; Colditz, G.A.; Stampfer, M.J.; Willett, W.C.; Gillman, M.W.; Hennekens, C.H.; Speizer, F.E. & Manson, J.E. (1999). Birthweight and the risk for type 2 diabetes mellitus in adult women . *Ann Intern Med,*Vol. 130(4 Pt 1): 278 – 84 .

Rode, L.; Hegaard, H.K.; Kjaergaard, H.; Moller, L.F.; Tabor, A. & Ottesen, B. (2007). Association between maternal weight gain and birth weight. *Obstet Gynecol*, Vol. 109(6): 1309-15.

Saenger, P.; Czernichow, P.; Hughes, I. & Reiter, E.O. (2007). Small for gestational age: short stature and beyond. *Endocr Rev*, Vol. 28(2): 219-51.

Saldana, T.M.; Siega-Riz, A.M. & Adair, L.S. (2004). Effect of macronutrient intake on the development of glucose intolerance during pregnancy. *Am J Clin Nutr*, Vol. 79(3): 479-86.

Schieve, L.A.; Cogswell, M.E. & Scanlon, K.S. (1998). Trends in pregnancy weight gain within and outside ranges recommended by the Institute of Medicine in a WIC population. *Matern Child Health J*, Vol. 2(2): 111-6.

Schmidt, I.M.; Chellakooty, M.; Biosen, K.A.; Damgaard, I.N.; Mau Kai, C.; Olgaard, K. & Main, K.M. (2005). Impired kidney growth in low-birth-weight children: Distinct effects of maturity and weight for gestational age. *Kidney Int*, Vol. 68(2): 731-40.

Stotland, N.E.; Caughey, A.B.; Breed, E.M. & Escobar, G.J. (2004). Risk factors and obstetric complications associated with macrosomia. *Int J Gynaecol Obstet*, Vol. 87(3): 220-6.

Surkan, P.J.; Hsieh, C.C.; Johansson, A.L.; Dickman, P.W. & Cnattingius, S. (2004). Reasons for increasing trends in large for gestational age births. *Obstet Gynecol*, Vol. 104(4): 720-6.

Susser, M.; Marolla, F.A. & Fleiss, J. (1972). Birth weight, fetal age and perinatal mortality. *Am J Epidemiol*, Vol. 96(3): 197-204.

Ward, C.; Lewis, S. & Coleman, T. (2007). Prevalence of maternal smoking and environmental tobacco smoke exposure during pregnancy and impact on birth weight: restrospective study using Millennium Cohort. *BMC Public Health*, Vol. 7: 81.

Watanabe, H.; Fukuoka, H.; Inoue, K.; Koyasu, M.; Nagai, Y. & Takimoto, H. (2007). Restricting weight gain during pregnancy in Japan: a controversial factor in reducing perinatal complications. *Eur J Obstet Gynecol Reprod Biol*, Vol. 133(1): 53-9.

Weiss, J.L.; Malone, F.D.; Emig, D.; Ball, R.H.; Nyberg, D.A.; Comstock, C.H.; Saade, G.; Eddleman, K.; Carter, S.M.; Craigo, S.D.; Carr, S.R. & D'Alton, A.E. (2004). Obesity, obstetric complications and cesarean delivery rate-a population-based screening study. *Am J Obstet Gynecol*, Vol. 190(4): 1091-7.

Whincup, P.H.; Kaye, S.J.; Owen, C.G. & Anazawa, S. (2008). Birth weight and risk of type 2 diabetes: a systematic review. *JAMA*, Vol.300(24): 2886-97.

Wilcox, A.J. & Skjaerven, R. (1992). Birth weight and perinatal mortality: the effect of gestational age. *Am J Public Health*, Vol. 82(3): 378-382.

Wiles, N.J.; Peters, T.J.; Leon, D.A. & Lewis, G. (2005). Birth weight and psychological distress at age 45-51 years: Results from the Aberdeen Children of the 1950s cohort study. *Br J Psychiatry*, Vol. 187: 21-8.

6

Post Abortion Care Services in Nigeria

Echendu Dolly Adinma
Department Of Community Medicine, Faculty Of Medicine,
College Of Health Sciences, Nnamdi Azikiwe University,
Nnewi Campus, Nnewi,
Anambra State,
Nigeria

1. Introduction

Abortion, whether spontaneous or induced, may be associated with complications that constitute global public health challenge especially in developing countries. In many such countries, abortion is often both unauthorized and unsafe. Only the wealthy and more educated women have access to safe procedures, leaving the poor and often marginalized women to suffer disproportionately, on account of illegal, or restrictive abortion laws (Bankole et al., 2006; Faúndes & Barzelatto, 2006). In countries with restrictive abortion laws, due to the absence of legal abortion services, women attempt to end unwanted pregnancies through clandestine means. Such women terminate pregnancy by themselves, and sometimes in collaboration with quacks in unhygienic environments (Bankole et al., 2006). The techniques used in most cases are likely to cause morbidities such as genital track trauma, haemorrhage, and infection, or even outright maternal deaths (Ahiadeke, 2001; Rogo, 1993). To compound the problem, when most women in developing countries miscarry or suffer potentially life-threatening complications from unsafe abortion, they rarely have access to prompt treatment (Rogo, 1993). Whereas a woman's life time risk of dying from complications of pregnancy or childbirth in Europe is 1 in 600, it is outrageously high in Africa with figures as high as one in 7 in Ethiopia, for example, with more than half of those deaths attributable to unsafe abortion (WHO, 2001). The risk of death from unsafe abortion in developing countries is the highest in the world with a case fatality rate of 0.7 % for sub-Saharan Africa (WHO, 1998).

Post abortion care (PAC) is a global approach towards solving the problem of maternal mortality and morbidity arising from abortion complications from both spontaneous and induced abortion. It consists of a series of medical and related interventions designed to manage the complications of abortion. Its overall aim is to reduce maternal morbidity and mortality from abortion and its complications, and to improve women's sexual and reproductive health and lives. A comprehensive post abortion care service has been identified to be useful in ameliorating the often adverse health consequences associated with unsafe abortion in regions with restrictive abortion laws.

This chapter reviews the magnitude of abortion problems together with the place of PAC in the combat of abortion related maternal morbidity and mortality.

2. Magnitude of abortion problem

Abortion is one of the most important direct medical causes of maternal mortality, accounting for 12-40 % of overall global maternal deaths (WHO, 1994; Fatusi & Ijadunola, 2003). World Health Organization estimates that 46 million induced abortions occur annually the world over (WHO, 1998). To attest to the enormity of this global abortion problem, Henshaw et al., 1998, in a comprehensive review of data on abortion further deduced that one out of every four pregnancies the world over is voluntarily terminated. Conservative estimate from Henshaw et al review of induced abortion indicates that 20 million induced abortions are performed under unsafe circumstances, causing the death of over 80,000 women annually (Henshaw, 1990; Henshaw et al., 1998; Henshaw et al., 1999. This, however, has regional variations, with rates as low as 2 per 1000 occurring in developed countries and as high as 28 per 1000 taking place in developing countries where restrictive abortion laws abound in great proportions (Ahman & Shah, 2002). In Nigeria with restrictive abortion law for example, Centre for Reproductive Rights reported maternal mortality of 34,000 attributable to abortion in 2008 alone (Centre for Reproductive Rights, 2008)!

Unsafe abortion has human, social and economic costs. While the human cost is related to physical complications that lead to the death of the woman, or associated long term sequelae, the social cost is related to the long-term physical limitations such as infertility, or from moral, legal or cultural stigma that women who abort may suffer. The economic cost is related to the reduction of health resources that would have been used for the management of critical health problems being diverted towards the treatment of abortion complications especially in developing countries (Faúndes & Barzelatto, 2006).

Every year, more than 4.2 million African women undergo unsafe abortion with an estimated 38,000 of them dying from the experience, leaving countless others with severe morbidities (Henshaw, 1990). These numbers represent over 50 % of all women globally who die from abortion-related causes (WHO, 1998). Amongst those surviving the ordeal, several thousands experience various forms of short- and long-term morbidities. The morbidities include uterine perforation, chronic pelvic pain, and secondary infertility. Victims of unsafe abortion may in addition suffer stigma and isolation forced on them by their families and communities.

Considering the huge contribution of unsafe abortion to the very high maternal mortality in most countries, it is apparent that efforts to reduce maternal mortality and improve maternal health without addressing the issue of unsafe abortion will not succeed.

Only 40 % of the population in the world lives in countries where abortion laws are unrestrictive such that abortion is permissible at the woman's request. The remaining 60 % live in areas with abortion laws of varied restrictions, and most of these are in developing countries (Rahman et al., 1997; Cooks et al., 1999). With only a few exceptions, the abortion law in African countries are based on very restrictive 19th century European penal code permitting legal abortions only to save the life of the woman (Henshaw, 1990; Cooks et al., 1999). For example, in Nigeria, abortion law is restrictive and encoded in the portions of the Criminal and Penal codes related to miscarriage, culled from the "British Offence against the persons" Act of 1861 and annotated by S. S. Richardson in 1933, excerpts of which is as follows:

3. Criminal code act

This is applicable mainly in Southern Nigeria and includes Sections 228, 229, 230, 297 and 328 of the Criminal code.

3.1 Section 228

Any person who, with intent to procure miscarriage of a woman whether she is or is not with child, unlawfully administers to her or causes her to take any poison or other noxious thing, or uses any force of any kind, or uses any other means whatever, is guilty of a felony, and is liable to imprisonment for fourteen years.

3.2 Section 229

Any woman who, with intent to procure her own miscarriage, whether she is or is not with child, unlawfully administers to herself any poison or other noxious thing, or uses any force of any kind, or uses any other means whatever, or permits any such thing or means to be administered or used to her, is guilty of a felony, and is liable to imprisonment for seven years.

3.3 Section 230

Any person who unlawfully supplies to or procures for any person any thing whatever, knowing that it is intended to be unlawfully used to procure the miscarriage of a woman, whether she is or is not with child, is guilty of a felony, and is liable to imprisonment for three years.

3.4 Section 297

A person is not criminally responsible for performing in good faith and with reasonable skill a surgical operation upon any person for his benefit, or upon an unborn child for the preservation of the mother's life, if the performance of the operation is reasonable, having regard to the patient's state at the time and to all the circustances of the case.

3.5 Section 328

Any person who, when a woman is about to be delivered of a child, prevents the child from being born alive by any act or omission of such a nature that, if the child had been born alive and had then died, he would be deemed to have unlawfully killed the child, is guilty of a felony, and is liable to imprisonment for life.

4. Penal code

This is applicable to Northern Nigeria:

4.1 Section 232 – Causing a woman to miscarry

Whoever voluntarily causes a woman with child to miscarry shall, if such miscarriage be not caused in good faith for the purpose of saving the life of the woman, be punished with imprisonment for a term which may extend to fourteen years or with fine or with both.

4.2 Section 233 – Causing death of a woman with the intent of causing her miscarriage

Whoever with intent of causing the miscarriage of a woman whether with child or not does any act which causes the death of such woman, shall be punished:

a. with imprisonment for a term which may extend to fourteen years and shall also be liable to fine and
b. if the act is done without the consent of the woman, with imprisonment for life, or for any less term and shall also be liable to fine.

4.3 Section 234 – Using force on a woman to cause her miscariage

Whoever uses force to any woman and thereby unintentionally causes her to miscarry, shall be punished:

a. with imprisonment for a term which may extend to three years or with fine or with both and
b. if the offender knew that the woman was with child, he shall be punished with imprisonment for a term which may extend to five years or with fine or with both.

4.4 Section 235 – Preventing a child from being born alive

Whoever before the birth of any child does any act with the intention of thereby preventing that child from being born alive or causing it to die after its birth, shall if such act be not caused in good faith for the purpose of saving the life of the mother, be punished with imprisonment for a term which may extend to fourteen years or with fine or with both.

4.5 Section 236 – Causing the death of unborn child

Whoever does any act in such circumstances that, if he thereby caused death , he would be guilty of culpable homicide, and does by such act cause the death of a quick unborn child shall be punished with imprisonment for life or for a less term and shall also be liable to fine (http://annualreview.law.harvard.edu/population/abortion/NIGERIA. abo.htm).

It is clear from these Codes that the performance of induced abortion in most cases, except when the life of the woman is at risk, in Nigeria constitutes felony punishable with jail terms that my even be as severe as life sentences! The effect of this no doubt is that abortion practice is driven underground creating the enabling environment for the clandestine activities of quacks to flourish.

5. Evolution of post abortion care

Post Abortion Care (PAC) was developed to stem the maternal mortality and morbidity arising from unsafe abortions especially in countries with restrictive abortion laws. It is defined as an approach for reducing mortality and morbidity from incomplete and unsafe abortion and resulting complications, and for improving women's sexual and reproductive health and lives (Post abortion Care Consortium Community Task Force, 2002). It was first articulated by Ipas, US based non-governmental organization, in 1991, and later published by the Post Abortion Care Consortium in 1995. However, the role of safe abortion services in the improvement of women's health was recognized in the 1994 International Conference on Population and Development (ICPD). At this conference, participants agreed that "in circumstances where abortion is not against the law, such abortion should be safe. In all cases women should have access to quality services for the management of complications arising from abortion" (ICPD, 1994).

6. Elements of post abortion care

The original PAC model consisted of three elements drawn specifically from health care delivery providers perspective without taking due cognizance of the need to accommodate the psychological and physical feelings of the client as well as the community who are the beneficiaries of the services. The three elements of the original PAC model include the following:

1. Emergency treatment services for complications of spontaneous or unsafe induced abortions;
2. Post abortion family planning counseling and services; and
3. Links between emergency abortion treatment services and comprehensive reproductive health care provider perspective.

However in 2001, the PAC Community Task Force expanded the model to five elements, tailored to provide the necessary ingredients for sustainable PAC services by making them more client-oriented. The five elements are:

1. Community and service providers partnership for prevention of unwanted pregnancy and unsafe abortion, together with the mobilization of resources and ensuring that services reflect and meet community expectations and needs;
2. Counseling to identify and respond to women's emotional and physical health needs and other concerns;
3. Treatment of incomplete and unsafe abortion and its complications including the use of manual vacuum aspirator (MVA);

4. Contraceptive and family planning services to help women prevent an unwanted pregnancy or practice birth spacing; and
5. Linkage to reproductive and other health services that are preferably provided on-site or via referrals to other accessible facilities in the providers' networks.

Women centered post abortion care was developed in 2005 as a step forward from the original PAC. It is a comprehensive approach to meeting each woman's medical and psychosocial needs at the time of treatment for abortion complications. In course of providing women centered post abortion care by health care workers, factors influencing women's need for and access to care such as personal circumstances and living conditions are taken into cognizance to ensure quality service delivery.

PAC has found wide acceptability in developing countries as a very important tool in the combat of maternal mortality from abortion. In countries like Nigeria and Ghana, and many other developing countries of Asia, middle level providers especially Nurse-Midwives have been trained on PAC and have been employed widely in the provision of abortion treatment services especially in rural areas. In Nigeria, Medical Practitioners and Nurse-Midwives both in the private and public health facilities are being trained on the practice of PAC with tremendous success. PAC has also been incorporated by the Nursing and Midwifery Council of Nigeria into the training curriculum of midwifery in Nigeria. PAC training programmes however still need to be better streamlined and more intensified. In a recent survey of 437 health practitioners in southeastern Nigeria, comprising mostly of Doctors and Nurse-Midwives, as high as 75.5% of the respondents were aware of PAC, although only 35.5% used manual vacuum aspirator (MVA) (Adinma et al., 2010). In a related survey of 431 health care professionals in the same area, only 41% had been trained on PAC counseling (Adinma et al., 2010a, 2010b). These attest to the need for the intensification of PAC training programmes to widen the provision of PAC services to all parts of the country.

7. Conclusion

The contribution of abortion to high maternal mortality in countries with restrictive abortion laws has made PAC services increasingly relevant particularly in these areas. PAC, for its individualized approach and simplicity of application have been found to be attractive even to middle level health care providers who are readily available in rural areas without the benefit of the services of Medical Doctors. The impact of PAC towards maternal mortality reduction is likely to become evident when a wide coverage of the services is achieved in countries where they are needed. This can be possible when such countries put in place a well packaged PAC training programme made available to all health care practitioners treating abortion to ensure quality services.

8. References

Adinma, JIB., Ikeako, L., Adinma, ED., Ezeama, CO., & Ugboaja, JO. (2010). Awareness and practice of post abortion care services among health care professionals in southeastern Nigeria. *The Southeast Asian J of Tropical Medicine and Public Health*, 41, 3, 696-704.

Adinma, JIB., Ikeako, L., Adinma, ED, Ezeama, C., & Eke, NO. (2010). Post abortion care counseling practiced by health professionals in southeastern Nigeria. *International Journal of Gynecology and Obstetrics*, 111, 53-56.

Ahiadeke, C. (2001).Incidence of induced abortion in southern Ghana. *International Family Planning Perspectives*, 27, 2, 96-101.

Ahman, E., & Shah, I. (2002). Unsafe abortion: worldwide estimates for 2000. *Reprod. Health Matters*, 10, 13-17.

Bankole, A., Oye-Adeniran, BA., Singh, S., Adewole, IF., Wulf, D., Sedgh, G., & Hussain, R. (2006).Unwanted pregnancy and induced abortion in Nigeria: causes and consequences, Guttmacher Institutes, 4.

Centre for Reproductive Rights regarding maternal mortality in Nigeria – universal periodic review of Nigeria, August 29 2008: 5.

Cooks, RJ., Dickens, BM., & Bliss, LE. (1999). International developments in abortion laws from 1988-1998, *American Journal of Public Health*, 89, 579-586.

Fatusi, AO., & Ijadunola, KT. (2003). National study on emergency obstetrics care facilities in Nigeria, UNFPA/Federal Ministry of Health, Abuja, Nigeria. 2003.

Faúndes, A., & Barzelatto, JS. (Eds). (2006). *Consequences of unsafe abortion – The human drama of abortion*, Vanderbilt University Press, USA, 35.

Henshaw, SK. (1990). Induced abortion: a world review. *International Family Planning Perspectives*, 22, 76-89.

Henshaw, SK., Singh, S., Oye-Adeniran, BA., Adewole, IF., Iwere, N., & Cuca, YP. (1998). The incidence of induced abortion in Nigeria. *International Family Planning Perspectives*, 24, 156-164.

Henshaw, SK., Singh, S., & Haas, T. (1999). The incidence of abortion worldwide. *International Family Planning Perspectives*, 24, 30-38.

Post abortion Care Consortium Community Task Force. (2002). Essential elements of post abortion care: An expanded and updated model. *PAC in Action 2*, Special Supplement, September 2002.

Programme of Action adopted at the International Conference on Population and Development, Cairo, 1994. Paragraph 8.25.

Rahman, A., Katzive, L., & Henshaw, SK. (1998). A global review of laws on induced abortion, 1985-1997. *International Family Planning Perspective*, 24, 56-64.

Richardson, SS. (1933). Nigeria abortion law, In: *http://annualreview.law.harvard.edu/population/abortion/NIGERIA.abo.htm.* (Accessed July 15, 2011).

Rogo, KO. (1993). Induced abortion in sub-Saharan Africa. *East African Medical Journal*, 70, 6, 386-395.

World Health Organization. (2001). Maternal Mortality in 1995: Estimates developed by WHO, UNICEF and UNFPA. WHO/MSM/01.9 Geneva: WHO, 2001.

World Health Organization.(1998). Unsafe Abortion. Global and Regional estimates of incidence and mortality due to unsafe abortion with a listing of available Country data. Geneva: WHO, 1998.

World Health Organization. (1994). Mother-Baby-Package: implementing safe motherhood in countries. Practical Guide. Maternal health and safe motherhood programmes, Division of Family Health, WHO, Geneva. 1994.

7

Medical and Surgical Induced Abortion

Dennis G. Chambers

Queen Elizabeth Hospital Pregnancy Advisory Centre, Adelaide,
Australia

1. Introduction

No method of contraception is 100% effective; over half the women seeking an abortion are using contraception (Jones et al., 2002). It has been estimated that 42 million abortions are carried out every year, and half of these are illegal and unsafe (Sedgh et al., 2007). A proportion of women of all backgrounds with an unintended pregnancy are going to seek an abortion, legal or illegal, irrespective of the risks involved (Rosenfield, 1994) . Unplanned pregnancies are a problem that faces all societies; the Guttmacher Institute in New York determined that 49% of all pregnancies occurring in the USA in 1994 were unintended, 54% of these ending in abortion, and 48% of women aged 15-44 had had at least one unintended pregnancy at some point in their lives (Henshaw, 1998). The United Nations estimated that in 2008 of the 208 million pregnancies worldwide 41% were unintended (Singh et al., 2010). The Guttmacher Institute estimates that 30% of American women will have an abortion by the age of 45 (Jones & Kavanagh, 2011).

Access to abortion varies around the world from completely free access in some developed countries to total prohibition in some undeveloped countries. In developing countries there is often a lack of training and equipment that leads to termination of pregnancies by the outdated procedure of sharp curettage, with consequent higher injury and complication rates (Henshaw, 1990). Rehan, (2011) states that the treatment of unsafe abortion complications consumes a large portion of O&G hospital budgets in developing countries. Shah & Ahman (2010) reported estimates from the World Health Organisation that there were 21.6 million unsafe abortions worldwide in 2008. Rasch (2011) in an overview found that globally an estimated 66,500 women die every year as a result of unsafe abortions, and in Sub-Saharan African states unsafe abortion rates are 18-39 per 1,000 women. Srinil (2011) surveyed complication rates in 170 women treated for unsafe abortion and found incidences of haemorrhage requiring blood transfusion 66.6%, shock 63%, acute renal failure 22.2%, sepsis with disseminated intravascular coagulation 7.4%, and 2 deaths. Shaw (2011) highlighted the dilemma facing many Muslim women because of the fact that there was little knowledge or open discussion of the view that Islam permits the termination of pregnancy for serious abnormality within 120 days of conception.

Where women have no access to legal abortion self administration of misoprostol commonly occurs with women accessing misoprostol from a pharmacy or through the internet. A Google search of "buy mifepristone and/or misoprostol online" produces over 2,000 hits. Before 1970 when the legalisation of abortion began to spread around the world menstrual extraction by manual vacuum aspiration was used to circumvent abortion prohibition (Potts et al., 1977). Menstrual regulation continued to be used in government funded clinics in some developing countries where abortion has never been legalised because it occurs technically without verification of the presence of a pregnancy (Dixon-Mueller, 1988). A report on the menstrual regulation policy in Bangladesh states that the provision of menstrual regulation averts unsafe abortion and associated maternal morbidity and mortality, and on a per capita basis, saves scarce health system resources (Johnson et al., 2010).

Son preference and sex-selective abortion is another major problem found in some Asian countries. Zhou et al., (2011) report that in China the sex ratio at birth is 120 male births to 100 females. Jha et al., (2011) estimate that in China selective abortion of girls totalled about 4.2 -12.1 million per year from 1980-2010.

Women worldwide want to control the timing and number of their children, not just for personal and family reasons, but in the interest of being able to provide adequately for a child at the point in time in question. Whilst first trimester abortion is accessible to some degree in most western countries, access to second trimester abortion tends to be very restricted. This is despite there being a constant proportion over the years of approximately 12% of legal abortions occurring after 12 weeks gestation (Gamble et al., 2008), most of these being for psycho-social reasons, and a small but increasing proportion being for suspected or confirmed foetal anomaly. Teenagers in all countries seek abortions later; approximately 30% of abortions in girls under 15 years of age take place in the second trimester (Jones et al., 2002}. This delay is due to teenagers having little or no experience at recognising pregnancy symptoms, a lack of general knowledge, and the problems associated with emotional immaturity. At any age delay in seeking an abortion may be due to periods normally being irregular, bleeding during pregnancy being mistaken for periods, a past history of infertility, menopausal symptoms, having been conscientiously using contraception, ambivalence due to conflicting beliefs, sudden financial stress, breakdown of a relationship, domestic violence, disorganised or chaotic life associated with substance abuse, delaying by medical attendants with mis-diagnosis of the pregnancy, or obstruction by health advisers with anti-abortion views.

2. Medical abortion to 63 days gestation

Medical abortion has several advantages over surgical abortion in that the overall cost is usually lower, medical staff with surgical skills are not required, and in terminations below 9 weeks gestation no hospital admission is required. Medical abortion virtually eliminates the risks of surgery and anaesthesia, and allows more flexible timing, with out-patient treatment, and the convenience of completion in the home environment; also women feel more in control and many feel that an induced miscarriage is a more natural process. Disadvantages of medical compared with surgical abortion are a higher failure rate, more prolonged bleeding, and a higher risk of retained products of conception complicating recovery.

2.1 Mifepristone and misoprostol

The gold standard of medical abortion is the combination of mifepristone followed by misoprostol. Mifepristone is a potent antiprogestogen with antiglucocorticoid activity; it acts at the level of the progesterone receptor being a competitive progesterone antagonist, and in combination with a prostaglandin is effective for medical abortion at all gestations (Ashok et al., 2002). The effects of mifepristone on the pregnant uterus are induced contractility, decidual necrosis with bleeding (Garfield et al., 1988), and cervical softening. Oral mifepristone achieves peak serum concentrations in pregnant women in 2 hours, with a half life of 24-29 hours (Heikinheimo, 1989). Contraindications to the use of mifepristone are adrenal failure and hereditary porphyria. Misoprostol is a synthetic prostaglandin E1 analog which regulates various immunologic cascades (Davies et al., 2001). It is a potent uterotonic drug, but its use in obstetrics and gynaecology is in all countries apart from France an off-label use as it is only marketed for the prevention and treatment of peptic ulcer disease. It has been used widely in obstetrics and gynaecology practice because of its effectiveness, low cost, stability in light and hot climate conditions, and ease of administration compared with its licensed counterparts dinoprostone and gemeprost (Song, 2000). Misoprostol is marketed as a 200 mcg tablet that is rapidly absorbed by the vaginal, rectal, oral, sublingual and buccal routes. The sublingual route results in the highest serum peak concentration levels and the highest bioavailability; the vaginal route has the lowest peak concentrations, but the longest duration of peak levels (Tang et al., 2002; 2009). Nevertheless measures of uterine contractility have shown similar effects for both routes (Tang et al., 2007).

Misoprostol has uterotonic and cervical priming actions; its advantage over other prostaglandins is that it is cheap, can be administered through any mucosal surface, can be used by asthmatics, and can be stored at room temperature for years. Misoprostol is a very safe and well tolerated drug. Pre-clinical toxicological studies indicate a safety margin of at least 500-1000 fold between lethal doses in animals and therapeutic doses in humans (Kotsonis et al., 1985). The misoprostol 200 mcg tablet is tolerated even in relatively high dosage; attempted suicide with high single dosage has failed with 30 tablets but succeeded with 60 tablets (Henriques et al., 2007). No clinically significant haematological, endocrine, biochemical, immunological, respiratory, ophthalmic, platelet, or cardiovascular effects have been found with misoprostol; diarrhoea is the major adverse reaction that has been reported consistently with misoprostol, but it is usually mild and self-limiting; nausea and vomiting may also occur and will resolve in 2-6 hours; fever and chills are common with high doses (Tang et al., 2007). Chambers et al., (2009) reported that in 1,000 women taking one misoprostol 200 mcg tablet orally three hours before suction termination of pregnancy the side effects were cramps: mild 52.2%, moderate 4%, severe 0.7%; nausea: mild 28.3%, moderate 4.9%, severe 1.4%; bleeding mild 8.6%, moderate 1.7%, severe 0.1%; diarrhoea: mild 3.8%, moderate 0.2%, severe 0% (Fig. 2).

2.2 Preparation for abortion

A consultation requirement is the completion of a health check questionnaire by the woman of her present and past medical and surgical history including allergies. A health worker should then interview the woman alone, without the presence of her partner or friends, to determine that her decision to terminate her pregnancy is her own and that she is not being unduly influenced by others. If the health worker feels a woman has not made a clear decision she should be offered an appointment with a counsellor for supportive decision making counselling to assist her to clarify her ambivalence. Specialised genetic counselling should be offered to all women seeking termination of pregnancy (TOP) for foetal anomaly.

The different methods of abortion that the clinic can offer are then explained, with the advantages and disadvantages of each method being detailed. It is important to determine the number of weeks' gestation of the woman as medical abortion past 9 weeks (63 days) gestation needs closer medical supervision and it is generally considered that it is not good practice to terminate these pregnancies on an out-patient basis. Bracken et al., (2011) have shown that reliance on a woman's report of her last menstrual period together with a bimanual pelvic examination is almost as accurate as ultrasound examination and therefore safe in determining eligibility for medical abortion at home.

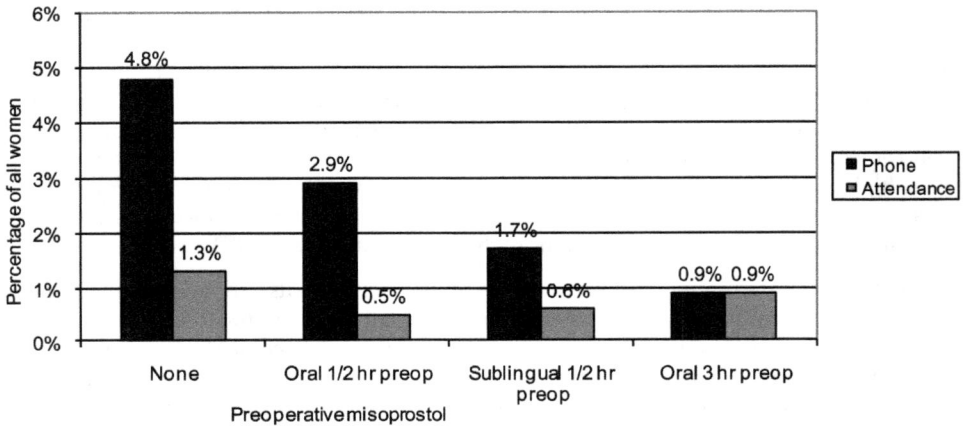

Fig. 1. The percentage of all women making contact by phone or attendance with pain and bleeding following first trimester surgical termination of pregnancy with varying misoprostol single 200mcg tablet regimens (Chambers et al., 2009).

The dosage regimens of the drugs to be used should be explained along with the clinic attendances that will be required. Bleeding with the passage of clots, and cramping of variable intensity, will occur as the expulsion of the pregnancy from the uterus occurs, usually 2-4 hours after the initial dose of misoprostol. Strong analgesic drugs including codeine, tramadol and ibuprofen should be prescribed to ease the severity of the cramping pains; antiemetic metoclopramide tablets should also be prescribed. Bleeding may continue for up to 2 weeks, and occasionally up to 4 weeks. Possible side effects of nausea, vomiting, diarrhoea, chills or mild fever are discussed. The risk of birth defects if the woman decides to continue the pregnancy after taking the abortion drugs should be emphasised. The possible complications of retained products of conception, heavy bleeding, infection and continuing pregnancy should be discussed. An emergency 24 hour contact number should be given for the woman to seek help if bleeding is heavier than soaking a pad an hour for 2 hours or if there is a persistent temperature over 38⁰C. Blood testing for blood group, haemoglobin and quantitative beta-human chorionic gonadotrophin (hCG} should be performed. Medical abortion is contraindicated if the haemoglobin level is less than 9.5 g/dl. Previous caesarean section operations are not a contraindication; the incidence of caesarean scar rupture from misoprostol uterine contraction stimulation is extremely low. Explain that Rh(D) negative women with no anti-D antibodies will need anti-D immune globulin in a dose of 50 mcg (250 IU) under 13 weeks and 300 mcg (1500 IU) over 13 weeks (Lubusky et al., 2010). The risk of an ectopic pregnancy should be explained if relevant; pelvic ultrasound examination and repeat quantitative beta-hCG should be ordered if an ectopic pregnancy has not been excluded. Kaneshiro et al., (2011) state that medical abortion can be provided in a safe and effective manner up to 63 days gestation without the routine use of ultrasound. It is important to discuss contraceptive methods that can be offered: a prescription for the oral contraceptive pill; long acting slow release progesterone intrauterine device (IUD) or implant – the latter should be inserted with the misoprostol dose not the mifepristone dose as this reduces the efficacy of the mifepristone (Church et al., 2010). Immediate IUD insertion after abortion has been shown to result in higher rates of IUD use at 6 months than delayed insertion, without an increased risk of complications (Bednarek et al., 2011). It is important to ensure that informed consent is given in writing for all procedures before any treatment is commenced.

2.3 Induction with mifepristone and misoprostol

The initial medication is one oral tablet of mifepristone 200 mg. It has been shown that increasing the dosage of mifepristone beyond this level markedly increases the cost with no additional benefit in outcomes (Shannon et al., 2005). The optimal time interval before the administration of misoprostol 800 µg is 48 hours. My personal experience of over 2000 women with the use of a 48 hour interval is a success rate of 99.9%. Ashok et al (1998) reported a success rate of 99.4% in 2000 women. Alternatives to the 48 hour interval are immediate with no interval, or a 24-36 hour interval; although the success rates for these are lower they are still in the high nineties (Goel et al., 2011). The highest success rates for stimulating expulsive uterine contractions are with the woman, after washing her hands and wetting the tablets with a quick dip in water, inserting the four misoprostol 200 mcg tablets vaginally. An alternative route of administration is bucally with a success rate almost as high. The misoprostol may be administered by the woman in the clinic or at home, providing there is no legal restriction of this. Prospective cohort studies have shown no difference in effectiveness of acceptability between home-based and clinic based medical abortion across countries (Ngo et al., 2011). It has been demonstrated that early first-trimester abortion provided by certified nurses and auxiliary nurse midwives is as safe and effective as that provided by doctors (Warriner et al., 2011). Women should be provided with strong analgesic tablets to use, commencing with the first dose one hour before the administration of misoprostol. I have found that adding a home dosage of one sublingual misoprostol 200 mcg tablet three times a day on the two days following the initial misoprostol dose reduces the incidence of surgical intervention for complications.

Follow up two weeks later is essential to exclude the rare event of a continuing pregnancy. Grossman and Grindlay (2011) have reviewed the various alternatives to ultrasound and concluded that the most promising modalities include serum hCG measurement (a fall of at least 50%), standardised assessment of women's symptoms, low-sensitivity urine pregnancy testing and telephone consultation. Although ultrasound reliably detects the removal of a previously detected gestation sac, it has been shown to be unreliable in determining completion or otherwise of the abortion process, the serum hCG level being a more reliable indicator of the amount of any retained tissue. The commonest complication of medical abortion is retained products of conception causing prolonged bleeding. Published D&C

rates for retained products vary from 0.9% (Clark et al., 2010) to 18.9% (Odeh et al., 2010) and 25.3% (Liao et al., 2010). These wide variations reflect the varying sensitivity thresholds of clinicians for diagnosing the need for surgical intervention. The highest figure is from China where the authors state that post-abortion curettage would be performed if the client continues to have vaginal bleeding 2 weeks after administration of mifepristone; this figure corresponds with my experience that approximately 25% of women are still bleeding at 2 weeks. The lower figure corresponds with my experience that most women with retained products will settle if given more time, surgery being reserved for persistent heavy bleeding. Although bleeding ceases in the majority of women in less than two weeks, some women will bleed for up to four weeks. Further treatment with misoprostol is a reasonable option for persistent or heavy bleeding, its efficacy having been shown in treating retained products following spontaneous miscarriage (Bui, 2011) and in retained products following surgical termination of pregnancy (Chambers & Mulligan, 2009). Using my experience of treating retained products of conception following surgical abortion with misoprostol the effective dosage has been determined as being four misoprostol 200 mcg tablets vaginally or buccally followed by two tablets sublingually or buccally four times a day for the next two days. Lower doses are ineffective, the non-pregnant uterus being much less responsive to misoprostol than the pregnant uterus, and the woman can be reassured that even this much higher dosage will not result in strong cramping pains.

The convenience of medical abortion has to be balanced against a higher complication rate than surgical abortion. Ninimäki et al., (2009) reported on the comparative complication rates in two cohorts of over 20,000 women each in Finland and found that the overall incidence of adverse events was fourfold higher in the medical compared with surgical abortion cohort, 20.0% compared with 5.6%.; haemorrhage 15.6% compared with 2.1%, incomplete abortion 6.7% compared with 1.6%, surgical (re)evacuation 5.9% compared with 1.8%.There was no difference in infection rates, both being 1.7%. Operative complications occurred in 0.03% of medical and 0.6% of surgical cohorts. In a smaller South Australian study of women requiring hospital treatment for complications Mulligan & Messenger (2011) concluded that complication rates of early medical abortion compared favourably to early surgical abortion: haemorrhage 0.5% medical compared with 0.03% surgical, and admission for sepsis 0.2% medical compared with 0.06% surgical. It is noteworthy that no prophylactic antibiotics were used in either the medical or surgical cohorts in this study. Whilst doxycycline antibiotic infection prophylaxis is commonly used, Achilles & Reeves (2011) note that the universal requirement for such treatment has not been established, and Fjerstad et al., (2011) conclude there is no evidence that it offers any benefit, a finding that I concur with (Chambers et al.,2009).

2.4 Induction with misoprostol alone

When the cost of mifepristone which is up to 100 times that of misoprostol, precludes its use, misoprostol alone in the single dosage of 800 mcg vaginally has been widely used. Prasad et al., (2008) reported a complete abortion rate of 94.2% with this method. However Salakos et al., (2008) reported a success rate of only 85.2% with the same single dose method. Fekih et al., (2010) used a regimen of sublingual misoprostol 800mcg four hourly to a maximum of three doses with a success rate of 92.1%. Cheng et al., (2010) have reported a 100% success rate in terminating second trimester pregnancies with oral misoprostol alone given at doses of 200 mcg/hr for the first 12 hours and 400 mcg/hr after 12hours until delivery; the most common side effect was diarrhoea, which was easily relieved by medication. This paper illustrates the safety of higher doses of misoprostol than previously used, with a much higher success rate that should be replicable in the first trimester. Whenever misoprostol is used it is essential that women are warned of the possible adverse consequences for the foetus of deciding to continue the pregnancy after already commencing misoprostol. Barbero et al., (2011) have reported that they have found a significant association between prenatal exposure to misoprostol and the occurrence of major congenital anomalies.

3. Medical abortion beyond 63 days gestation

Late first trimester and second trimester medical termination of pregnancy is more challenging than early first trimester medical abortion and should only take place in an in-patient setting, either in a hospital, or in a day clinic that can stay open for extended hours. Although second trimester termination by D&E can take place in a day-surgery clinic in a shorter time, and has been shown to have a lower complication rate than medical abortion (Bryant et al., 2011}, there are many institutions that do not have the facilities, specialised equipment, or staff with the required expertise to offer a D&E service. Medical termination can be performed with a lower level of staff training. The mifepristone and misoprostol combination is the method of choice, but where mifepristone is not available induction with misoprostol alone can be used.

3.1 Induction with mifepristone and misoprostol

The priming dose of mifepristone is one 200 mg tablet administered orally 48 hours before admission for misoprostol induction. If the woman is nauseous an anti-emetic should be administered first. Hou et al., (2010) have compared one and two day intervals and have determined that a 2-day mifepristone–misoprostol interval resulted in fewer incomplete abortions than a 1-day interval for second trimester termination of pregnancy. Misoprostol historically has been administered vaginally in the second trimester, but a meta-analysis of published randomised controlled trials that compared sublingual and vaginal routes concluded that the sublingual route shortened the induction-foetal expulsion interval and was the route preferred among women and staff (Cabrera et al., 2011). No statistically significant differences between treatment groups were observed for placental retention or for side effect except for fever, which was more common in the vaginal group; the preferred route is therefore sublingual. Brouns et al., (2010) have compared misoprostol 200 mcg or 400 mcg given at 4 hour intervals, with a maximum of 10 administrations in 48 hours, until the foetus was delivered. They found that both regimens were equally effective, but the time to delivery of the foetus was significantly longer in the 200 mcg group; they concluded that the misoprostol 400 mcg four-hourly regimen is the one of choice.

3.2 Induction with misoprostol alone

Where mifepristone is not available misoprostol alone can be used. Cheng et al., (2010) have reported a 100% success rate in gestation up to 25 weeks with a regimen of oral misoprostol given in a dose of 200 mcg hourly for the first 12 hours and 400 mcg hourly after 12 hours until delivery. The median induction to delivery interval was 12.0 hours, with a range of 6.3 to 30.9 hours. Delivery occurred within 24 hours in 81.3% of women. The median dosage of misoprostol was 2,600 mcg (13 misoprostol 200 mcg tablets). The most common side effect was diarrhoea which was easily relieved by medication.

3.3 Complications of medical abortion

The three main complications of second trimester medical abortion are placental retention, infection and haemorrhage. A large retrospective study of misoprostol induced terminations by Green et al., (2007) reported that the retained placenta rate needing surgical intervention was 6%; in 59% of women the placenta was expelled naturally within one hour of the delivery of the foetus, and expectant management did not increase the haemorrhage rate. In another large retrospective study by Ashok et al., (2004) the infection rate was 2.6% and the haemorrhage requiring transfusion rate was less than 1%. Lavoué et al., (2011) have performed a retrospective study of a medical abortion series at 12 to 14 weeks gestations and reported that the secondary manual revision or vacuum aspiration rate was 41%. Bryant et al., (2011) have compared the complication rates of medical and surgical termination of second trimester pregnancies for foetal anomalies or foetal death. In this retrospective cohort study they found that labour-induction abortions had higher complication rates and lower effectiveness than did D&E. They reported that 24% of women undergoing labour induction experienced one or more complications, in contrast to 3% undergoing D&E. They concluded that D&E is significantly safer and more effective than labour induction for second-trimester abortion for foetal indications and women should be offered a choice of method.

4. Surgical induced abortion

The surgical abortion method varies according to the gestation. In early gestations the procedure is done mainly by suction curettage. In very early gestations vacuum aspiration is commonly used. In later gestations the products of conception are too large and too rigid to be all evacuated through a suction curette and manual removal with forceps is required for at least some of the products of conception. The cut off point is traditionally 12–13 weeks, with the operation before this being a suction or vacuum termination of pregnancy (STOP or VTOP) and the operation after that point being a dilatation and evacuation (D&E). For abortion statistics therefore the second trimester is calculated from the 13th week.

4.1 Misoprostol cervical priming

Having now used preoperative misoprostol routinely before surgical termination of pregnancy for the last 17 years I have no doubt that it should be standard procedure before every operation. Misoprostol in the correct dose for the gestation, and at the optimum time interval preoperatively, is highly effective in softening and dilating the cervix in order to minimise the need for rigid dilator use. The most effective dosage regimen for each gestation has been determined by incremental changes over the years and they are detailed in Table 1. The optimal effect on the cervix from administering misoprostol is achieved after 3 hours (Tang et al., 2002) so whenever possible I use a regimen with an interval as close to 3 hours as the time frame will allow. This is most difficult when women are scheduled for operation the same day as the initial consultation. Therefore only women whose residence is a long distance from the clinic are scheduled for same day surgery. All other women are seen at a clinic consultation on a day prior to their surgery and given a misoprostol tablet to take home and use 3 hours before their operation appointment. Satisfactory cervical priming is achieved in first trimester gestations up to 9 weeks gestation with one misoprostol 200 mcg tablet taken orally. The oral route is preferred to minimise side effects occurring before the woman arrives for surgery, distressing cramping being more likely to occur with the sublingual, buccal or vaginal route (Aronsson et al., 2004).

Chambers et al., (2009) surveyed the number of women making either a phone or an attendance contact with pain and bleeding after surgical termination of a first trimester pregnancy following four different regimens. The first regimen included no misoprostol priming, in the second regimen oral misoprostol 200 mcg was administered 30 minutes preoperatively, in the third regimen sublingual misoprostol 200 mcg was administered 30 minutes preoperatively, and in the fourth regimen oral misoprostol 200 mcg was administered 3 hours preoperatively. All women receiving preoperative misoprostol also were administered misoprostol 200 mcg vaginally at the end of the operation. Figure 1 shows the results of the survey: each new regimen led to an approximate halving of the number of women making contact with symptoms of retained products of conception.

The results of a survey (Chambers et al., 2009) of side effects occurring in 1,000 women taking one oral tablet of misoprostol 200 mcg at home 3 hours before surgery are shown in Figure 2.

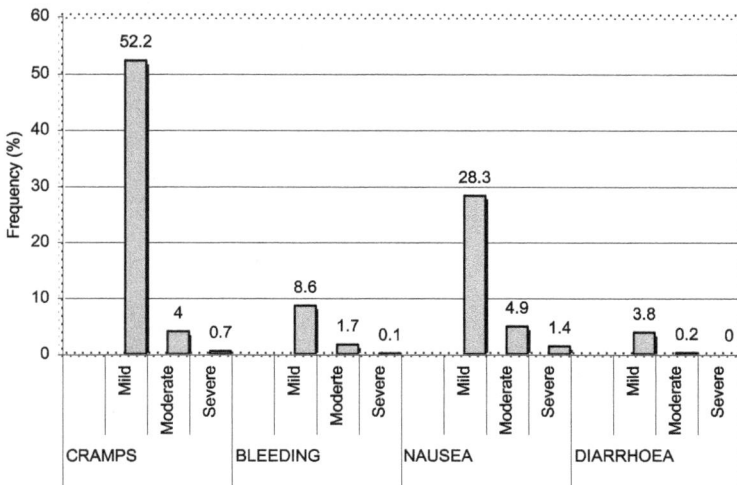

Fig. 2. Side effects in 1,000 women taking one misoprostol 200µg tablet orally 3 hours before surgery (Chambers et al., 2009).

The only significant side effect was mild cramping in 52.2% of women. Mild nausea was reported in 28.3% of women, but this was difficult to separate from pregnancy morning sickness. If the operator wishes to avoid mechanical dilatation completely then a higher dose of misoprostol should be used; 2 or 3 misoprostol 200 mcg tablets sublingually can be used, but this will be at the expense of women requiring strong analgesics prescribed for the relief of strong uterine cramping pains and therefore needing to be admitted to the clinic for a longer period preoperatively. It has been shown that there is no advantage in administering the misoprostol vaginally as was once common practice (Parveen et al., 2011) and both women and clinic staff prefer other routes to the vaginal one. For gestations beyond 9 weeks a single tablet of misoprostol does not produce reliably adequate cervical priming and the dose required increases incrementally as shown in Table 1. Adequate cervical priming at higher gestations is essential; inadequate priming followed by difficult mechanical dilatation has been shown to be one of the prime causes of cervical laceration and perforation of the uterus (Pridmore & Chambers, 1999). At 10 weeks the dose should be doubled to 2 misoprostol 200mcg tablets. At higher gestations than 10 weeks the total dose required is more than two tablets and the dosage is then split into ½ hourly doses as administering more than two tablets together produces too may side effects with the risk of excessively strong contractions and the risk of uterine rupture. At 11 weeks gestation the dose is 3 misoprostol 200 mcg tablets, at 12 to 13 weeks gestation the total dose is 5 tablets, and at 14 to 16 weeks the total dose is 7 tablets. Whenever possible a single dose of one oral tablet of misoprostol 200 mcg taken 3 hours before admission at gestations up to 16 weeks enhances the priming effect on the cervix , greatly improving the ease and safety of the operation.

GESTATION	MISOPROSTOL
5-9 weeks prebooked client	200 mcg orally at home 3 hours before admission
5-9 weeks same day service	200 mcg sublingually with theatre ½ - 1 hour later
10 weeks	200 mcg orally at home 3 hours before admission + 200 mcg sublingually on admission with theatre ½ hour later
11 weeks	200 mcg orally at home 3 hours before admission + 2x200 mcg sublingually on admission with theatre ½ hour later
12-13 weeks	200 mcg orally at home 3 hours before admission + 2 doses 2 x 200 mcg ½ hourly on admission with theatre 1-2 hours later
14-16 weeks	200 mcg orally at home 3 hours before admission + 3 doses 2 x 200 mcg ½ hourly on admission with theatre 3 hours later
17-22 weeks before osmotic dilator procedure on day 2	2x200 mcg sublingually at home at 7am + 2 doses 2 x 200 mcg ½ hourly after admission with theatre ½ -1 hour after last dose.
17-22 weeks after osmotic dilator and before D&E	2 x 200mcg PR at end osmotic dilator operation + 4 doses 200mcg sublingual ½ hourly with D&E 3 hours after the last dose.

Table 1. Misoprostol dosage regimens at each gestation for cervical priming before surgical termination of pregnancy (Chambers et al., 2009).

Pridmore & Chambers (1999) found that although previous caesarean section was a risk factor for perforation in the second trimester, it was not a risk factor in the first trimester. Misoprostol should be routinely administered at the end of every surgical abortion procedure to tone the uterus; this has been proved to reduce the incidence of postoperative bleeding and retained products of conception as shown in Figure 1 (Chambers et al., 2009). In the first trimester one misoprostol 200mcg tablet should be inserted into the posterior fornix of the vagina; in the second trimester two tablets should be inserted into the rectum. If for any reason misoprostol cannot be administered in the theatre other research (Mulayim et al., 2009) has shown that similar benefits can be achieved by administering one misoprostol 200 mcg tablet sublingually immediately after every first trimester procedure.

4.2 Manual vacuum aspiration

Manual vacuum aspirators (MVA) are widely used in developing countries where cost barriers prohibit the use of the more sophisticated and expensive electrical suction pumps. However there has been an increase in their use in developed countries in recent years, particularly in the first 9 weeks of pregnancy. These hand held pumps consist of a large syringe cylinder with a valve mechanism that allows a negative suction pressure to be built up as the plunger is withdrawn against closed valves. A sterile suction cannula is then attached and suction is generated by releasing the valves. The process can be repeated as often as necessary to empty the uterus and the aspirator can generate a suction pressure of up to 60 mm Hg. The MVA has the advantage of not only cheapness, but portability because of the small size and light weight. They are also very quiet in action compared to electric pumps which many women appreciate when the procedure is carried out under a local anaesthetic. Aspirators do not need to be sterilised, but the reusable models do need to be dismantled and thoroughly cleansed and disinfected between uses.

4.3 Surgical abortion in the first trimester

Anaesthesia can be either local, general or a combination of both. The woman is placed in the lithotomy position on the operating table and if ultrasound is available in the theatre it is useful to do a preoperative vaginal probe ultrasound to confirm the gestation and assess the position of the uterus. The pudendal area and vagina are then cleaned with an antiseptic solution such as povidone-iodine or chlorhexidine. An alternative is to only cleanse the cervix and use prophylactic antibiotic cover with doxycycline. I prefer the preparation of the whole operative field and the use of a sterile drape. A no-touch technique is used throughout the operation, the surgeon avoiding touching the parts of instruments that will enter the uterine cavity, and clean instruments are kept separate from used ones on the instrument trolley. With this approach antibiotic cover has never been used in clinics I have operated in and the resulting infection rate has been no higher than that reported for clinics where routine antibiotics are always prescribed. If ultrasound is not used in the theatre a bimanual pelvic examination should be carried out to determine the size and position of the uterus. Determining the lie of the uterus is very important; the commonest cause of perforation of the posterior wall of the uterus is failure to recognise the presence of an acutely anteverted uterus, and perforation of the anterior wall occurs when an acute retroversion is not detected. There is a wide choice of vaginal specula that are available and operator preferences vary. I prefer a single bladed Sim's speculum that rests on the perineum as it allows more room to manipulate instruments than does the bi-valve speculum; this is important in avoiding damage to the anterior or posterior wall of a uterus that is acutely flexed forwards or backwards. The anterior lip of the cervix is then grasped with either vulsellum forceps or a tenaculum. I do not like the single tooth tenaculum as it can tear the cervix and it partially obstructs access to the cervical canal. I prefer to use two multi-tooth vulsellum forceps side by side as they do not tear the cervix if they do slip off and they improve access to the cervical canal. Where the cervix is small and conical applying even a single forceps to the small anterior lip can obstruct access to the external os; in this situation one forceps should be applied laterally on each side of the cervix.

Local anaesthetic of lignocaine with adrenaline or vasopressin is now injected whether or not a general anaesthetic is being used. The addition of a local anaesthetic to a propofol general anaesthetic means less propofol is required and the vasoconstrictor greatly reduces blood loss. In all women over 6 weeks gestation I routinely use 5-10 mls of 2% lignocaine with adrenaline 1:200,000 injected bilaterally directly into the cervix at the level of the internal os through a 1½" 21 gauge needle passed up the cervical canal. This measure greatly reduces blood loss, removes the need for deep general anaesthesia, and gives some pain relief post-operatively. I prefer the intracervical to the paracervical block as it is quicker acting. For gestations 4-6 weeks I use lignocaine without adrenaline because in these very early gestations the uterine arteries are still small and there is a risk of prolonged vasospasm and tissue necrosis if adrenaline is used.

The cervical canal is now gently explored with the smallest metal dilator or uterine sound to determine its direction; this is a crucial step in the dilating process as if any force is used at this stage a false canal can easily be made which with further dilatation can easily perforate the wall of the uterus. If the direction of the cervical canal into the uterus cannot be found a bimanual examination should be performed to determine the position of the body of the uterus above the cervix. A common cause of difficulty is an acutely anteverted uterus; if this is detected as the problem a nurse assistant should be asked to apply manual suprapubic pressure to push the uterus backwards, when cannulation of the cervical canal can then usually be easily achieved. If the problem is an acutely retroverted uterus cannulation should be done with a curved dilator or sound with the curvature directed posteriorly. Problems with cannulation of the cervical canal are greatly reduced by ensuring adequate priming with misoprostol; when the problem persists, the procedure should be rescheduled with priming with a larger dosage of misoprostol and a minimum time interval of 3 hours between the last dose and the operation.

Dilatation of the cervix with graded dilators should not commence until the direction of the canal has been determined with certainty, and a small dilator has been passed with ease into the uterine cavity. The cervix should then be dilated to the number of weeks gestation converted to millimetres. The safest and easiest to use dilators are the well tapered dilators such as the Pratt or Hawkin-Ambler. The much cheaper but blunter Hegar dilators are often the only ones available and these are adequate provided sufficient misoprostol priming of the cervix has occurred. The Pratt dilators have the French circumferential system of sizing and need to have the size divided by 3 (π) to determine the millimetre dilatation being achieved. If Hegar dilators are the ones routinely available it is very helpful to have a set of Pratt or Hawkin-Ambler dilators held in reserve for the occasional very tight cervix. If a point is reached in dilatation where resistance increases and a degree of force has to be used, the dilator shaft should be guarded with a finger at a length from the tip less than the length of the cervico-uterine canal to avoid the risk of perforating the uterine wall. Perforation of the uterus is most likely to occur when there is difficulty dilating the cervix; perforation is usually recognised by an instrument passing endlessly with no sensation of stopping at the expected level of the fundus. Perforation by a dilator alone rarely causes a problem, but if it is not recognised and a suction curette is then passed through the perforation damage to viscera is then a risk. When a perforation is suspected of having occurred, the woman should be observed for 3-4 hours post-operatively to ascertain that there are no signs of peritoneal irritation before she is discharged. If peritonism is present at this time the woman will require transfer to an in-patient facility for further observation.

The size of suction curette used will correspond to the dilatation achieved. The two main types of suction curette used are flexible and rigid and operators have their own preferences. The main disadvantage of the rigid curette is that it has a terminal bevelled orifice that is relatively sharp compared with the blunt end of the flexible curette, and it is therefore the only one likely to be at risk of causing a perforation. To avoid this risk the rigid curette should be introduced very gently up to the fundus of the uterus and then withdrawn in a rotating spiral manner. The flexible curette being blunt ended can safely be used with a rapid in and out motion, achieving quicker evacuation; the disadvantage of the flexible curette is that it cannot be steered into the cornual angles where tissue may be missed. The rigid curette can be either straight or curved, and the curved is the one I prefer for the very reason that the angle allows the cornual recesses to be adequately suctioned. In summary, a combination of use of the two types is the ideal solution. A minimum suction pressure of 60 mm Hg is required by either a manual vacuum aspirator of electric suction. Electric suction has the advantage of greater speed, particularly if set at 75 to 90 mm Hg suction pressure. From 10 to 12 weeks gestations solid placental tissue may lodge in the cervical canal and require removal with a small forceps. At 12 weeks gestation solid tissue may not be removable from the body of the uterus by suction alone and the use of ovum forceps may be needed to evacuate all products of conception. To complete the evacuation of the pregnancy a sharp curette should be gently used to explore the uterine cavity to ensure that no small pieces of tissue have been missed; when the whole amniotic sac has been evacuated the feel of scraping the uterine wall changes from a smooth to a rough gritty sensation. It is important to avoid any vigorous use of the sharp curette as this can lead to removal of the basal layer of the endometrium and risk the formation of intrauterine synechial adhesions and the consequent development of Asherman's syndrome with amenorrhoea or hypomenorrhoea and pelvic pain which will require treatment by hysteroscopic division of the adhesive bands (March, 2011).

The commonest post-operative complication of suction termination of pregnancy is bleeding and cramping from retained products of conception, and in the majority of cases where this occurs the missed tissue is located in a retroverted uterus. In all women where the uterine cavity on curettage is defined as not being anteverted, it is important not to assume that the position of the body of the uterus is midline without excluding a retroflexed position. This is done by exploring with a sharp curette along the posterior wall of the uterus, and as the fundus is approached applying posterior pressure whilst angling the curette to point backwards. It is surprising how often this manoeuvre suddenly reveals a missed collection of tissue in an acutely retroflexed uterus, the curette passing backwards at almost 90 degrees to the line of the utero-cervical canal to reach the fundus.

The use of the intravenous uterotonic oxytocin has been shown to have no value in the first trimester (Nygaard et al., 2011), and similarly methylergometrine is of no value in the first trimester. The value of the routine postoperative use of the uterotonic misoprostol 200 mcg inserted into the posterior fornix of the vagina at the conclusion of first trimester surgical abortion has been researched and established by Chambers et al., (2009); its routine introduction was found to have led to a marked decrease in the number of women contacting the clinic post-operatively with bleeding and cramping due to retained products of conception as shown in Fig. 1.

If ultrasound is available in the theatre a check with the ultrasound vaginal probe will confirm that the pregnancy has been completely evacuated and that a possible twin pregnancy sac has not been missed; if a twin sac remains in a bicornuate uterus, the abdominal ultrasound should be used to guide the operator as the uterus is re-explored for the twin sac. If ultrasound is not available the evacuated products should be examined to confirm completion of the procedure. Some clinics routinely use laboratory histological confirmation, but there is a possible problem here in that confirmation of the presence of trophoblastic material can be taken as evidence of completion when only a small portion of trophoblastic material has been removed and there is actually a continuing pregnancy. Examination of products in the theatre after each case is routine in many clinics. The evacuated tissue is floated in a small amount of water in a backlit glass dish; magnification is used to identify the transparent gestational sac, the frond like chorionic villi, clear decidual tissue and small foetal parts at gestations over 8 weeks. If evacuation of a pregnancy cannot be confirmed the woman should be investigated for the possible presence of an ectopic pregnancy, particularly if the serum beta-hCG is over 1,500 IU/ml.

Scheduling all women for a follow-up appointment has been shown to have no value in improving outcomes. What is important is that all women on discharge should be given a 24 hour telephone contact number they can use to discuss any post-operative symptoms they are concerned about. Most symptoms will only require reassurance, and the minority with possible symptoms of concern can be given an appointment to return to the clinic for examination. Perriera et al., (2010) have reported that telephone follow-up combined with urine pregnancy testing is a feasible alternative to routine ultrasound or serial hCG measurements after medical abortion. The commonest complication requiring investigation and treatment after surgical abortion is persistent bleeding and cramping; that these symptoms are due to the presence of retained products of conception can be confirmed with an ultrasound examination. The simplest treatment in this situation is the administration of misoprostol 200 mcg sublingually three times a day for 2 days. Chambers & Mulligan (2009) have reported this regimen to be 93% effective in the first week following the operation; in the second week a higher dosage is required of 4 misoprostol 200 mcg tablets initially vaginally, sublingually or bucally followed by 2 tablets four times a day sublingually for 2 days. Figure 3 shows the marked reduction in the repeat D&C rate following the introduction of this treatment for retained products in their clinic.

4.4 Surgical abortion at 13 to 16 weeks

Approximately 9% of all pregnancy terminations occur at 13-16 weeks gestation. In the first four weeks of the second trimester termination of pregnancy can reliably be performed as a one stage procedure with D&E performed in one day after adequate cervical priming with misoprostol (Chambers et al., 2011a). As shown in Table 1, the dosage of misoprostol required increases with the gestation. At 12-13 weeks for a same day service client 2 sublingual doses of misoprostol 400 mcg are given 30 minutes apart with D&E 1 to 2 hours after the last dose. For a prebooked client this dosage regimen is preceded by one oral dose of misoprostol 200 mcg at home 3 hours before admission to the clinic, with D&E ½ to 1 hour after the last dose. At 14-16 weeks an additional third sublingual dose of misoprostol 400 mcg is given 30 minutes after the second sublingual dose, with D&E 3 hours after the last dose. A retrospective study I performed with colleagues (Chambers et al., 2011a) showed that the simple addition of one oral tablet of misoprostol 200 mcg at home 3 hours before admission to the regimen of 2 tablets ½ hourly for two or three doses on admission increased the probability of all women at 13-16 weeks gestation completing a termination of pregnancy in one day with a single D&E procedure to 100%, and with a reduced theatre time, the operators noting operations to be easier to perform with the extra priming from the one oral tablet taken 3 hours before admission.

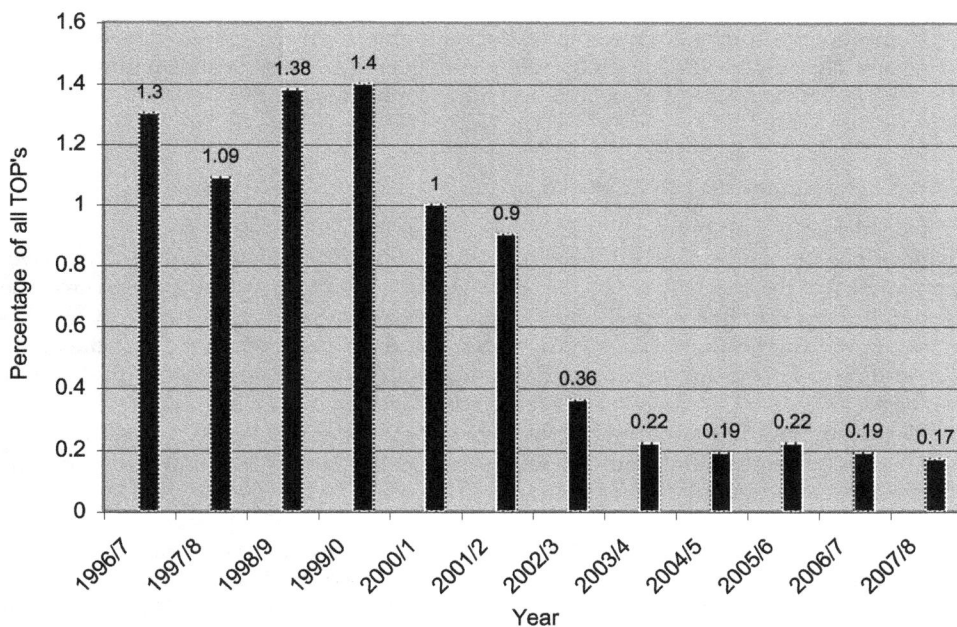

Fig. 3. Percentage repeat D&C rate per 12 months period for retained products of conception following suction TOP. The routine use of misoprostol for treatment of retained products began in 2002 (Chambers & Mulligan, 2009).

Preparation of the woman in the theatre is as in first trimester up to dilatation of the cervix. Dilatation again should be equal to the number of weeks' gestation in millimetres. Bierer type forceps of a size appropriate the dilatation are then used to evacuate the contents of the uterus, the manual removal of tissue being supplemented by the use of a rigid suction curette. My preference is for the use of a 12 mm curved rigid suction curette for all second trimester gestations, but curettes up to 16 mm are available and preferred by some operators. Real time ultrasound guidance is very useful when available, a nurse assistant using the abdominal ultrasound probe to show the operator where the end of his/her instrument is working and the location of tissue still to be evacuated. The evacuation of the uterus is concluded by checking with a large size 3 or 4 sharp curette, and a 12mm curved rigid suction curette followed by an 8mm flexible suction curette to determine that the uterus is completely empty. An intravenous injection of uterotonic oxytocin 5-10 units is given. Finally two misoprostol 200 mcg tablets should be inserted into the posterior fornix of the vagina for further prolonged uterotonic effect.

The commonest difficulty met performing a D&E at these gestations is the foetal head being trapped in the cornual recess on one side of the fundus. A moderately large size 3 or 4 sharp curette can often be used to prise the head out of its trapped position, allowing forceps to grasp and extract it. Alternatively a suction curette can be used to draw the head down. If the problem persists administering sevoflurane will often relax the uterus enough to free the trapped foetal part. When all these measures fail, rather than persisting and risking perforating the uterus, 2 misoprostol 200 mcg tablets should be inserted into the posterior vaginal fornix or rectum and the woman returned to the ward where 4 sublingual doses of misoprostol 200 mcg are administered at 30 minute intervals. The woman is returned to the theatre 2-3 hours later when the foetal head will be found lying in the lower segment of the uterine cavity.

4.5 Surgical abortion at 17 to 22 weeks

Approximately 4% of all pregnancy terminations occur at 17 to 22 weeks gestation. At these gestations it becomes increasingly difficult to safely terminate the pregnancy in one day. Safety is proportional to the ease with which the cervix can be dilated to an extent appropriate to the gestation before D&E. It is cervical trauma from excessive mechanical dilatation of a cervix that has been scarred from previous gynaecological or other pelvic surgery that is the prime factor leading to tearing and perforation of the uterus in second trimester D&E (Pridmore & Chambers, 1999). As it is not possible to predict which women will be easy to dilate I prefer to treat all women from 17 weeks gestation as having the potential for difficulty in dilatation so use a multistage regimen for them all. The first stage on day 1 consists of two parts, the insertion of osmotic cervical dilators and the injection of a foeticide under a short intravenous propofol anaesthetic. After induction of the anaesthetic the woman is prepared as described for surgical abortion at 13-16 weeks. When the cervix has been secured with vulsellum forceps at 17-19 weeks gestation one 4 mm x 65 mm Dilapan-S™ osmotic dilator is inserted into the cervical canal and at 20-22 weeks two Dilapan-S™ dilators are inserted. Dilapan-S™ is a hydrophilic polymer rod manufactured from a proprietary hydrogel, which is hygroscopic and expands radially more rapidly, consistently and to a greater degree than the seaweed preparation laminaria tents, with the result that fewer Dilapan-S™ can be inserted for shorter periods of time (Lohr, 2008). A povidone–iodine soaked pack is inserted into the vagina to prevent expulsion of the dilators before swelling has occurred.

The foeticide digoxin 1 mg is then injected into the chest or head of the foetus under ultrasound guidance if available. Molaei et al., (2008) have reported that the injection of digoxin into either the foetus or amniotic fluid without ultrasound guidance has a high success rate. Consent for the digoxin injection is included on the operation consent form and the woman is informed that the injection causes progressive slowing of the foetal heart until it stops; the advantages of the procedure are that it averts the risk of the foetus being inadvertently born alive, with the possibility of resuscitation attempts being made, and that maceration of the foetal tissues produces softening of the ligaments which facilitates easy and safe evacuation of the foetus from the uterus (Hern, 2001).

The woman is discharged home with anti-emetic metoclopramide 10 mg tablets, analgesic tramadol 50 mg tablets, sleeping sedative temazepam 10 mg tablets, and antibiotic tablets azithromycin 1 g and tinidazole 2 g to be taken that evening. The next morning she takes 2 misoprostol 200 mcg tablets sublingually at home at 7am, the dose is repeated on arrival back at the clinic a 7.45am and a third dose of two tablets sublingually is give 30 minutes later. She is also given 5-10 mg of oxycodone orally, this being by far the most effective analgesic in this situation in my experience. Half to one hour after this last dose the woman is taken to theatre and intravenous propofol anaesthesia induced. Preparation for the operation is as before. The general anaesthetic is augmented with an intracervical injection of 10 to 15 ml of 2% lignocaine with 1:200,000 adrenaline. The osmotic dilators are removed and the amount of dilatation achieved is measured by passing Hegar dilators until the first resistance is met. This measurement determines whether there is sufficient dilatation for an immediate safe D&E or whether further dilatation is required. Table 2 shows the amount of dilatation required for safe D&E at each gestation.

Gestation in weeks	16	17	18	19	20	21	22
Cervical dilators	14	15	16	17	18	19	20
D&E	16	18	20	22	24	26	28

Table 2. Minimum mm dilatations required before insertion of cervical dilators and before D&E (Chambers et al., 2011b).

Table 2 also shows the amount of dilatation that is required at each gestation before the insertion of further osmotic dilators if the woman is to be safe for return for D&E the same day. These safe limits have been determined by me from 17 years experience performing late second trimester terminations. It has been determined from a review of women with complications that it is cervical trauma from excessive mechanical dilatation of a cervix that has been scarred from previous gynaecological or other pelvic surgery that is the prime factor leading to tearing and perforation of the uterus in second trimester D&E (Pridmore & Chambers, 1999). In this review I also analysed in each case the amount of mechanical dilatation that was used before tearing occurred and the parity of each woman with tearing. With this information I have been able to draw up some guidelines for the mechanical dilatation limits for safe dilatation. My survey found that no primiparous woman had ever sustained a second trimester peroration of the uterus, with mechanical dilatation up to 10 mm being used beyond the point of first resistance in several women. Survey of the parous women with perforations revealed that that for each pregnancy of a woman's parity the perforation occurred after approximately 2 mm less mechanical dilation. The rough guideline that I use therefore is that a limit of 10 mm of mechanical dilatation beyond the point of first resistance should not be passed in primiparous women and this limit should be reduced by 2mm for each pregnancy of parity. This guideline should only be used in combination with the high total dose misoprostol cervical priming described. High total dose misoprostol regimens have been proved to be very effective and safe, even in women with caesarean scars (Malapati et al., 2011).The dilatation at which first resistance occurred having been determined, if this plus minimal rigid dilatation equals the minimum dilatation for safe D&E at the woman's gestation, which increases from 17 mm at 17 weeks to 28 mm at 22 weeks, as in Table 2, the pregnancy can be terminated forthwith by D&E as for 13-16 weeks gestation.

If the minimum dilatation for safe D&E has not been achieved the cervix is dilated with Hawkin Ambler or Pratt dilators to a dilatation equal to the weeks gestation minus 2 mm as in Table 2. In parous women, and women with a history of previous gynaecological surgery, the protocol described above limiting mechanical dilatation is applied. The membranes should be ruptured routinely at this stage, and all liquor is expressed by abdominal pressure, with a small forceps being used to displace the presenting foetal part to allow free drainage. If part of the umbilical cord prolapses it should be excised. The cervical canal is then filled with 3 to 5 Dilapan-S™ synthetic hygroscopic dilators dipped in an antiseptic solution such as povidone-iodine. The number of dilators is recorded on the operation sheet. A vaginal pack is soaked in the antiseptic solution and placed in the vagina to hold the laminaria in place until they start swelling. At the end of the procedure an indomethacin or diclofenac 100 mg suppository and a prochlorperazine 25 mg suppository are placed in the rectum along with 2 moistened misoprostol200 mcg tablets if the woman is to be returned to theatre for D&E the same day; 98% of women are suitable for same day D&E. The woman is returned to the ward where she is administered 1 misoprostol 200 mcg tablet sublingually at half hour intervals for four doses. She is returned to theatre 3 hours after the last dose or earlier if delivery is imminent. I have found that 1-2% of women are extremely poor responders to misoprostol (Chambers et al., 2009) and in these women the D&E will not be the same day. Because the membranes will be ruptured for 24 hours a single dose of intravenous antibiotics is injected, amoxycillin 2 g (or a third generation cephalosporin if there is allergy to amoxicillin) and gentamycin 160 mg and the post-operative misoprostol regimen as described for same day return for D&E is omitted.

4.5.1 D&E technique 17-22 weeks

The vaginal pack and cervical dilators are removed and the number checked. If either the pack or dilators are not visible, the posterior fornix should be explored for them by bimanual examination at the end of the procedure rather than assuming that they had been passed spontaneously. Further mechanical dilatation is carried out if required to reach the target dilatation for safe D&E at that gestation listed in Table 2; the amount of mechanical dilatation should again be limited by the guidelines for women with risk factors as previously detailed. A nurse assistant should hold the vulsellum forceps handles through the sterile drape to leave both hands of the operator free. The uterus is evacuated at 17 to 18 weeks with 11 x ¾" Sopher forceps, at 19 to 20 weeks with the 11' x ½" Bierer forceps and at 21 - 22 weeks with the 11 x ¾" Bierer forceps. The Sopher forceps are used at smaller gestations as they have smaller teeth and are less likely to catch the uterine wall; the Bierer forceps are heavier with larger teeth and are used at later gestations to enable a better grip to be obtained on the larger foetal parts. The foetal head can usually be decompressed by crushing with forceps, using 2 hands if necessary. If at 21-22 weeks the cervix is widely dilated the presenting head may be tightly engaged in the cervical canal, in which case the base of the skull or presenting part should be punctured with a pointed size 11 disposable scalpel or scissors and decompressed by suction of the cranial contents with a 6 mm rigid suction curette.

When delivering an intact foetus body first, the arms must be brought down from alongside the head individually by hooking a finger in each axilla in turn. When the body delivers first it is rotated so that the back is uppermost, and traction is applied through the body; a scalpel or scissors is then used to puncture the occiput via the back of the neck, and the head decompressed by suction as described above.

Second trimester D&E procedures should be carried out under ultrasound control when this is available, a nurse assistant positioning the abdominal probe in the sagittal plane under the sterile drape. Observing the foetal image moving when forceps are rotated confirms that the forceps are grasping the foetus and not the uterine wall, which can happen with the Bierer forceps that have much more prominent teeth on the blades than the Sopher forceps. The Sopher forceps cannot be used in later gestations because the small teeth will not grip onto larger foetal parts without slipping. Intravenous oxytocin 5-10 units should be given as soon as all major foetal parts and the placenta have been delivered. The uterine cavity is then suction curetted with a 12 mm curved rigid suction curette. A size 3 or 4 sharp curette is used to check the emptiness of the uterus and the continuity of the utero-cervical wall, particularly after difficult evacuations. A final suction with an 8mm flexible curette is carried out.

At the conclusion of the operation, to confirm that the uterus is completely empty, a trans-vaginal probe ultrasound examination may be carried out if there was any difficulty obtaining a good view of the uterus with the abdominal probe, particularly if the woman is obese. If ultrasound has not been used all the tissues removed must be examined to ensure that all the major parts of the foetus and the whole placenta have been evacuated. Two moistened tablets of misoprostol 200 mcg and an indomethacin 100 mg suppository are then inserted through the anus. Alternatively the misoprostol tablets may be placed in the posterior fornix of the vagina for a more rapid effect. For 20-22 weeks gestations in parous women whose uterus is lacking in tone at the end of the procedure 40 units of oxytocin in 500 ml of IV fluid is run in over 1-2 hours post-operatively. When bleeding occurs in the immediate post operative period it should be treated by administering to the woman 2 sublingual tablets of misoprostol 200 mcg every 30 minutes until the bleeding stops. If there is no slowing of the blood loss after three doses of misoprostol the woman will need to be returned to theatre to exclude retained products in the uterus, a cervical or uterine laceration, or a spurting arteriole on the surface of the cervix. Published rates for serious D&E complications are Hern (2001) 0.0%, Patel et al., (2006) 0.45%, Chambers et al., (2011b) 0.0%. A Cochrane review by Newmann et al., (2010) concluded that mifepristone does not appear to be useful for cervical preparation in the second trimester because of the high rates of pre-procedural expulsions. I have trialled the addition of mifepristone to misoprostol and osmotic dilators in late second trimester terminations to enhance cervical dilatation, but after 21 cases the use of mifepristone was ceased due to one overnight delivery at home and excessive softening of the cervix causing a 19% incidence of cervical laceration (Chambers et al., 2011b).

4.6 Intact D&E beyond 22 weeks

Most clinics offering second trimester surgical terminations have a gestation limit of 22 weeks. A very small number of women seek termination of pregnancy beyond 22 weeks for mental health and social reasons. Hospital clinics offering medical terminations beyond 22 weeks are predominantly there for the treatment of women with either foetal death or severe foetal anomaly; these clinics are usually not prepared to accept women for termination of pregnancy for mental health and social reasons. A limited number of private clinics will accept these women. The technique used is injection of a foeticide, serial osmotic cervical dilators over 2-3 days followed by induction of labour with an oxytocin drip and evacuation of the uterus by intact D&E under a general anaesthetic when delivery is imminent. Chasen et al., (2004) have reported a series comparing D&E with intact D&E for terminations of pregnancy at 20 weeks gestation and over, and found that complication rates were the same, being approximately 5% for all complications in each of the two groups, with no difference in procedure time or estimated blood loss.

5. References

Achilles, SL; & Reeves, MF. (2011). Prevention of infection after induced abortion. *Contraception*, Vol. 83, No. 4, (Apr 2011), pp. 295-309, ISSN 0010-7824 Ashok, PW; Penney, GC; Flett, GM; & Templeton, A. (1998). An effective regimen for early medical abortion: a report of 2000 consecutive cases. *Hum Reprod*, Vol. 13, No. 10, (Oct 1998), pp.2962-5, ISSN 0268-1161

Aronsson, A; Bygdeman, M; & Gemzell-Danielsson, K. (2004). Effects of misoprostol on uterine contractility following different routes of administration. *Hum Reprod*, Vol.19, No. 1, (Jan 2004), pp. 81-4, ISSN 0269-1161

Ashok, PW; Templeton, A; Wagaarachchi, PT; & Flett, GM. (2004). Midtrimester medical termination of pregnancy: a review of 1002 consecutive cases. *Contraception*, Vol. 69, No. 1, (Jan 2004), pp.51-58, ISSN 0010-7824

Ashok, PW; Wagaarachchi, PT; & Templeton, A. (2002). The antiprogestogen mifepristone: a review. *Curr Med Chem Immunol Endocr Metab Agents*, Vol 2, (2002), pp.71-90, ISSN 1568-0134

Barbero, P; Liascovich, R; Valdez, R; & Moresco, A. (2011). Misoprostol teratogenicity: a prospective study in Argentina. *Arch Argent Pediatr*. Vol. 109, No. 3, (Jun 2011), pp.226-231, ISSN 0325-0075

Bednarek, PH; Creinin, MD; Reeves, MF; Cwiak, C; Espey, E; & Jensen, JT. (2011). Immediate versus delayed IUD insertion after uterine aspiration. *N Engl J Med*, Vol. 364, No. 23, (Jun 2011), pp.2208- 17, ISSN 0028-4793

Bracken, H; Clark, W; Lichtenberg, ES; Schweikert, SM; Tanenhaus, J; Barajas, A; Alpert, L; & Winikoff, B. (2011). Alternatives to routine ultrasound for eligibility assessment prior to early termination of pregnancy with mifepristone-misoprostol. *BJOG*. Vol. 118, No. 1, (Jan 2011), pp.17-23, ISSN 1470- 0328

Brouns, JF; van Wely, M; Burger, MP; & van Wijngaarden, WJ. (2010). Comparison of two dose regimens of misoprostol for second-trimester pregnancy termination. *Contraception*. Vol. 82, No. 3, (Sept 2010), pp.266-75, ISSN 0010-7824

Bryant, AG; Grimes, DA; Garrett, JM; & Stuart GS. (2011). Second-trimester abortion for fetal anomalies or fetal death: labor induction compared with dilatation and evacuation. *Obstet Gyneccol*. Vol. 117, No. 4, (Apr 2011), pp.788-92, ISSN 0029-7844

Bui, Q. (2011). Management options for early incomplete miscarriage. *Am Fam Physician*. Vol. 83, No. 3, (Feb 2011), pp.258-60, ISSN 0002-838X

Cabrera. Y; Fernández-Guisasola, J; Lobo, P; Gámir, S; & Alvarez, J. (2011). Comparison of sublingual versus vaginal misoprostol for second-trimester pregnancy termination:

a meta-analysis. *Aust N Z J Obstet Gynaecol.* Vol. 51, No. 2, (Apr 2011), pp.158-65, ISSN 0004-8666

Chambers, DG; & Mulligan, EC. (2009). Treatment of suction termination of pregnancy-retained products with misoprostol markedly reduces the repeat operation rate. *Aust N Z J Obstet Gynecol.* Vol. 49, No. 5, (Oct 2009), pp.551-553, ISSN 0004-8666

Chambers, DG; Mulligan, EC; Laver, AR; Weller,BK; Baird, JK; & Herbert, WY. (2009). Comparison of four perioperative misoprostol regimens for surgical termination of first-trimester pregnancy. *Int J Gynaecol Obstet.* Vol. 107, No. 3, (Dec 2009), pp.211-5, ISSN 0020-7292

Chambers, DG; Willcourt, RJ; Laver, AR; Baird, JK; & Herbert, WY. (2011a). Comparison of two misoprostol regimens for cervical priming before surgical pregnancy termination at 13 to 16 weeks gestation. *Open J Obstet Gynecol,* Vol. 1, No. 4 (Dec 2011), pp.187-190, ISSN 2160-8792

Chambers, DG; Willcourt, RJ; Laver, AR; Baird, JK; & Herbert, WY. (2011b). Comparison of Dilapan- S and laminaria tents for cervical priming before surgical pregnancy termination at 17 to 22 weeks' gestations. *Int J Womens' Health,* Vol.3, No. 1, (Oct 2011), pp. 347-52, ISSN 1179-1411

Chasen, ST; Kalish, RB; Gupta, M; Kaufman, JE; Rashbaum, WK; & Chervenak, FA . (2004). Dilatation and evacuation at > or = 20 weeks: comparison of operative techniques. *Am J Obstet Gynecol.* Vol. 190, No. 5, (May 2004), pp.1180-1183, ISSN 0002-9378

Cheng, SY; Hsue, CS; Hwang, GH; Tsai, LC; & Pei, SC. (2010). Hourly oral misoprostol administration for terminating midtrimester pregnancies: a pilot study. *Taiwan J Obstet Gynecol.* Vol. 49, No. 4, (Dec 2010), pp.438-41, ISSN 1028-4559

Church, E; Sengupta, S, & Chia, KV. (2010). The contraceptive implant for long acting reversible contraception in patients undergoing first trimester medical termination of pregnancy. *Sex & Reprod Healthcare.* Vol. 1, No. 3, (Aug 2010), pp.105-9, ISSN 1877-5756

Clark, W; Bracken, H; Tanenhaus, J; Schweikert, S; Lichtenberg, ES; & Winikoff, B. (2010). Alternatives to a routine follow-up visit for early medical abortion. *Obstet Gynecol* Vol. 115, No. 2 Pt1, (Feb 2010), pp.264-72, ISSN 0029-7844

Davies, NM; Longstreth, J; & Jamali, F. (2001 Jan). *Pharmacotherapy.* Vol. 21, No. 1, (Jan 2001), pp.60-23, ISSN 0277-0008

Dixon-Mueller, R (1988). Innovations in reproductive health care: menstrual regulation policies and programs in Bangladesh. *Stud Fam Plann.* Vol. 19, No. 3, (May-Jun 1998), pp.129-140, ISSN 0039- 3665

Fekih, M; Fathallah, K; Ben Regaya, L; Bouguizane,S; Chaieb, A; Bibi, M; & Khairi, H . (2010). Sublingual misoprostol for first trimester termination of pregnancy. *Int J Gynaecol Obstet.*Vol. 109, No. 1, (Apr 2010), pp.67-70, ISSN 0020-7292

Fjerstad, M; Trussell, J; Lichtenberg, ES; Sivin, I; & Cullins, V. (2011). Severity of infection following the introduction of new infection control measures for medical abortion. *Contraception.* Vol. 83, No. 4, (Apr 2011), pp.330-5, ISSN 0010-7824

Gamble, SB; Strauss, LT; Parker, WY; Cook, DA; Zane, SB; & Hamdan, S (2008). Abortion surveillance – United States, 2005. *MMWR Surveill Summ.* Vol. 57, No. 13, (Nov 2008), pp.1-32, ISSN 1546-0738

Garfield, RE; Blennerhassett, MG; & Miller. SM. (1988). Control of myometrial contractility: role and regulation of gap junctions. *Oxf Rev Reprod,Biol.* Vol. 10, (1988), pp.436-490, ISSN 0260-0854

Goel, A; Mittal, S; Taneja, BK; Singal, N; & Attri, S. (2011). Simultaneous administration of mifepristaone and misoprostol for early termination of pregnancy: a randomized controlled trial. *Arch Gynecol Obstet.* Vol. 283, No. 6, (Jun 2011), pp.1409-13, ISSN 0932-0067

Green, J; Borgatta, L; Sia, M; Kapp, N; Saia, K; Carr-Ellis, S; & Vragovic, O (2007). Intervention rates for placental removal following induction abortion with misoprostol. *Contraception.* Vol. 76, No. 4, (Oct 2007), pp.310-313, ISSN 0010-7824

Grossman, D; & Grindlay, K. (2011). Alternatives to ultrasound for follow-up after medication abortion: a systematic review. *Contraception.* Vol. 83, No. 6, (Jun 2001), pp.504-10, ISSN 0010-7824

Henriques, A; Lourenço, AV; Ribeirinho, A; Ferreira, H; & Graça, LM. (2007). Maternal death related to misoprostol overdose. *Obstet Gynecol.* Vol. 109, No. 2 Pt2, (Feb 2007), pp.489-90, ISSN 0029-7844

Henshaw, SK. (1990). Induced abortion: a world review. In: *Abortion, medicine, and the law.* Butler, JD; & Walbert, DF, (Ed.), pp.406-436, Facts on File, ISBN, New York

Henshaw, SK. (1998). Unintended pregnancy in the United States. *Fam Plann Perspect.* Vol. 30, No. 1, (Jan- Feb 1998), pp.24-9, 46, ISSN 0014-7354

Heikinheimo, O. (1989). Pharmacokinetics of the antiprogesterone RU486 in women during multiple dose administration. *J Steroid Biochem.* Vol. 32, No. 1A, (Jan 1989), pp.21-5, ISSN 0022-4731

Hern, WM. (2001). Laminaria, induced fetal demise and misoprostol in late abortion. *Int J Gynaecol Obstet.* Vol. 75, No. 3, (Dec 2001), pp.279-286, ISSN 0020-7292

Hou, S; Zhang, L; Chen, Q; Fang, A; & Chang, L. (2010). One- and two-day mifepristone-misoprostol intervals for second trimester termination of pregnancy between 13 and 16 weeks of gestation. *Int J Gynaecol Obstet.* Vol. 111, No. 2, (Nov 2010), pp.126-30, ISSN 0020-7292

Jha, P; Kesler, MA; Kumar, R; Ram, F; Ram,U; Aleksandrowicz, L; Bassani, DG; Chandra, S; & Banthia, JK. (2011) Trends in selective abortions of girls in India: analysis of nationally representative birth histories from 1990 to 2005 and census data from 1991 to 2011. *Lancet.* Vol. 377, No. 9781, (Jun 4 2011), pp.1921-1928, ISSN 0140-6736

Johnson, HB; Oliveras, E; Akhter, S; & Walker, DG. (2010). Health system costs of menstrual regulation and care for abortion complications in Bangladesh. *Int Perspect Sex Reproduct Health.* Vol. 36, No. 4, (Dec 2010), pp.197-204, ISSN 1944-0391

Jones, RK; Darroch, JE; & Henshaw, SK. (2002). Contraceptive use among U.S. women having abortions in 2000-2001. *Perspect Sex Reproduct Health.* Vol. 34, No. 6, (Nov-Dec 2002), pp.294-303, ISSN 1538- 6341

Jones, RK; & Kavanaugh, ML. (2011). Changes in abortion rates between 2000 and 2008 and lifetime incidence of abortion. *Obstet Gynecol.* Vol. 117, No. 6, (Jun 2011), pp.1358-66, ISSN 0029-7844

Kaneshiro, B; Edelman, A; Sneeringer, RK; & Ponce de Leon, RG. (2011). Expanding medical abortion: can medical abortion be effectively provided without the routine use of ultrasound? *Contraception.* Vol. 83, No. 6, (Mar 2011), pp.194-201, ISSN 0010-7824

Kotsonis, FN; Dodd, DC; Regnier, B; Kohn, FE. (1985). Preclinical toxicology profile of misoprostol. *Dig Dis Sci.* Vol. 30, No. 11 Suppl, (Nov 1985), pp.142S-146S, ISSN 0163-2116

Lavoué, ÃV; Vandenbroucke, L; Grouin, A; Briand, E; Bauville, E; Boyer, L; Lemeut, P; Bernard, O; Poulain, P; & Morcel, K. (2011). Medical abortion from 12 through 14 weeks' gestation: a retrospective study with 126 patients. *J Gynecol Obstet Biol Reprod (Paris).* Vol. 40, No. 7, (Nov 2011), pp.626-32. ISSN 0368-2315

Liao, H; Wei, Q; Duan, L; Ge, J; Zhou, Y; & Zeng, W. (2010). Repeated medical abortions and the risk of preterm birth in the subsequent pregnancy. *Arch Gynecol Obstet.* Vol. 284, No. 3, (Sep 2011), pp. 579-86, ISSN 0932-0067

Lohr, PA. (2008). Surgical abortion in the second trimester. *Reprod Health Matters.* Vol. 16, No. 31, (May 2008 Suppl), pp.151-161, ISSN 0968-8080

Lubuský, M; Procházka, M; Simetka, O; & Holusková, I. (2010). Guideline for prevention of RhD alloimmunization in RhD negative women. *Ceska Gynecol* . Vol. 75, No. 4, (Aug 2010), pp.323-4, ISSN 1210-7832

Malapati, R; Villaluna, G; & Nguyen, TM. (2011). Use of misoprostol for pregnancy termination in women with prior classical cesarean delivery: a report of 3 cases. *J Reproduct Med.* Vol. 56, No. 1-2, (Jan- Feb 2011), pp.85-6, ISSN 0024-7758

March, CM. (2011). Asherman's syndrome. *Semin Reproduct Med.* Vol. 29, No. 2, (Mar 2011), pp.83-94, ISSN 1526-8004

Molaei, M; Jones, HE; Weiselberg, T; McManama, M; Bassell, J; & Westhoff , CL. (2008). Effectiveness and safety of digoxin to induce fetal demise prior to second-trimester abortion. *Contraception.* Vol. 77, No. 3, (Mar 2008), pp.223-5, ISSN 0010-7824

Mulayim, B; Celik, NY; Onalan G; Zeyneloglu, HB; & Kuscu, E, (2009). Sublingual misoprostlol after surgical management of early termination of pregnancy. *Fertil Steril.* Vol. 92, No. 2, (Aug 2009), pp.678–81, ISSN 0015-0282

Mulligan, E; & Messenger, H. (2011). Mifepristone in South Australia - the first 1343 tablets. Aust Fam Physician. Vol. 40, No. 5, (May 2011), pp.342-5, ISSN 0004-8666

Newmann, SJ; Dalve-Endres, A; Diedrich, JT; Steinauer, JE; Meckstroth, K; & Drey, EA. (2010). Cervical preparation for second trimester dilatation and evacuation. *Cochrane Database Syst Rev.* Vol. 4, No. 8, (Aug 2010) pp.CD007310, ISSN 1469-493X

Ninimäki, M; Pouta, A; Bloigu, A; Gissler, M; Hemminki, E; Suhonen, S; & Heikinheimo, O. (2009). Immediate complications after medical compared with surgical termination of pregnancy. *Obstet Gynecol.* Vol. 114, No. 4, (Oct 2009), pp.795-804, ISSN 0029-7844

Ngo, TD; Park, MH; Shakur, H; & Free, C. (2011). Comparative effectiveness, safety and acceptability of medical abortion at home and in a clinic: a systematic review. *Bull World Health Organ.* Vol. 89, No. 5, (May 1 2011), pp.360-70, ISSN 0042-9686

Nygaard, IH; Valbø, A; Heide, HC; & Kresovic, M. (2011). Is oxytocin given during surgical termination of first trimester pregnancy useful? A randomised controlled trial. *Acta Obstet Gynecol Scand.* Vol. 90, No. 2, (Feb 2011), pp. 174-8, ISSN 0001-6349

Odeh, M; Tendler, R; Sosnovsky, K; Kais, M; Ophir, E; & Bornstein, J. (2010). The effect of parity and gravidity on the outcome of medical termination of pregnancy. *Isr Med Assoc J.* Vol. 12, No. 10, (Oct 2010), pp. 606-8, ISSN 1565-1088

Parveen, J; Khateeb, ZA; Mufti, SM; Shah, MA; Tandon, VR; Hakak, S; Singh, Z; Yasmeen, S; Mir, SA; Tabasum, R; & Jan, N. (2011). Comparison of sublingual, vaginal, and oral misoprostol in cervical ripening for first trimester abortion. *Indian J Pharmacol.* Vol. 43, No. 2, (Apr 2011), pp. 172-5, ISSN 0253-7613

Patel, A; Talmont, E; Morfesis, J; Pelta, M; Gatter, M; Momtaz, MR; Piotrowski, H; & Cullins, V. (2006). Adequacy and safety of buccal misoprostol for cervical preparation prior to termination of second-trimester pregnancy. *Contraception.* Vol. 73, No. 4, (Apr 2006), pp. 420-30, ISSN 0010-7824

Perriera,LK; Reeves, MF; Chen, BA; Hohmann, HL; Hayes, J; & Creinin, MD. (2010). Feasibility of telephone follow-up after medical abortion. *Contraception.* Vol. 81, No. 2, (Feb 2010), pp. 143-9, ISSN 0010-7824

Potts, M; Diggory, P; & Peel J (1997). *Abortion.* Cambridge University Press, ISBN, Cambridge, UK Prasad, S; Kumar, A; & Divya, A. (2009). Early termination of pregnancy by single-dose 800 microg misoprostol compared with surgical evacuation. *Fertil Steril.* Vol. 91, No. 1, (Jan 2009), pp. 28-31, ISSN 0015-0282

Pridmore, BR; & Chambers, DG. (1999). Uterine perforation during abortion: a review of diagnosis, management and prevention. *Aust N Z J Obstet Gynaecol.* Vol. 39, No. 3, (Aug 1999), pp.349-353, ISSN 0004-8666

Rasch V. (2011) Unsafe abortion and postabortion care – an overview. *Acta Obstet Gynecol Scand.* Vol. 90, No. 7, (Jul 2011), pp.692-700, ISSN 0001-6349

Rehan, N. (2011). Cost of treatment of unsafe abortion in public hospitals. *J Pak Med Assoc.* Vol. 61, No. 12, (Feb 2011), pp.169-72, ISSN 0030-9982

Rosenfield, A. (1994). Abortion and women's reproductive health. *Int J Gynaecol Obstet.* Vol. 46, No. 2, (Aug 1994), pp.173-179, ISSN 0020-7292

Salakos, N; Iavazzo, C; Bakalianou, K; Gregoriou, O; Poltoglou, G; Kalmantis, K; & Botsis, D. (2008). Misoprostol use as a method of medical abortion. *Clin Exp Obstet Gynecol.* Vol. 35, No. 2, (2008), pp.130-2, ISSN 0390-6663

Sedgh, G; Henshaw, SK; Singh, S; Ahman, E; & Shah, IH. (2007) Induced abortion: estimated rates and trends world wide. *Lancet.* Vol. 370, No. 9595, (Oct 13 2007), pp.1338-45, ISSN 0140-6736

Shah, I; & Ahman, E. (2010). Unsafe abortion in 2008: global and regional levels and trends. *Reprod Health Matters.* Vol. 18, No. 36, (Nov 2010), pp.90-101, ISSN 0968-8080

Shannon, CS; Winikoff , B; Hausknecht, R; Schaff, E; Blumenthal, PD; Oyer, D; Sankey, H; Wolff, J; & Goldberg, R.(2005). Multicenter trial of a simplified mifepristone medical abortion regimen. *Obstet Gynecol.* Vol. 105, No. 2, (Feb 2005), pp.345-351, ISSN 0029-7844

Shaw, A. (2011) 'They say Islam has a solution for everything, so why are there no guidelines for this?' Ethical dilemmas associated with the births and deaths of infants with fatal abnormalities from a small sample of Pakistani Muslim couples in Britain. *Bioethics.* 2011 Jun 7. Epub ahead of print. ISSN 0269-9702

Singh, S; Sedgh, G; Hussain, R (2010). Unintended pregnancy: worldwide levels, trend, and outcomes. *Stud Fam Plann.* Vol. 41, No. 4. (Dec 2010), pp.241-50, ISSN 0039-3665

Song, J. (2000). Use of misoprostol in obstetrics and gynecology. *Obstet & Gynecol Survey.* Vol. 55, No. 8, (Aug 200), pp.503-510, ISSN 0029-7828

Srinil, S. (2011) Factors associated with severe complications in unsafe abortion. *J Med Assoc Thai.* Vol. 94, No. 4, (Apr 2011), pp.408-14, ISSN 0125-2208

Tang OS; Gemzell-Danielsson, K; & Ho, PC. (2007). Misoprostol: pharmacokinetic profiles, effects on the uterus and side effects. *Int J Gynaecol & Obstet.* Vol. 99, No. Suppl 2, (Dec 2007), pp.S160-7, ISSN 0020-7292

Tang, OS; Schweer, H; Lee, SW; & Ho PC. (2009). Pharmacokinetics of repeated doses of misoprostol. *Hum Reprod.* Vol. 24, No. 8, (Aug 2009), pp.1862-9, ISSN 0268-1161

Tang, OS; Schweer,H; Seyberth, HW; Lee, SW; & Ho PC. (2002). Pharmacokinetics of different routes of misoprostol. *HumReprod.* Vol. 17, No. 2, (Feb 2002), pp.332-6, ISSN 0268-1161

Warriner, I; Wang, D; Huong, N; Thapa, K; Tamang, A; Shah, I; Baird, DT; & Meirik, O. (2011). Can midlevel health-care providers administer early medical abortion as safely and effectively as doctors? A randomised controlled equivalence trial in Nepal. *Lancet.* Vol. 377, No. 9772, (Apr 2 2011), pp.1155-61, ISSN 0140-6736

Zhou, C; Wang, XL; Zhou, XD; Hesketh, T. (2011). Son preference and sex-selective abortion in China: informing policy options. *Int J Public Health.* 2011 Jun 17. Epub ahead of print. ISSN 1661-8556

8

Renal Function and Urine Production in the Compromised Fetus

Mats Fagerquist

North Elfsborg County Hospital, Trollhattan
Sweden

1. Introduction

Fetal urine production begins in the first trimester. Autopsy findings of filled urinary bladders in human fetuses have been reported from 11 gestational weeks (Abramovich, 1968). In 1970, the first report on ultrasound investigations of the fetal urinary bladder was published (Garrett et al., 1970). Three years later, a method for estimating fetal urine production was introduced (Campbell et al., 1973).

In this paper, a short summary of amniotic fluid turnover is presented. Moreover, fetal renal development, artery flow velocity and urine production in normal and compromised fetuses are dealt with. The gradual development of the 2D ultrasound technique for estimating of the fetal urine production rate (HFUPR) is described. In addition, some confounding factors are mentioned. Finally, two important clinical questions, which must be taken into consideration when utilising the HFUPR for fetal surveillance, are identified.

2. Amniotic fluid

The volume of amniotic fluid increases during pregnancy (Queenan et al., 1972). In general, the secretion of liquid by the kidneys and from the fetal lungs and oro-nasal cavity is balanced by the removal of equal amounts of liquid (Flack et al., 1995). The main clearance pathway is the swallowing of fluid by the fetus. Additionally, albeit to a lesser degree, fluid passes from the amniotic lumen via the surfaces of the placenta and umbilical cord into the fetal blood circulation (the intramembranous pathway) and into the mother's circulation (the transmembranous pathway) via the uterine wall through the surface of the amniotic sac outside the placental border.

2.1 Abnormal amounts of amniotic fluid

Oligohydramnios (reduced volume < 300 mL) is found in 3-5% (Hansmann, 1985; Volante et al., 2004). Rupture of the membranes is the most common cause of oligohydramnios. A reduction in amniotic fluid volume is of particular concern when it occurs in conjunction with structural fetal anomalies, fetal growth restriction, kidney abnormalities, postdate pregnancies and maternal disease. In these high-risk conditions, it is associated with a poor perinatal outcome (Camanni et al., 2009; Hill et al., 1983). Early onset of oligohydramnios adversely affects fetal lung development, resulting in pulmonary hypoplasia, which might lead to death from severe respiratory insufficiency (Nicolini et al., 1989). However, numerous factors complicate the ultrasonographic diagnosis of oligohydramnios. They include the lack of a complete and detailed understanding of the physiology of the dynamics of oligohydramnios. For example, in 40%, the oligohydramnios occurs without any high-risk conditions and the current available data support the expectant non-interventional management of these cases complicated by isolated oligohydramnios (Sherer, 2002).

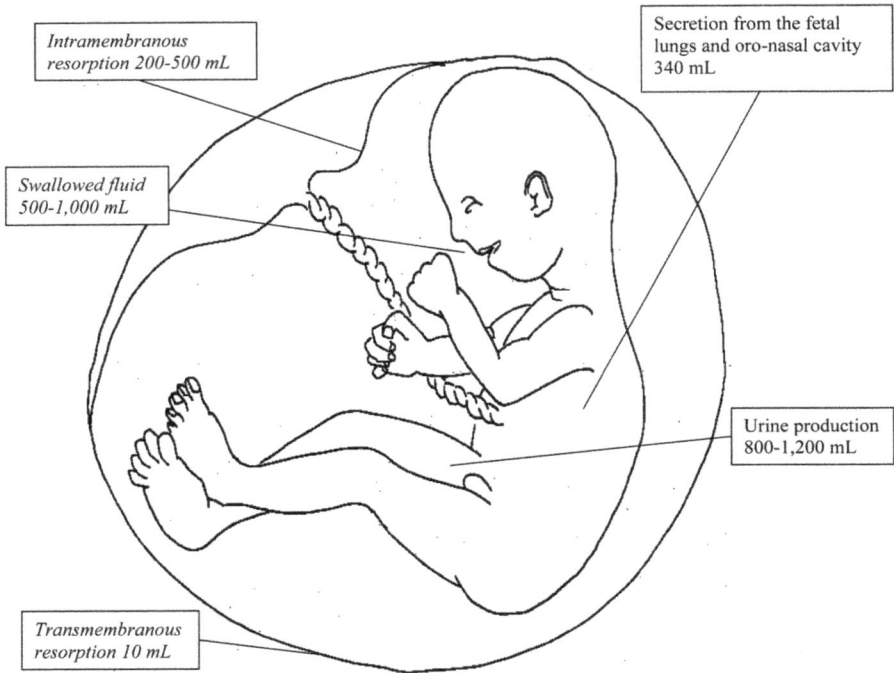

Data: Gilbert WM och Brace RA. Amniotic fluid volume and normal flows to and from the amniotic cavity. Semin Perinatol. 1993; 17: 150-157

Fig. 1. The amniotic fluid turnover at term. Half the secreted liquid from the fetal lungs and oro-nasal cavity reaches the amniotic sack and the other half is swallowed. The clearance pathways are denoted in italics.

Polyhydramnios (increased volume > 2,000 mL) is found in 1-3% (Volante et al., 2004). The underlying cause of excessive amniotic fluid volume is obvious in some clinical conditions in some clinical conditions and in cases of an minor an minor increase in amniotic fluid volume, the perinatal outcome is good. However, maternal kidney disease, diabetes type 2 and fetal conditions, such as chromosomal abnormalities, most commonly trisomy 21, followed by trisomy 18 and trisomy 13, might be causes (Hill et al., 1987). Moreover, polyhydramnios can be the result of oesophageal atresia and defects in the fetal CNS (Barkin et al., 1987; Kimble et al., 1998).

In cases with abnormal amniotic fluid volume, prenatal ultrasonography has been recommended for the evaluation of fetal anatomy and growth, swallowing patterns, blood flow velocity in different vessels and repeated estimation of the amount of fluid.

3. Fetal urine production

During the filling phase, the increasing volume of the urinary bladder can be observed, documented and assessed by ultrasound scans.

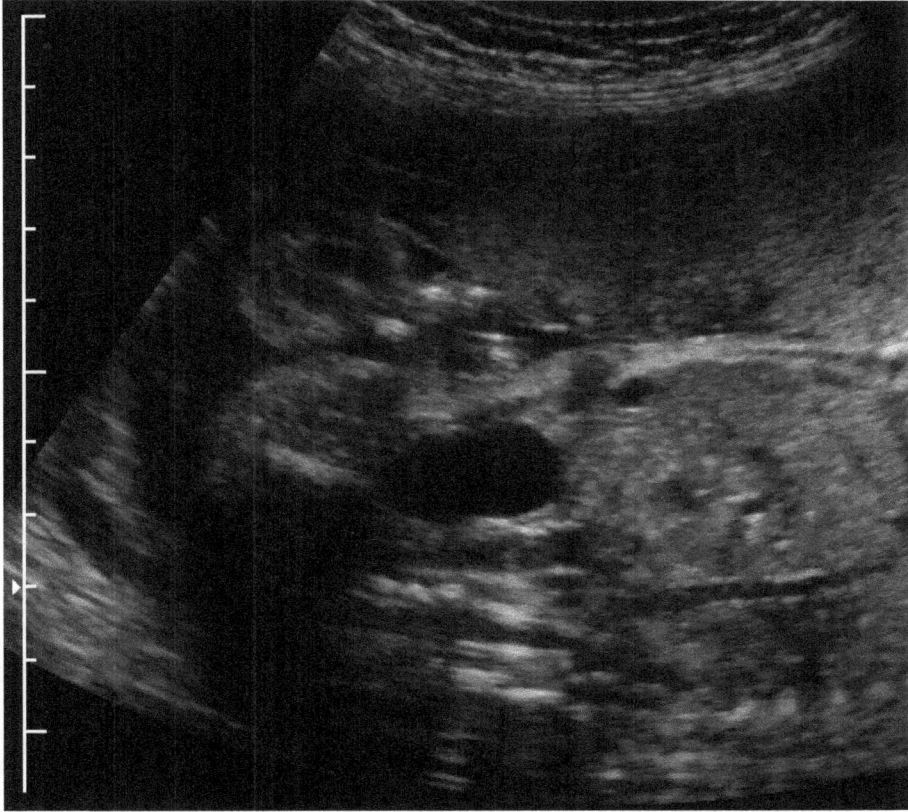

Fig. 2. This figure shows an appropriate longitudinal bladder image. The 2D ultrasound image on the ultrasound screen was documented on a CD and the volume was calculated in a computer.

The Hourly Fetal Urine Production Rate (HFUPR) can be estimated by regression analysis of calculated bladder volumes documented at different time points within one filling phase (Campbell et al., 1973; Fagerquist et al., 2001; Groome et al., 1991; Nicolaides et al., 1990; Rabinowitz et al., 1989; van Otterlo et al., 1977; Wladimiroff and Campbell, 1974), or by the difference between the maximum and minimum volumes divided by the time interval (Deutinger et al., 1987; Shin et al., 1987; Takeuchi et al., 1994).

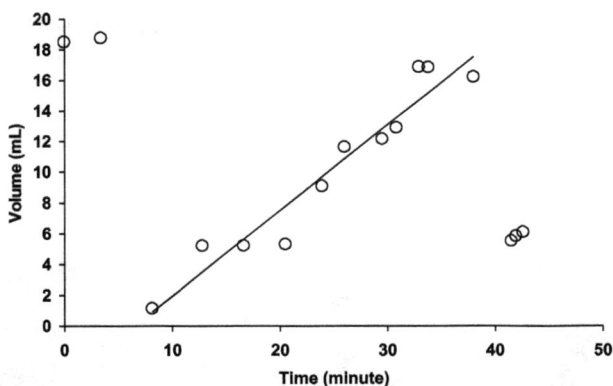

Fig. 3. The Hourly Fetal Urine Production Rate (HFUPR) estimation was based on the increase in bladder volume during a filling phase and extrapolated to a time span of one hour.

The filling and emptying dynamics of the fetal urinary bladder have been investigated in detail. The mean time for the bladder-filling phase was 25 minutes (range 7-43 minutes) and it was not significantly influenced by gestational age (Rabinowitz et al., 1989).

Gestational age (weeks)	Maximum volumes (mL)	HFUPR (mL/hour)
20	1	5
21	2	6
22	2	7
23	3	8
24	4	9
25	5	10
26	6	11
27	7	13
28	9	14
29	10	16
30	11	18
31	13	20
32	14	22
33	16	25
34	18	27
35	20	30
36	22	33
37	24	37
38	27	41
39	30	46
40	32	51

(Rabinowitz R, Peters MT, Vyas S, Campbell S, Nicolaides KH. Measurement of fetal urine production in normal pregnancy by real-time ultrasonography. Am J Obstet Gynecol 1989;161(5):1264-6)

Table 1. The maximum bladder volumes before emptying and HFUPR at different gestational ages were calculated by the author according to formulas in the reference article.

3.1 Urine production in the intra-uterine growth-restricted fetus

When comparing Intra-Uterine Growth-Restricted (IUGR) fetuses with Appropriate weight for Gestational Age (AGA) fetuses at the same gestational age, the HFUPR was significantly lower for IUGR fetuses (Nicolaides et al., 1990; Takeuchi et al., 1994; van Otterlo et al., 1977; Wladimiroff and Campbell, 1974). However, there were no significant differences when the IUGR fetuses were compared with controls of corresponding body weights but with lower gestational ages (Wladimiroff and Campbell, 1974). It was assumed that the reduced urine production rate for IUGR fetuses reflected renal hypoplasia, due to growth retardation. Although different investigations have presented various normal values, the HFUPR in IUGR fetuses compared with fetuses of normal size (AGA) has generally been reported to be lower (Nicolaides et al., 1990; Takeuchi et al., 1994; van Otterlo et al., 1977).

4. Fetal kidneys

In a human 2D ultrasound study comprising IUGR and AGA fetuses, the volume of fetal kidneys, as well as the urine production rate, was estimated (Deutinger et al., 1987). In IUGR fetuses, both the volume of the kidneys and the HFUPR were significantly reduced when compared with the AGA fetuses. In agreement with this study, the growth of fetal kidneys was significantly slower in Small for Gestational Age (SGA) vs. AGA fetuses when it came to the anterio-posterior diameter and transverse circumference of the kidneys (Konje et al., 1997). This divergence was most marked after 26 weeks of gestation.

The fetal kidneys gradually increase in volume with gestational age (Hansmann, 1985). Renal weight as an autopsy finding is, however, often compromised and associated with a coefficient of variation as large as 50%, due to oedema and passive venous engorgement. Renal functional capacity depends on the number of nephrons, but no known relationship exists between renal weight and the number of glomeruli (Hinchliffe et al., 1991). For many years, estimates of glomerular numbers have therefore been derived using a variety of methods (Bendtsen and Nyengaard, 1989). Unfortunately, these methods have been shown to have some degrees of bias. However, a new stereological dissector technique permits the direct, unbiased estimation of glomerular numbers (Hinchliffe et al., 1992). This new dissector method was used to estimate the number of nephrons in fetuses. The number was 15,000 per kidney in human fetuses at 15 gestational weeks and between 740,000 and 1,060,000 at term.

The total number of nephrons was estimated in a comparative investigation of six IUGR stillbirths of known gestational age with controls comprising eleven stillbirths with a birth weight greater than the 10th percentile (prenatal period) and eight liveborn IUGR infants, who died within a year of birth, with a control group of seven appropriately grown infants who also died within a year of birth (postnatal period). The number of nephrons for five of the six IUGR stillborn children and all the growth-retarded children who died within one year was significantly reduced compared with the controls (Hinchliffe et al., 1992). Moreover, in animal models, growth restriction has been associated with a reduced number of nephrons (Bauer et al., 2002; Bauer et al., 2003). It has been suggested that the mechanism underlying the reduced number of nephrons in IUGR fetuses is increased apoptosis due to changes in the levels of apoptosis-related proteins (Pham et al., 2003).

4.1 Renal artery flow velocity and urine production in fetuses with hypoxemia

The HFUPR was determined by 2D ultrasound immediately before cordocentesis for blood gas analysis in 27 Small for Gestational Age (SGA) and 101 AGA fetuses (Nicolaides et al., 1990). The HFUPR was reduced in the group of SGA fetuses in comparison with AGA fetuses. Furthermore, the reduction in urine production for the SGA fetuses was correlated with the degree of fetal hypoxemia, while the degree of fetal hypoxemia did not correlate with the degree of fetal smallness.

Several studies demonstrate associations between increased impedance in the fetal renal arteries and factors suggestive of compromised fetal conditions and, in some studies, also reduced urine production rates (Mikovic et al., 2003; Miura, 1991; Stigter et al., 2001; Vyas et al., 1989). In one study, the renal artery flow-velocity wave forms were examined in normal and hypoxemic human fetuses (Vyas et al., 1989). The Pulsatility Index (PI), which is peak systolic velocity minus end diastolic velocity over mean velocity, was higher in SGA than in AGA fetuses. Furthermore, using cordocentesis in the SGA fetuses, a significant, direct correlation was found between blood oxygen deficit and increased renal artery PI (Vyas et al., 1989). Moreover, in a study of 35 IUGR fetuses, the PI in the fetal renal arteries was significantly increased (Mikovic et al., 2003). In studies of fetal urine production, it was demonstrated that the PI in the renal artery was higher in IUGR than in AGA fetuses and that it displayed a negative correlation with the urine production rate and the amniotic fluid volume (Miura, 1991). In spite of varying results regarding the PI in fetal renal arteries (Silver et al., 2003; Stigter et al., 2001), the data suggest that, in fetal hypoxemia, there is a redistribution of blood flow, with a decrease in renal blood perfusion and a decrease in HFUPR. These findings may be important, as it would be of great clinical interest to detect whether or not a particular fetus with growth restriction is further compromised.

5. Confounding factors

A highly significant diurnal rhythm was observed in an on-line, computerised study of sheep (Brace and Moore, 1991). In that study, the urine flow rate was measured continuously over a period of days. In 8/9 animals, the peak flow rate occurred at around 9 pm, while it occurred at 9.30 am in the remaining sheep fetus. The maximum urine flow was $28 \pm 5\%$ above the 24-hour mean. Although this significant diurnal variation was demonstrated in an animal model, it is important not to disregard a possible diurnal variation in human fetal urine production as well.

The urine production rate was estimated two hours before and two hours after maternal breakfast in 25 AGA and 15 IUGR fetuses. After breakfast, the HFUPR increased in AGA fetuses but did not change in IUGR fetuses (Yasuhi et al., 1996). The PI of the fetal renal artery was significantly reduced after maternal food ingestion in uncomplicated pregnancies (Yasuhi et al., 1997). To our knowledge, no conflicting reports have been published and, to avoid the confounding variation due to diurnal variation and maternal meal ingestion, it is recommended that the estimation of fetal urine production should be performed under standardised conditions. Also, maternal water ingestion might influence the fetal urine production rate (Flack et al., 1995; Oosterhof et al., 2000).

6. Methods for estimating the volume of the fetal urinary bladder

Calculated bladder volumes cannot be validated in living human fetuses, as the true fetal urinary bladder volumes are not known. The reliability of the estimated bladder dimensions, on the other hand, has been evaluated using the 2D ultrasound technique (Fagerquist et al., 2001; Fagerquist et al., 2003; Fagerquist et al., 2002). The calculation of the measurement error was based on the variability in repeated estimations of identical bladder volumes. Standard deviation (SD) was used because the variation was normally distributed. Furthermore, there was a linear relationship between bladder volume and the measurement error, which has been thoroughly documented in three previous studies (Fagerquist et al., 2001; Fagerquist et al., 2003; Fagerquist et al., 2002). This is a prerequisite for using a linear regression function (Skrepnek, 2005).

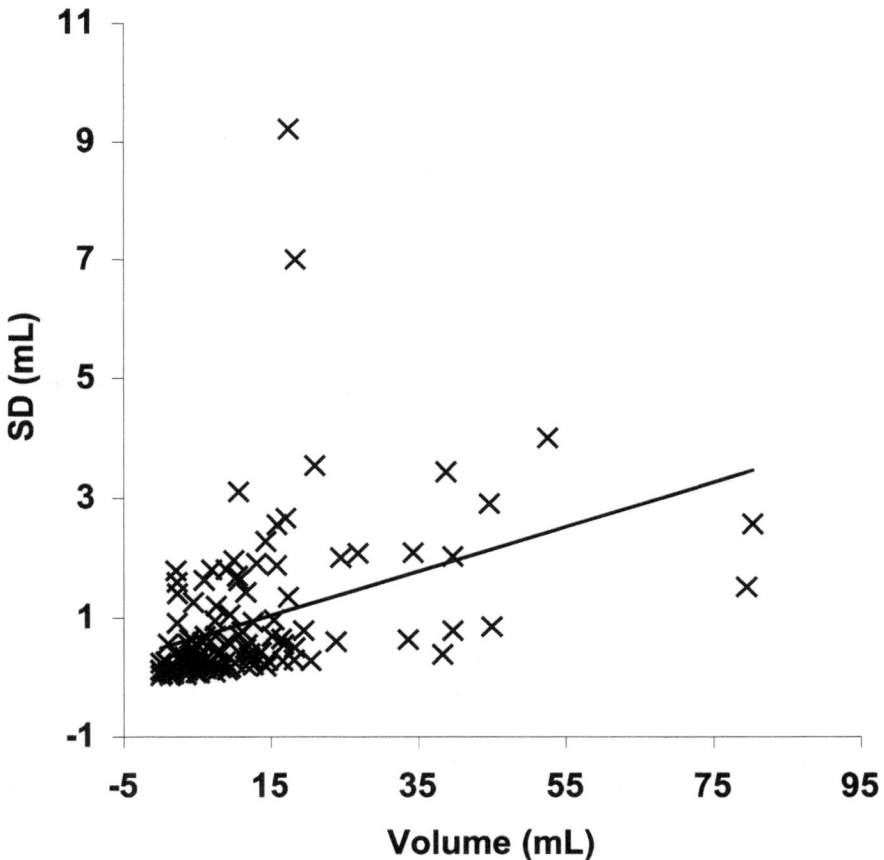

Fig. 4. The SD was calculated when estimating the bladder volume of 120 fetuses. Different methods were used and this gave rise to 222 relationships between SD and bladder volume. The maximum and minimum bladder volumes were 80.5 mL and 0.1 mL respectively. The distribution of the SDs supports a linear relationship (correlation coefficient 0.36).

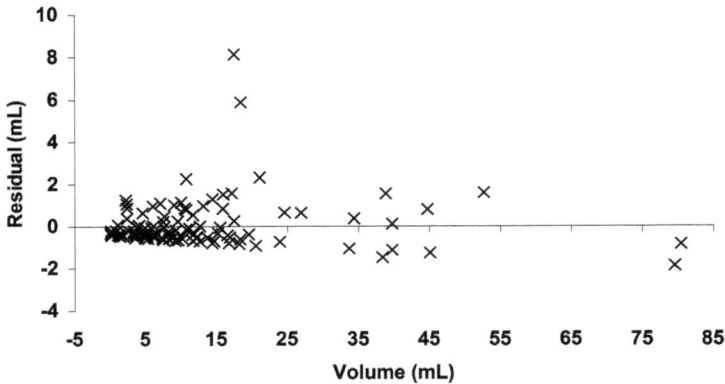

Fig. 5. The distribution of the residuals supports a linear relationship between the SD and bladder volume based on 222 relationships between the SD and bladder volume. The maximum and minimum of the residuals were 8.2 mL and -1.9 mL respectively. The mean was 0.00 mL and the median -0.37 mL.

One important finding was that the fetal urinary bladder can be regarded as a rotational body. This means that an appropriate 2D longitudinal image of the fetal bladder has all the information that is needed for volume calculation. This discovery simplifies the way the volume can be calculated.

The method for estimating the volume of the fetal urinary bladder was gradually developed in order to reduce the SD for volume estimation. In the first paper, the volume measurement errors (SD) when using the conventional method and the ellipsoid formula were analysed (Fagerquist et al., 2001). The SD for the measurement error was 17.3-10.9% for bladder volumes of 5-40 mL.

By introducing the sum-of-cylinders method, the SD was significantly reduced to 8.8-3.5% (p=0.0032) (Fagerquist et al., 2003).

6.1 The 2D technique and the sum-of-cylinders method

Before volume computation, the operator performed an interactive process using the Microsoft-Paint and Microsoft Excel computer programs. The bladder image documented in the Microsoft-Paint format and the data of calibration in an Excel sheet were activated in the MathCad computer program.

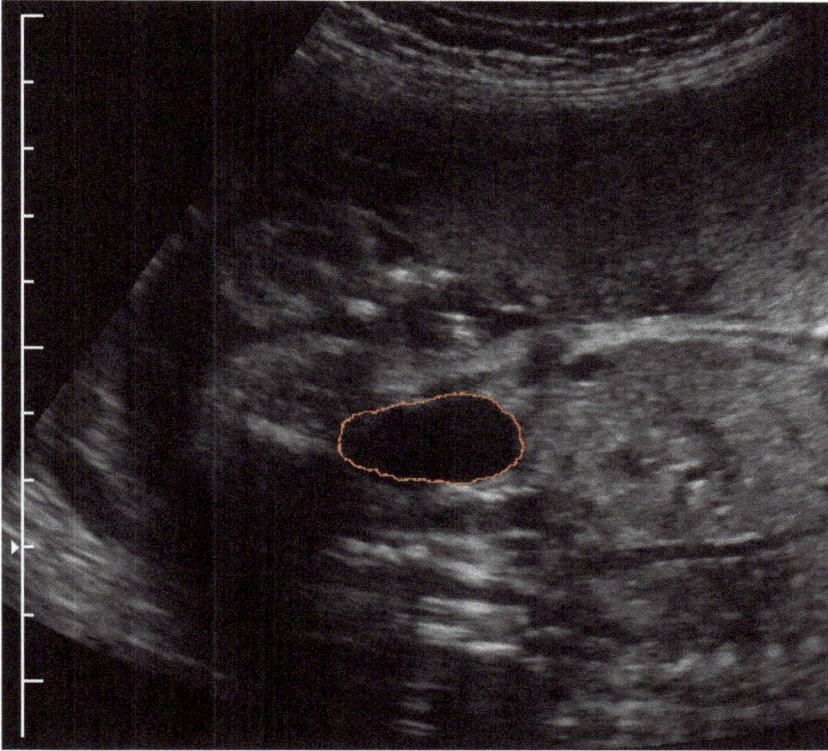

Fig. 6. The image that was going to be used for volume computation according to the sum-of-cylinders method was created in an interactive process. Firstly, the operator traced the bladder borders with a red digital marker on the computer screen using the Microsoft-Paint computer program.

The software determines the co-ordinates for the bladder boundary pixels. The image was analysed by the software and each column of pixels was scanned 1) from left to right on the screen, moving from top of the image to bottom in each column to identify the red marked top pixel of the bladder border and 2) from right to left on the screen, moving from bottom of the image to top in each column to identify the red marked bottom pixel of the bladder border. The length of each vertical strip (from top to bottom red pixels in each column) perpendicular to the long axis was computed. The length of each strip was regarded as the diameter of a cylinder, one pixel high. The total bladder volume was calculated by adding all the cylinders.

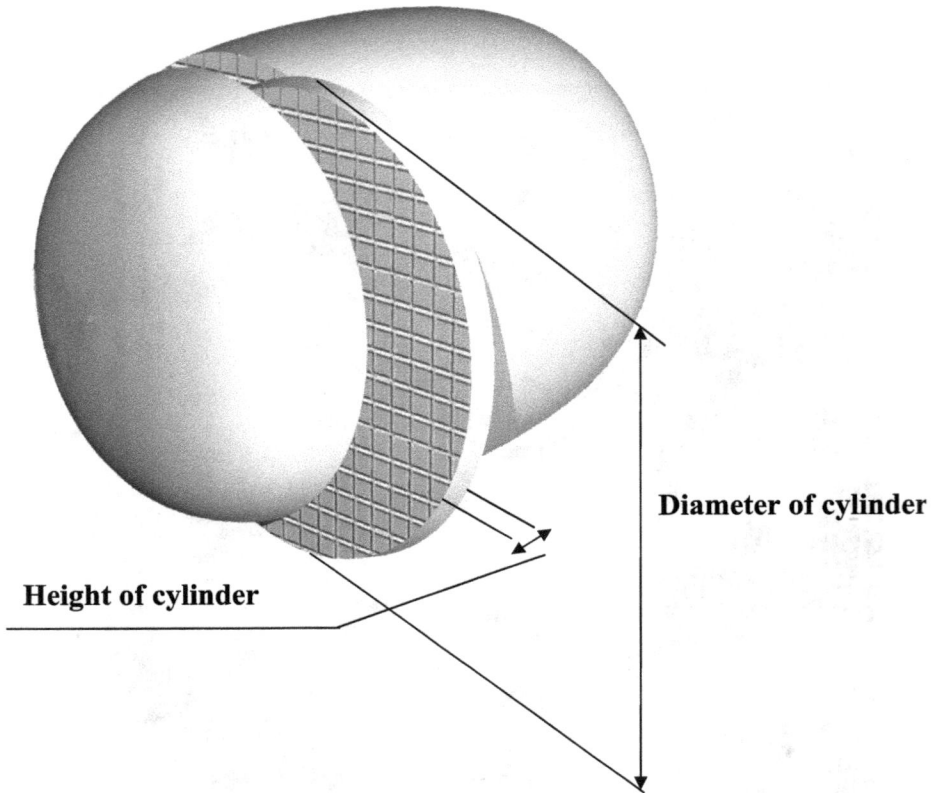

Fig. 7. Using the MathCad computer programs, the vertical distances between marked pixels included in the bladder border was estimated. The bladder image was then electronically subdivided in vertical cylinders and the sum of these cylinders with the height of one pixel equals the bladder volume.

6.2 The 3D ultrasound technique

The 3D ultrasound technique and integrated software, such as the "Virtual Organ Computer-aided AnaLysis" system (VOCAL™), are already available for volume estimation and measurements in the in vitro setting and are both reliable and valid (Raine-Fenning et al., 2003). Moreover, this technique has been applied to the fetal urinary bladder (Lee et al., 2007; Touboul et al., 2008). Unfortunately, the 3D technique is prone to the same types of problem encountered in 2D ultrasound imaging, plus others unique to volume acquisition and visualisation (Nelson et al., 2000). When selecting the initial bladder image, the operator can avoid shadows from the fetal pelvis. However, according to the VOCAL system, the subsequent process for volume estimation is automatic and disturbing shadows are not avoided. Furthermore, in this program, only 40 electronic points are available for the contour marking, which is another disadvantage.

On the other hand, when using the 2D ultrasound technique, the operator can avoid disturbing shadows by selecting an appropriate longitudinal bladder image. The bladder is defined by the operator who electronically marks the pixels, which are included in the bladder contour. Typically, this corresponds to 200-300 pixels in the boundary. In this way, the technical limit for optimal precision, one pixel, is reached; this is the smallest unit of display resolution.

7. The measurement error when estimating the HFUPR

When estimating the HFUPR, the measurement error is made when assessing the volume of the bladder, and that SD has been estimated for the 2D technique and the sum-of-cylinders method. There are some other factors that influence the HFUPR measurement error, the magnitude of the HFUPR and the number and time points of bladder image capture. To date, no information relating to the SD for bladder volume estimation by 3D ultrasound, which is a prerequisite for the subsequent analysis of estimation accuracy, is available.

When utilising the HFUPR for fetal surveillance, it is necessary to know whether the estimated HUFPR is pathologically low, i.e. below the 5th percentile point. It is therefore necessary to answer the question: 1) What is the risk of false readings at the 5th percentile point, for example, even though the true HFUPR is at a higher percentile point? Furthermore, it is necessary to answer the question: 2) How much of an observed HFUPR change (for example, during daily controls) can be explained exclusively by measurement error? The implication of the volume measurement error was demonstrated in detail in a publication publication concerning the 2D technique and the sum-of-cylinders method. (Fagerquist et al., 2010).

8. Conclusion

The data suggest that, in fetal hypoxemia, there might be a redistribution of blood flow, with a reduction in both renal perfusion and fetal urine production rate, which can be estimated by ultrasound. These findings may be important, as it would be of great clinical interest to determine whether or not a particular fetus with growth restriction is further compromised. To utilise the HFUPR, for fetal surveillance, a program is available for estimating the risk of false readings at a low percentile point, even though the true HFUPR is at a higher percentile point, and the degree to which an observed HFUPR change can be explained exclusively by measurement error.

9. Acknowledgments

I would like to thank Ingemar Kjellmer, Professor at the Department of Pediatrics, Sahlgrenska University Hospital, Gothenburg, for his enthusiasm and encouragement, Anders Odén, Adjunct Professor of Biostatistics, Chalmers University of Technology, Gothenburg, for his patience, and Ulf Fagerquist, Tech Lic, my brother and friend, who created the computer programs, which gave us the opportunity to approach the true volume of the fetal urinary bladder.

Moreover, I would like to express my sincere thanks to Hans Steyskal, Professor and Mathematics Consultant, Concord, MA, USA, for his advice, and Sture G. Blomberg, MD, PhD, for his valuable criticism and support.

10. References

Abramovich DR. 1968. The volume of amniotic fluid in early pregnancy. J Obstet Gynaecol Br Commonw 75(7):728-731.

Barkin SZ, Pretorius DH, Beckett MK, Manchester DK, Nelson TR, Manco-Johnson ML. 1987. Severe polyhydramnios: incidence of anomalies. AJR Am J Roentgenol 148(1):155-159.

Bauer R, Walter B, Bauer K, Klupsch R, Patt S, Zwiener U. 2002. Intrauterine growth restriction reduces nephron number and renal excretory function in newborn piglets. Acta Physiol Scand 176(2):83-90.

Bauer R, Walter B, Brust P, Fuchtner F, Zwiener U. 2003. Impact of asymmetric intrauterine growth restriction on organ function in newborn piglets. Eur J Obstet Gynecol Reprod Biol 110 Suppl 1:S40-49.

Bendtsen TF, Nyengaard JR. 1989. Unbiased estimation of particle number using sections--an historical perspective with special reference to the stereology of glomeruli. J Microsc 153 (Pt 1):93-102.

Brace RA, Moore TR. 1991. Diurnal rhythms in fetal urine flow, vascular pressures, and heart rate in sheep. Am J Physiol 261(4 Pt 2):R1015-1021.

Camanni D, Zaccara A, Capitanucci ML, Brizzi C, Mobili L, Giorlandino C, Mosiello G, De Gennaro M. 2009. Acute oligohydramnios: antenatal expression of VURD syndrome? Fetal Diagn Ther 26(4):185-188.

Campbell S, Wladimiroff JW, Dewhurst CJ. 1973. The antenatal measurement of fetal urine production. J Obstet Gynaecol Br Commonw 80(8):680-686.

Deutinger J, Bartl W, Pfersmann C, Neumark J, Bernaschek G. 1987. Fetal kidney volume and urine production in cases of fetal growth retardation. J Perinat Med 15(3):307-315.

Fagerquist M, Fagerquist U, Oden A, Blomberg SG. 2001. Fetal urine production and accuracy when estimating fetal urinary bladder volume. Ultrasound Obstet Gynecol 17(2):132-139.

Fagerquist M, Fagerquist U, Oden A, Blomberg SG. 2003. Estimation of fetal urinary bladder volume using the sum-of-cylinders method vs. the ellipsoid formula. Ultrasound Obstet Gynecol 22(1):67-73.

Fagerquist M, Fagerquist U, Steyskal H, Oden A, Blomberg SG. 2002. Accuracy in estimating fetal urinary bladder volume using a modified ultrasound technique. Ultrasound Obstet Gynecol 19(4):371-379.

Fagerquist MA, Fagerquist UO, Oden A, Blomberg SG, Mattsson LA. 2010. Derivations that enable the testing of fetal urine production as a method of fetal surveillance. Arch Gynecol. Obstet. 282(5): 481-6.

Flack NJ, Sepulveda W, Bower S, Fisk NM. 1995. Acute maternal hydration in third-trimester oligohydramnios: effects on amniotic fluid volume, uteroplacental perfusion, and fetal blood flow and urine output. Am J Obstet Gynecol 173(4):1186-1191.

Garrett WJ, Grunwald G, Robinson DE. 1970. Prenatal diagnosis of fetal polycystic kidney by ultrasound. Aust N Z J Obstet Gynaecol 10(1):7-9.

Groome LJ, Owen J, Neely CL, Hauth JC. 1991. Oligohydramnios: antepartum fetal urine production and intrapartum fetal distress. Am J Obstet Gynecol 165(4 Pt 1):1077-1080.

Hansmann M. 1985. Ultrasound Diagnosis in Obstetrics and Gynecology. Springer-Verlag Berlin.

Hill LM, Breckle R, Thomas ML, Fries JK. 1987. Polyhydramnios: ultrasonically detected prevalence and neonatal outcome. Obstet Gynecol 69(1):21-25.

Hill LM, Breckle R, Wolfgram KR, O'Brien PC. 1983. Oligohydramnios: ultrasonically detected incidence and subsequent fetal outcome. Am J Obstet Gynecol 147(4):407-410.

Hinchliffe SA, Lynch MR, Sargent PH, Howard CV, Van Velzen D. 1992. The effect of intrauterine growth retardation on the development of renal nephrons. Br J Obstet Gynaecol 99(4):296-301.

Hinchliffe SA, Sargent PH, Howard CV, Chan YF, van Velzen D. 1991. Human intrauterine renal growth expressed in absolute number of glomeruli assessed by the disector method and Cavalieri principle. Lab Invest 64(6):777-784.

Kimble RM, Harding JE, Kolbe A. 1998. Does gut atresia cause polyhydramnios? Pediatr Surg Int 13(2-3):115-117.

Konje JC, Okaro CI, Bell SC, de Chazal R, Taylor DJ. 1997. A cross-sectional study of changes in fetal renal size with gestation in appropriate- and small-for-gestational-age fetuses. Ultrasound Obstet Gynecol 10(1):22-26.

Lee SM, Park SK, Shim SS, Jun JK, Park JS, Syn HC. 2007. Measurement of fetal urine production by three-dimensional ultrasonography in normal pregnancy. Ultrasound Obstet Gynecol 30(3):281-286.

Mikovic Z, Mandic V, Djukic M, Egic A, Filimonovic D, Cerovic N, Popovac M. 2003. [Longitudinal analysis of arterial Doppler parameters in growth retarded fetuses]. Srp Arh Celok Lek 131(1-2):21-25.

Miura H. 1991. [Evaluation of fetal renal arterial blood flow waveforms with pulsed Doppler flowmetry and the correlation to estimated fetal body weight, fetal urine production rate and amniotic fluid volume]. Nippon Sanka Fujinka Gakkai Zasshi 43(12):1647-1652.

Nelson TR, Pretorius DH, Hull A, Riccabona M, Sklansky MS, James G. 2000. Sources and impact of artifacts on clinical three-dimensional ultrasound imaging. Ultrasound Obstet Gynecol 16(4):374-383.

Nicolaides KH, Peters MT, Vyas S, Rabinowitz R, Rosen DJ, Campbell S. 1990. Relation of rate of urine production to oxygen tension in small-for-gestational-age fetuses. Am J Obstet Gynecol 162(2):387-391.

Nicolini U, Fisk NM, Rodeck CH, Talbert DG, Wigglesworth JS. 1989. Low amniotic pressure in oligohydramnios--is this the cause of pulmonary hypoplasia? Am J Obstet Gynecol 161(5):1098-1101.

Oosterhof H, Haak MC, Aarnoudse JG. 2000. Acute maternal rehydration increases the urine production rate in the near-term human fetus. Am J Obstet Gynecol 183(1):226-229.

Pham TD, MacLennan NK, Chiu CT, Laksana GS, Hsu JL, Lane RH. 2003. Uteroplacental insufficiency increases apoptosis and alters p53 gene methylation in the full-term IUGR rat kidney. Am J Physiol Regul Integr Comp Physiol 285(5):R962-970.

Queenan JT, Thompson W, Whitfield CR, Shah SI. 1972. Amniotic fluid volumes in normal pregnancies. Am J Obstet Gynecol 114(1):34-38.

Rabinowitz R, Peters MT, Vyas S, Campbell S, Nicolaides KH. 1989. Measurement of fetal urine production in normal pregnancy by real-time ultrasonography. Am J Obstet Gynecol 161(5):1264-1266.

Raine-Fenning NJ, Clewes JS, Kendall NR, Bunkheila AK, Campbell BK, Johnson IR. 2003. The interobserver reliability and validity of volume calculation from three-dimensional ultrasound datasets in the in vitro setting. Ultrasound Obstet Gynecol 21(3):283-291.

Sherer DM. 2002. A review of amniotic fluid dynamics and the enigma of isolated oligohydramnios. Am J Perinatol 19(5):253-266.

Shin T, Koyanagi T, Hara K, Kubota S, Nakano H. 1987. Development of urine production and urination in the human fetus assessed by real-time ultrasound. Asia Oceania J Obstet Gynaecol 13(4):473-479.

Silver LE, Decamps PJ, Korst LM, Platt LD, Castro LC. 2003. Intrauterine growth restriction is accompanied by decreased renal volume in the human fetus. Am J Obstet Gynecol 188(5):1320-1325.

Skrepnek GH. 2005. Regression Methods in the Empiric Analysis of Health Care Data. J Manag Care Pharm 11(3):240-251.

Stigter RH, Mulder EJ, Bruinse HW, Visser GH. 2001. Doppler studies on the fetal renal artery in the severely growth-restricted fetus. Ultrasound Obstet Gynecol 18(2):141-145.

Takeuchi H, Koyanagi T, Yoshizato T, Takashima T, Satoh S, Nakano H. 1994. Fetal urine production at different gestational ages: correlation to various compromised fetuses in utero. Early Hum Dev 40(1):1-11.

Touboul C, Boulvain M, Picone O, Levaillant JM, Frydman R, Senat MV. 2008. Normal fetal urine production rate estimated with 3-dimensional ultrasonography using the rotational technique (virtual organ computer-aided analysis). Am J Obstet Gynecol.

van Otterlo LC, Wladimiroff JW, Wallenburg HC. 1977. Relationship between fetal urine production and amniotic fluid volume in normal pregnancy and pregnancy complicated by diabetes. Br J Obstet Gynaecol 84(3):205-209.

Wladimiroff JW, Campbell S. 1974. Fetal urine-production rates in normal and complicated pregnancy. Lancet 1(7849):151-154.

Volante E, Gramellini D, Moretti S, Kaihura C, Bevilacqua G. 2004. Alteration of the amniotic fluid and neonatal outcome. Acta Biomed Ateneo Parmense 75 Suppl 1:71-75.

Vyas S, Nicolaides KH, Campbell S. 1989. Renal artery flow-velocity waveforms in normal and hypoxemic fetuses. Am J Obstet Gynecol 161(1):168-172.

Yasuhi I, Hirai M, Ishimaru T, Yamabe T. 1996. Change in fetal urine production rate in growth-restricted fetuses after maternal meal ingestion. Obstet Gynecol 88(5):833-837.

Yasuhi I, Hirai M, Oka S, Nakajima H, Ishimaru T. 1997. Effect of maternal meal ingestion on fetal renal artery resistance. Obstet Gynecol 90(3):340-343.

9

Recent Insights into the Role of the Insulin-Like Growth Factor Axis in Preeclampsia

Dimitra Kappou[1], Nikos Vrachnis[2] and Stavros Sifakis[1]
[1]Department of Obstetrics-Gynecology, University Hospital of Heraklion, Crete,
[2]2nd Department of Obstetrics & Gynecology, Aretaieion Hospital,
University of Athens, Athens,
Greece

1. Introduction

Preeclampsia, a hypertensive disorder that complicates approximately 3-5% of first pregnancies and is usually clinically manifested after 20 weeks of gestation, is a major cause of perinatal morbidity and mortality; also, neonates of preeclamptic mothers are prone to preterm birth, low birth weight for gestational age and fetal growth restriction [Goldman-Wohl & Yagel, 2002]. Although the pathophysiologic process of preeclampsia is not fully elucidated, abnormal placentation, shallow endovascular invasion, placental hypoxia, maternal insulin resistance and diffuse endothelial dysfunction seem to be interconnected key events that may precede the clinical onset of the disease by weeks or months [Davison et al., 2004]. In particular, impaired placental perfusion is evident even from the first trimester as it has been documented by the findings of both histologic and Doppler ultrasound findings of the uterine arteries and the altered levels of placental derived biochemical markers as pregnancy-associated plasma protein (PAPP-A) [Poon et al., 2009a; Poon et al., 2009b].

The insulin-like growth factor (IGF) system comprises the IGF peptides (IGF-I, IGF-II), the cellular IGF receptors (type I, type II), and a family of soluble high affinity IGF binding proteins (IGFBP-1 to IGFBP-6) which modulate the bioavailability and activity of the IGFs [Jones & Clemmons, 1994] (Figure 1). Since the discovery of the IGF system before 50 or so years, there is ample evidence for their role in cell proliferation, differentiation and migration and their anti-apoptotic properties as well; thus they are involved in several physiological and pathological processes during prenatal and postnatal life [Forbes & Westwood, 2008]. This review aims to critically evaluate the postulated role of IGF axis components in the pathogenesis of preeclampsia and to discuss the mechanisms through which these effects are mediated.

1.1 The IGF system in pregnancy

During pregnancy, several alterations are noted regarding the expression pattern and function of IGFs. According to a recent longitudinal study, the maternal serum levels of IGF-I remain stable until 20 weeks and then increase whereas IGF-II values do not relatively change throughout gestation [Olausson et al., 2008]. Though in non-pregnant-individuals,

IGF-I is primarily derived from the liver, during gestation its main source is decidua under the stimulatory action of a specific growth hormone placental variant (PGH) that is produced by syncytiotrophoblast and extravillous trophoblast from the 7th or 8th week of gestation and gradually replaces pituitary growth hormone (GH) in the maternal circulation. PGH is implicated in the physiological adjustment to gestation by stimulating gluconeogenesis, lipolysis and anabolism and exercises its effects either indirectly by regulating IGF-I levels or in an autocrine/paracrine manner [Sifakis et al., 2009]. In plasma during postnatal life, most of the IGFs (75%) exist in a 140-k Da heterotrimeric complex consisting of IGFBP-3 and an -85 kDa protein, the acid-labile (ALS); when this complex dissociates, IGFs form smaller, binary complexes with the other IGFBPs while less than 1% of IGFs circulate in free biologically active form [Baxter, 1994].

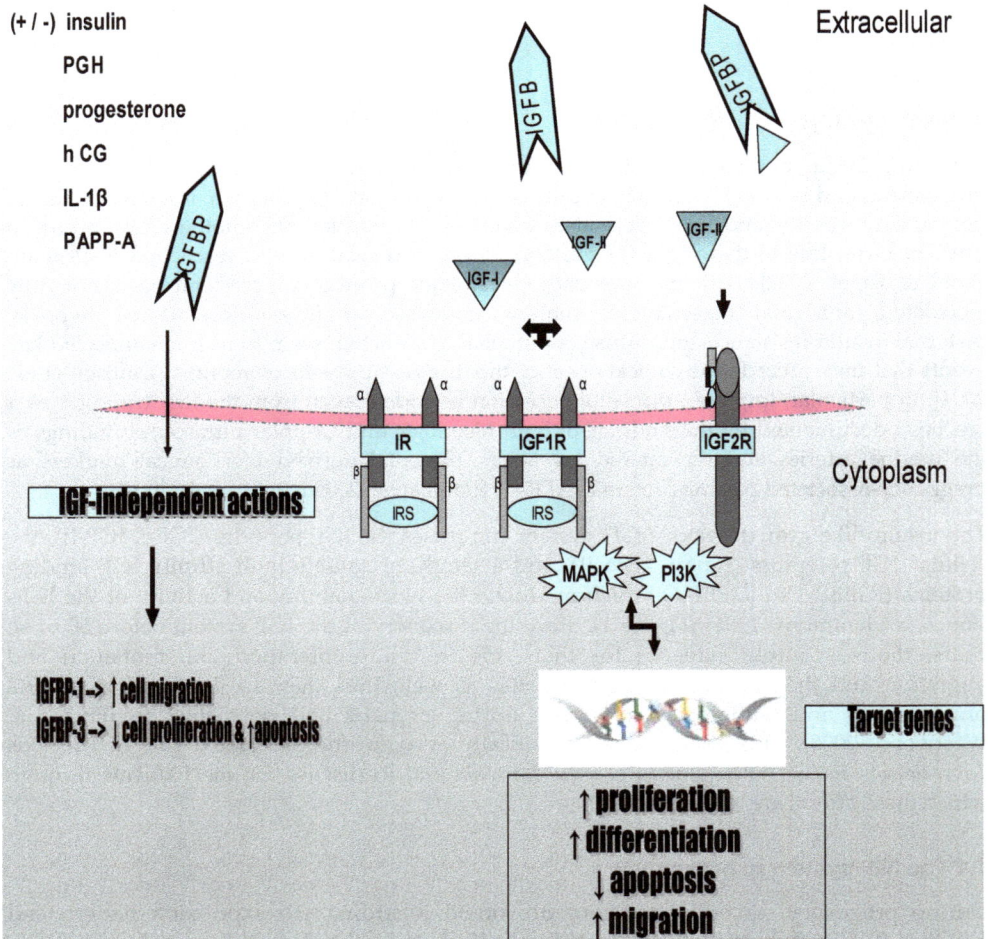

Fig. 1. A simplified model of the components of the IGF axis and their role in placental development

Despite many similarities, IGFBPs have distinctive properties concerning their exact function, their constant hormonal and metabolic regulation, their structural features and the tissue distribution of their expression during the various stages of development. Although in the non-pregnant state, IGFBP-I is mainly produced in the liver, during pregnancy its predominant site of synthesis is the decidualized endometrium [Forbes & Westwood, 2008]. In particular, IGFBP-1 is increasing rapidly in maternal serum so as to be abundant in second- and third-trimester concomitantly with the second wave of trophoblast invasion until 35 weeks and then decrease thereafter till term [Olausson et al., 2008]. IGFBP-3, the most abundant binding protein for IGFs, provides a circulating storage reservoir for IGFs although its affinity may be decreased in gestation period. An endogenous pregnancy-related serum IGFBP-3 proteolytic activity is considered a fundamental mechanism to increase bioactive IGFs [Lewitt et al., 1998]. Conflicting results have been reported regarding IGFBP-3 concentration throughout pregnancy probably as a result of different applied measurement methods; a recent longitudinal study reported that the maternal serum levels of IGFBP-3 remained stable and increased only after 35 weeks of gestation [Olausson et al., 2008]. The exact impact of IGFBPs also depends on the posttranslational modification of the protein (e.g. phosphorylation, glycosylation, altered proteolysis) which is under rapid and dynamic regulation [Forbes & Westwood, 2008]. Specifically, the IGFBP-I gene has multiple regulatory elements in its promoter that synergize or act independently and it is strongly regulated by insulin though IGFBP-3 is primarily determined by GH [Powell et al., 1995]. Besides, IGFBPs, particularly IGFBP-1, -3 and -5, carry out IGF-independent actions including inhibition of cell growth and induction of apoptosis; however their downstream effects need further investigation [Cohen et al., 1993; Jones et al., 1993].

The biological actions of both IGFs are mediated by binding to the two IGF receptors [Monzavi & Cohen, 2002]. The type I IGF receptor (IGF1R), a member of the protein tyrosine kinase receptor superfamily, is the main receptor for signal transduction and cellular action of the IGFs though the type II IGF receptor is identical to the mannose-6-phosphate receptor which shuttles lysosomal enzymes and binds IGF-II and (to a lesser extent) IGF-I [Monzavi & Cohen, 2002]. Another type of receptor which is also expressed in the placenta and binds to IGF-II in fetal tissues with similar affinity to IGF1R is the insulin receptor (IR) that is structurally similar to IGF1R but with a distinct signaling pathway mainly mitogenic [Frasca et al., 1999].

2. IGF system in fetal growth and preeclampsia

2.1 The role of the IGF system in fetal growth

An increasing wealth of literature including clinical and knockout studies in mice points to the crucial role of IGF axis in correct embryonic and placental development and growth. Regarding the role of IGF-I in fetoplacental growth, clinical studies based on the measurements in cord blood from healthy newborns demonstrated that birth weight is positively correlated with IGF levels and therefore, the levels are low and raised in small-for gestational-age (SGA) infants and large-for gestation-age (LGA) infants retrospectively [Giudice et al., 1995; Osorio et al., 1996; Boyne et al., 2003]. These clinical observations were further confirmed by studies using transgenic mice in which the mutation of the gene encoding either IGF-I or IGF-II resulted in restricted growth [Efstratiadis, 1998]. However, other research groups do not lend support to a relationship between total IGF-I and birth weight [Chellakooty et al., 2003]. Surprisingly, increased transcription of IGF-I and IGF-II not essentially associated with a corresponding increase in proteins levels have also been noted in IUGR pregnancies interpreted as a compensatory attempt against the inhibitory effect of either the enhanced level of IGFBPs and/or number of IGF2R or a response to impaired growth [Dalcik et al., 2001; Sheikh et al., 2001]. Alternatively, maternal diabetes seems to result in inverse changes of circulating fetal IGF-I and IGFBP-1 at birth leading to the proposal that a decrease in IGFBP-1 and to a lesser extent an increase in IGFs of cord blood samples may represent an important mechanism that contributes to macrosomia in these pregnancies [Lindsay et al., 2007].

Additionally, extensive data are available on the involvement of the IGFBPs in the abnormal fetal growth and maturity, chiefly highlighting the role of IGFBP-1 & IGFBP-3 in this process. Several research groups support that IGFBP-1 concentrations in amniotic fluid, maternal serum and fetal cord blood are predictive of newborn birth weight in both humans and mice; particularly, a striking inverse correlation between IGFBP-1 levels and fetal size is established although it is not clarified if an elevated level of circulating IGFBP-I is sufficient to cause fetal growth retardation or it depends on IGF-I mediated cell proliferation [Chard 1994; Crossey et al., 2002]. In contrast to IGFBP-1 and IGFBP-2 which correlate inversely with IGF-1 levels and birthweight, IGF-I and IGFBP-3 appear to be regulated in a coordinated manner, and show a significant positive relationship to parameters of fetal growth in both normal and complicated pregnancies despite the narrow reported conflicting results [Fant et al., 1993; Verhaeghe et al., 1993]. However, there are also reports of elevated IGFBP-3 levels in SGA infants and in low-birth weight offspring of mice over expressing the human IGFBP-3 gene [Holmes et al., 1997; Modric et al., 2001]. Also, disrupted IGF receptors' expression can also negatively affect fetal growth as it is demonstrated by a recent study reporting severe fetal growth restriction in two infants with a heterozygous missense mutation in the IGFIR gene [Walenkamp et al., 2006]. On the contrary, IGF-2R is thought to clear the IGF-II from the circulation and this is obviously supported by studies showing that mice lacking the IGF2R have greater birth weights than wild-type littermates [Lau et al., 1994; Efstratiadis, 1998].

2.2 The role of IGF system in preeclampsia

A central feature of preeclampsia is defective placentation expressed as shallow placental invasion limited to the superficial portion of decidua and abnormal remodeling of the endometrial vasculature due to failure of the conversion of the maternal spiral arteries into vessels of low resistance and high capacitance, as it has been supported by histological analysis of preeclamptic tissue specimens [Goldman-Wohl & Yagel, 2002]. Indirect evidence for impaired placental perfusion in pregnancies destined to develop preeclampsia has been provided by Doppler studies of the uterine arteries which showed increased pulsatility index (PI) from the first trimester of pregnancy [Martin et al., 2001; Poon et al., 2009b]. Immunohistochemical studies in human and animal placentas have meticulously demonstrated the placental synthesis of IGF system components; however, it is not accurate to draw conclusions for the development of human placenta based on animal models as the placenta is one of the very few organs that is unique to each species, both anatomically and functionally.

The evolutionary pattern of expression of IGFs, IGFBPs and IGF-1R genes in the developing human placenta and fetal membranes has been described from as early as 6 weeks' gestation to term in order to detect the exact expression cite of each peptide and the potential cite of its action [Han et al., 1996]. Functionally, IGF axis appears to be involved in many aspects of placental development and metabolism both in uncomplicated and preeclamptic pregnancies though the exact signaling pathways have yet to be determined [Hills et al., 2004]. Studies based on cultured human trophoblast cells and cell lines propose that IGFs promote proliferation, regulate trophoblast migration and the differentiation of cytotrophoblasts into syncytiotrophoblasts and extravillous cells, enhance the proliferation and survival of placental fibroblast, exhibit anti-apoptotic effect and mediate nutrient availability at the fetoplacental unit [Lacey et al., 2002; Smith et al., 2002; Miller et al., 2005].

To date, the majority of published studies carried out to describe the alteration profile of the components of the IGF axis in preeclampsia are based on assays in maternal serum specimens. The extracted results do not always reflect the placental expression of the studied factors as the liver is an additional source of circulating factors in maternal serum or other posttranscriptional and/or posttranslational modifications maybe involved as it has been proposed for FGR placentas [Shin et al., 2003]. Regarding the early stages of gestation, when preeclampsia is in a pre-symptomatic stage, the published results are mainly focused on IGFs, IGFBP-1 and IGFBP-3 and are limited compared to the later stages where there is also discrepancy but to a lesser extent. The comparative analysis of these studies is a challenging task for several reasons such as the conflicting results, the differences in the study design, the sampling weeks, the dissimilar distribution of the severity and the subtypes of preeclampsia analyzed, the selection of the study population, the portion of each factor measured (total, bounded or free form) and the limitations of each study. Differentiations in the sensitivity and specificity of assays applied and the adjustment for confounding factors may also account for some of the variations observed across studies.

2.3 IGFs

Several studies have accessed the interesting way in which the trophoblast-derived IGF-II and the decidual-derived IGFBP-I interact in the uterine environment in a paracrine manner and how this modulates trophoblast invasion in preeclampsia [Giudice et al., 1999; Irwin et al., 2001; Shin et al., 2003]. IGF-II m RNA is highly expressed by trophoblast with the greatest concentrations expressed at the invading front even from the 6th week of gestation, indicating a possible role of this peptide in cytotrophoblastic proliferation and the decidualization of the maternal stroma while IGFBP-I is the most plentifully expressed binding protein in the decidualized endometrium under the stimulatory effect of HCG and progesterone [Moy et al., 1996; Fowler et al., 2000]. Interestingly, the mean IGFBP-I m RNA and protein level were significantly elevated in preeclampsia compared with uncomplicated pregnancies in positive correlation with the severity of the disease [Shin et al., 2003]. In line with this observation, Giudice et al indicated the possible involvement of this protein in abnormal placentation and the same research group supported that the decidual derived IGFBP-I may lead to high maternal serum concentrations due to the increased vascular permeability of the leaky capillaries common in preeclampsia [Giudice et al., 1997]. As for the IGF-II, a significant decrease more profound in severe preeclampsia was confirmed both in m RNA and protein expression in preeclamptic placentas, by different research groups [Giudice et al., 1999; Shin et al., 2003]. Published data indicate that IGF-II stimulates proliferation and migration of cytotrophoblasts, regulates nutrient exchange but is not implicated in placental cell differentiation so the decreased levels of this factor may alter the invasive nature of cytotrophoblasts resulting in placental dysfunction [Shin et al., 2003]. On the contrary, Gratton et al. observed increased IGF-II m RNA abundance in the intermediate trophoblast surrounding placental infracts suggesting a role in placental repair or remodeling and decreased IGFBP-1 m RNA levels [Gratton et al., 2002]. Besides, in an in-vivo analysis of term placentas of gestations complicated by acute or chronic hypoxic ischemia, IGF-2 m RNA levels were elevated only in chronic hypoxia in contrast to IGF-I and PGH m RNA levels which did not significantly change, maybe as a part of a local metabolic adjustment [Trollmann et al., 2007].

IGF-II level in maternal serum is less investigated and up to now it seems not to significantly vary between preeclamptic and normotensive women [Giudice et al., 1997; Lewitt et al., 1998]. A possible explanation is that it does not share exactly the same regulation pattern with IGF-I as it is not primarily GH-dependent [Giudice et al., 1997]. On the contrary, there is a remarkable inconsistency among published results about the concentration of IGF-I in pregnancies destined to be preeclamptic. The only prospective cohort study that measured free rather than total IGF-I and IGFBP-1 levels and made adjustment for several confounding factors such as gestational age at blood collection, maternal age, parity, and prepregnancy adiposity, reported lower concentrations of these factors apparent in first trimester [Ning et al., 2004]. The attenuation of IGF-1 synthesis may result from impaired PGH synthesis as a consequence of the compromised placentation observed in preeclampsia [Ning et al., 2004]. Although several cross-sectional and longitudinal studies have found a positive correlation between serum PGH and IGF-1 values in pregnancies with fetoplacental unit disorders, our recent results do not provide support to the upper speculation as lower IGF-I levels but no alteration in PGH levels were observed in 11-13 weeks of gestation in pregnancies subsequently complicated by preeclampsia of either early or late onset [Sifakis et al., 2010; Sifakis et al. 2011a]. To elucidate this matter, it would be of special interest to investigate the range of the IGF-I levels in parallel with the change of PGH production throughout the disease transition from a latent preclinical stage to the clinically manifested preeclampsia.

Given that IGF-I acts positively on insulin sensitivity and the tissue availability of IGF-I is a significant determinant of insulin sensitivity in patients with essential hypertension, it could be presumed that decreased circulating levels of this factor would be responsible, at least in part, for insulin resistance in preeclampsia [Kocyigit et al., 2004]. However, Bartha et al. supported that increased insulin resistance is associated with gestational hypertension rather than preeclampsia and that there is no significant correlation between insulin sensitivity index and serum IGF-I levels [Bartha et al., 2002]. Also, there is no obvious explanation for the findings of other studies which recruited women before the clinical manifestation of the disease and reported that the maternal serum levels of IGF-I were either increased or not significantly altered [Hubinette et al., 2003; Vatten et al., 2008]. Based on a similar prospective approach, an increase in IGF-I from the first to second trimester and not within each trimester was associated with higher risk of preterm preeclampsia possibly interpreted as a compensatory mechanism to preserve fetal growth or/and a possible accelerated proteolysis of IGFBPs [Vatten et al., 2008]. Along with this thesis, a recent study demonstrated elevated second trimester levels of PGH in women, who later developed preeclampsia associated with intrauterine growth restriction leading to greater availability of nutrients for the fetoplacental unit [Papadopoulou et al., 2006]. However, we cannot offer an explanation for the apparent delay from first to second trimester for such a placental response.

Regarding the period that follows the clinical manifestation of preeclampsia, IGF-I levels seem to markedly decrease in preeclamptic subjects, particularly in the severe subtype of this disorder [Halhali et al., 2000; Ingec et al., 2004; Altinkaynak et al., 2003]. Even though it could be the result of the compromised production of placental PGH, relative studies based on a single point-in –time observations in preeclamptic pregnancies complicated further or not by fetal growth restriction are inconsistent and a longitudinal description of the correlation between IGF-I and PGH in different trimesters is lacking [Mittal et al., 2007; Schiessl et al., 2007] In contrast, two different research groups reported no difference between IGF-I values in preeclamptic women and normotensive controls, the one referred to preeclamptic women with late-onset disease and the other recruited women with preeclampsia of all subtypes [Lewitt et al., 1998].

2.4 IGFBPs

2.4.1 IGFBP-1

A lot of controversy exists regarding the role and the precise mechanisms of action of IGFBP-I at the maternal-fetal interface. On the one hand, IGFBP-I may act as a maternal restrain to trophoblast invasion via its inhibitory effect on mitogenic IGFs in decidual microenvironment [Ritvos et al., 1998]. On the other hand, Gleeson et al. doubt these results showing that IGFBP-I potentiates directly the human trophoblast migration by binding of its RGD domain (Arg-Gly-Asp) to the $\alpha5\beta1$ integrin/fibronectin receptor on invading trophoblast leading to activation of mitogen activated protein kinase (MAPK) pathway [Gleeson et al., 2001]. This hypothesis is consistent with the observation that the regulation of $\alpha3$, $\alpha5$, $\beta1$, $\beta4$ integrin subunits (classes of adhesion molecules receptors) in trophoblast cells is altered in preeclamptic pregnancies [Zhou et al., 1993]. In vivo, it is still questionable which pathway of IGFBP-1 action is deregulated resulting in net suppression on trophoblast invasion.

A possible source of this inconsistency is the altered post-translational modification of IGFBP-1 in pregnant women [Forbes & Westwood, 2008]. In the circulation of non-pregnant women, IGFBP-1 exists only in its phosphorylated state (p-IGFBP-1) with high affinity for IGFs whereas during pregnancy, IGFBP-1 is extensively dephosphorylated to non-phosphorylated and intermediately phosphorylated isoforms (np-IGFBP-I) with a 6-fold lesser binding affinity for IGF-I and similar affinity for IGF-II [Westwood et al., 1994]. The functional significance of this modification is highlighted by the finding that np-IGFBP-1 enhanced the metabolic actions of IGF-I in nutrient transport in contrast to the inhibitory phosphorylated isoform [Yu et al., 1998]. A more complete interpretation of the data requires consideration of the distribution of the phosphoisoforms of IGFBP-I accompanying preeclampsia in each trimester of pregnancy.

De Groot et al. were the first who evaluated the midtrimester plasma level of IGFBP-1 in pregnancies destined to develop mild/moderate preeclampsia and observed lower circulating levels possibly due to the defective placentation that could affect the vascular deportation of this protein and/or its reduced hepatic synthesis [De Groot et al., 1996]. A more recent study underlined the fact that in a subgroup of women with coexisted White A diabetes the concentration of the protein was especially low even before the clinical manifestation of the two diseases [Hietala et al., 2000]. This notification implies that hyperinsulinemia, an important factor in the pathogenesis of preeclampsia, may additionally affect the level of serum IGFBP-1 although their association is still enigmatic.

In non pregnant women, IGFBP-I is negatively regulated by insulin and prevents glucose uptake by muscle and hepatic cells, possibly through IGF-dependent pathways [Holly et al., 1998]. Therefore decreased IGFBP-I have been related to various states of hyperinsulinemia including women with hypertension and insulin resistance. The interconnection of these two distinct entities is underlined by a series of well established clinical observations as that pregnancy-induced hypertension is more common in women with impaired glucose tolerance, pregnant women with diabetes have a higher incidence of preeclampsia and hyperinsulinemia can be detected in women several years after their first preeclamptic pregnancy [Suhonen & Teramo, 1993]. Surprisingly, other investigators have reported normal insulin response to intravenous glucose tolerance tests in preeclamptic women or even that these women were more sensitive to insulin [Solomon et al., 1994]. It is theorized that the negative relationship between insulin and IGFBP-1, typical of non-pregnant state, persists throughout normal pregnancy but seems to be lost in the early stages of pregnancies destined to become preeclamptic and either insulin starts to have a stimulatory effect on IGFBP-1 or both are regulated by another factor associated to preeclampsia such as hypoxia [Anim-Nyame et al., 2003]. However, in a longitudinal study, the circulating IGFBP-1 concentrations were found to be lower in serial samples obtained from women destined to develop preeclampsia indicating that IGFBP-1 is unlikely to act via its IGF-mediated effect and may actually promote trophoblast function acting through a signaling IGF-independent pathway [Anim-Nyame et al., 2000]. Concurrently, relatively low concentrations of IGFBP-1 both in the first and second trimesters were related to higher risk of term and in a lesser extent for preterm preeclampsia as it is noted in non-pregnant women with a higher prevalence of metabolic syndrome [Vatten et al., 2008]. This differentiation may further reflect two distinct clinical entities, as preterm preeclampsia is a clinically more severe form often accompanied by fetal restricted growth due to the placental disease in contrast to term preeclampsia in which placental perfusion and fetal growth are often normal and the main pathophysiological processes resemble those of the metabolic syndrome with an increase in adipose tissue and impaired glucose and lipid metabolism.

In pregnancies with established disease, IGFBP-1 levels are grossly elevated in the majority of the research studies with older studies supporting a positive correlation with severity of the disease and recent studies the opposite [Giudice et al., 1997; Ingec et al., 2004). This fluctuation in serum levels in relation to the clinical onset of preeclampsia has also been reported for other placental proteins, such as PAPP-A. Elevated circulating peptide levels may reflect the increased synthesis of IGFBP-1 from decidual cells which in turn may play a role in the shallow implantation, characteristic of preeclampsia. In another prospective study, IGFBP-I concentration was found augmented at the time of delivery only in preeclampsia complicated further by IUGR demonstrating that this change may simply reflect low birthweight in these cases or alternatively the higher incidence of IUGR in severe preeclampsia [Wang et al., 1996].

2.4.2 Other IGFBPs

In addition to the decidua basalis and parietalis, IGFBP-3, IGFBP-4, and IGFBP-5 are expressed in fetal cells with IGFBP-3 being the most prominent [Han et al., 1996]. Interestingly, the cleavage of IGFBP-3 into fragments during pregnancy except from increasing the availability of IGFs may have additional significance as in the same time these fragments can exert IGF-independent biological activity [Firth & Baxter, 2002]. Concerning the role of IGFBP-3 in preeclampsia, a study designed to detect genes associated to increased apoptosis in preeclamptic placentas showed a strong down regulation pattern leading to lower IGF-mediated anti-apoptotic effect causing placental dysfunction [Han et al., 2006]. In future, the interaction of some IGFBPs with other placental-produced factors should be also investigated. PAPP-A, a useful early marker of preeclampsia, has been identified as protease to IGFBP-3 and -4 so its lower levels observed in preeclampsia might diminish the amount of IGFs being available for cell uptake and growth stimulation [Cowans et al., 2007].

IGFBP-3, the major carrier for IGFs in plasma during pregnancy is the only studied binding protein in maternal serum from preeclamptic pregnancies. The only so far published study that reported no change in IGFBP-3 levels in early stages of gestation is opposite to recent data that demonstrate an increase in IGFBP-3 concentration at 11-13 weeks in term but not in preterm preeclampsia not associated to uterine artery PI which is a known measure of impaired placental perfusion [Sifakis et al., 2011b]. Most likely, this finding could be the result of impaired glucose tolerance and increased insulin resistance as there is in vitro and in vivo evidence for a relationship between circulating IGFBP-3 levels and hyperglycemia and a IGFBP-3 potent insulin-antagonizing capability exerted either via IGF-independent pathways or by decreasing IGF-bioavailability. After the clinical establishment of preeclampsia, there is inconsistency among reported results as both a reduction and no change in its levels have been demonstrated [Altinkaynak et al., 2003; Wang et al., 1996].

3. Conclusion

Overall, it is still uncertain if the deregulation of the tuned balance among IGF system components possesses a crucial role in the pathogenesis of preeclampsia or is just a mere consequence of the disease. From this summary of relevant research, it is not yet plausible to determine the magnitude of possible associations, if any, between varying concentrations of IGFs and IGFBPs in maternal circulation and preeclampsia risk. Hopefully, the quantification of maternal plasma levels of the peptides of the IGF family may utilize as a predictive screening test to select pregnant women at increased risk for developing preeclampsia who may be favored from the administration of aspirin or other antiplatelet therapy or more intense sonographic surveillance, optimally as the only parameter or combined with other known independent indicators of preeclampsia risk. Clearly, much additional research is warranted including longitudinal studies with serial measurements of these factors and molecular clarification of the signaling pathways of each component intending to novel diagnostic interventions and to cast further light on the pathogenesis of preeclampsia as well.

4. References

Altinkaynak K, Aksoy H, Bakan E, Kumtepe Y. Seru IGF-I and IGFBP-3 in healthy pregnancies and patients with preeclampsia. Clin Biochem 2003;36:221-223.

Anim-Nyame N, Hills FA, Sooranna SR, Steer PJ, Johnson MR. A longitudinal study of maternal plasma insulin-like growth factor binding protein-1 concentrations during normal pregnancy and pregnancies complicated by preeclampsia. Hum Reprod 2000;15:2215-2219.

Anim-Nyame N, Hills FA, Sooranna SR, Steer PJ, Johnson MJ. The relationship between insulin and insulin-like growth factor binding protein-1 is modified by preeclampsia. Gynecol Endocrinol 2003;17:471-476.

Bartha JL, Romero-Carmona R, Torrejon-Cardoso R, Comino-Delgado R. Insulin, insulin-like growth factor-1, and insulin resistance in women with pregnancy-induced hypertension. Am J Obstet Gynecol 2002;187:735-740

Baxter RC. Insulin-like growth factor binding proteins in the human circulation: a review. Hormone Research 1994;42:140-44.

Boyne MS, Thame M, Bennett FI, Osmond C, Miell JP, Forrester TE. The relationship among circulating insulin-like growth factor (IGF)-I, IGF-binding proteins-1 and -2, and birth anthropometry: a prospective study. J Clin Endocrinol Metab 2003;88:1687-1691.

Chard T. Insulin-like growth factors and their binding proteins in normal and abnormal human fetal growth. Growth Regul 1994;4:91-100.

Chellakooty M, Vangsgaard K, Larsen T, Scheike T, et al. A longitudinal study of intrauterine growth and the placental growth hormone (GH)-insulin-like growth factor I axis in maternal circulation: association between placental GH and fetal growth. J Clin Endocrinol Metab 2003;89:384-391.

Cohen P, Lamson G, Okajima T, Rosenfold RG. Transfection of the human insulin-like growth factor binding protein-3 gene into Balb/c fibroblasts inhibits cellular growth. Mol Endocrinol 1993;7:380-386.

Cowans NJ, Spencer K. First-trimester ADAM12 and PAPP-A as markers for intrauterine fetal growth restriction through their roles in the insulin-like growth factor system. Prenat Diagn 2007;27:264-271.

Crossey PA, Pillai CC, Miell JP. Altered placental development and intrauterine growth restriction in IGF binding protein-1 transgenic mice. J Clin Invest 2002;110:411- 418.

Dalcik H, Yardimoglu M, Vural B, Dalcik C, Filiz S, Gonca S, Kokturk S, Ceylan S: Expression of insulin-like growth factor in the placenta of intrauterine growth-retarded human fetuses. Acta Histochem 2001;103:195-207.

Davison JM, Homuth V, Jeyabalan A, Conrad KP, et al. New aspects in the pathophysiology of preeclampsia. J Am Soc Nephrol 2004;15:2440-2448.

De Groot CJM, O'Brien TJ and Taylor RN. Biochemical evidence of impaired trophoblastic invasion of decidual stroma in women destined to have preeclampsia. Am J Obstet Gynecol 1996;175:24-29.

Efstratiadis A: Genetics of mouse growth. Int J Dev Biol 1998;42:955-976.

Fant M, Salafia C, Baxter RC, Schwander J, Vogel C, Pezzullo J, Moya F. Circulating levels of IGFs and IGF binding proteins in human cord serum: relationships to intrauterine growth. Regul Pept 1993;48:29-39.

Firth SM, Baxter RC: Cellular actions of the insulin-like growth factor binding proteins. Endocr Rev 2002; 23:824–854.

Forbes K, Westwood M. The IGF axis and placental function. Horm Res 2008;69:129-137.

Fowler DJ, Nicolaides KH, Miell JP. Insulin-like growth factor binding protein -1 (IGFBP-1): a multifactorial role in the human female reproductive tract. Hum Reprod Update 2000;6;495-504.

Frasca F, Pandini G, Scalia P, Sciacca L, Mineo R, Costantino A, Goldfine ID, Belfiore A, Vigneri R: Insulin receptor isoform A, a newly recognized, high-affinity insulinlike growth factor II receptor in fetal and cancer cells. Mol Cell Biol 1999;19:3278–3288.

Gleeson LM, Chakraborty C, McKinnon T, Lala PK. Insulin-like growth factor-binding protein 1 stimulates human trophoblast migration by signaling through alpha 5 beta 1 integrin via mitogen-activated protein kinase pathway. J Clin Endocrinol Metab 2001;86:2484-2493.

Giudice LC, de Zegher F, Gargosky SE, Dsupin BA, de las Fuentes L, Crystal RA, Hintz RL, Rosenfeld RG: Insulin-like growth factors and their binding proteins in the term and preterm human fetus and neonate with normal and extremes of intrauterine growth. J Clin Endocrinol Metab 1995;80:1548–1555.

Giudice LC, Martina NA, Crystal RA, Tazuke S, Druzin M. Insulin-like growth factor binding protein-1 at the maternal-fetal interface and IGF-I, IGF-II and IGFBP-1 in the circulation of women with severe preeclampsia. Am J Obstet Gynecol 1997;176:751-757.

Giudice LC, Irwin JG. Roles of the insulin-like growth factor family in non-pregnant human endometrium and at the decidual: trophoblast interface. Semin Reprod Endocrinol 1999;17:13-21.

Goldman-Wohl D, Yagel S. Regulation of trophoblast invasion: from normal implantation to preeclampsia. Mol Cell Endocrinol 2002;187:233-238.

Gratton RJ, Asano H, Han VKM. The regional expression of insulin-like growth factor II (IGF-II) and insulin-like growth factor binding protein-1 (IGFBP-1) in the placenta of women with preeclampsia. Placenta 2002;23:303-310.

Halhali A, Tovar AR, Torres N, Bourges H, Garabedian M, Larrea F. Preeclampsia is associated with low circulating levels of insulin-like growth factor I and 1,25-dihydroxyvitamin D in maternal and umbilical cord compartments. J Clin Endocrinol Metab 2000;85:1828-1833.

Han VKM, Bassett N, Walton J, Challis JRG. The expression of insulin-like growth factor (IGF) and IGF-binding protein (IGFBP) genes in the human placenta and membranes: evidence for IGF-IGFBP interactions at the feto-maternal interface. J Clin Endocrinol Metab 1996;81:2680-2693

Han JY, Kim YS, Cho GJ, Roh GS, et al. Altered gene expression of caspase-10, death receptro-3 and IGFBP-3 in preeclamptic placentas. Mol. Cells 2006;22:168-174.

Hietala R, Pohja-Nylander P, Rutanen EM and Laatikainen T. Serum insulin-like growth factor binding protein-1 at 16 weeks and subsequent preeclampsia. Obstet Gynecol 2000;95:185-189.

Hills FA, Elder MG, Chard T, Sullivan MH. Regulation of human villous trophoblast by insulin-like growth factors and insulin-like growth factor-binding protein-1. J Endocrinol 2004;183:487-496.

Holly JMP, Biddlecombe RA, Dunger DB et al. Circadian variation of GH- independent IGF-binding protein in diabetes mellitus and its relationship to insulin. A new role for insulin? Clin Endocrinol (Oxf) 1988;29:667-675.

Holmes R, Montemagno R, Jones J, Preece M, Rodeck C, Soothill P: Fetal and maternal plasma insulin-like growth factors and binding proteins in pregnancies with appropriate or retarded fetal growth. Early Hum Dev 1997;49:7-17.

Hubinette A, Lichtenstein P, Brismar K, Vatten L, Jacobsen G, Ekbom A, Cnattingius S. Serum insulin-like growth factors in normal pregnancy and in pregnancies complicated by preeclampsia. Acta Obstet Gynecol Scand 2003;82:1004-1009.

Ingec M, Gursoy HG, Yildiz L, Kumtepe Y, Kadanali S. Serum levels of insulin, IGF-I, and IGFBP-1 in preeclampsia and eclampsia. Int J Gynaecol Obstet 2004;84:214-219.

Irwin JC, Suen LF, Faessen GH, Popovici RM, Giudice LC. Insulin-like growth factor (IGF)-II inhibition of endometrial stroma cell tissue inhibitor of metalloproteinase-3 and IGF-binding protein-1 suggests paracrine interactions at the decidua: trophoblast interface during human implantation. J Clin Endocrionol Metab 2001;86:2060-2064.

Jones JL, Gockerman A, Busby WH, Jr, Wright G, Clemmons DR. Insulin-like growth factor binding protein 1 stimulates cell migration and binds to the alpha 5 beta 1 integrin by means of its Arg-Gly-Asp sequence. Proc Natl Acad Sci USA 1993;90:10553-10557.

Jones JI and Clemmons DR. Insulin-like growth factors and their binding proteins. Endocr Rev 1994;18:1-31.

Kocyigit Y, Bayhan G, Atamer A, Atamer Y. Serm leves of leptin, insulin-like growth factor-I and insulin-like growth factor binding protein-3 in women with pre-eclampsia, and their relationship to insulin resistance. Gynecol Endocrinol 2004;18:341-348.

Lacey H, Haigh T, Westwood M, Aplin JD: Mesenchymally-derived insulin-like growth factor 1 provides a paracrine stimulus for trophoblast migration. BMC Dev Biol 2002;2:5.

Lau MM, Stewart CE, Liu Z, Bhatt H, Rotwein P, Stewart CL: Loss of the imprinted IGF2/cation-independent mannose 6-phosphate receptor results in fetal overgrowth and perinatal lethality. Genes Dev 1994;8:2953-2963.

Lewitt MS, Scott FP, Clarke NM, Wu T, Sinosich MJ, Baxter RC. Regulation of insulin-like growth factor-binding protein-3 ternary complex formation in pregnancy. Journal of Endocrinology 1998;159:265-274.

Lindsay RS, Westgate JA, Beattie J, Pattison NS, Gamble G, Mildenhall LF, Breier BH, Johnstone FD. Inverse changes in fetal insulin-like growth factor (IGF)-1 and IGF binding protein-1 in association with higher birth weight in maternal diabetes. Clin Endocrinol 2007;66:322-328.

Martin AM, Bindra R, Curcio P, Cicero S, Nicolaides KH. Screening for pre-eclampsia and fetal growth restriction by uterine artery Doppler at 11-14 weeks of gestation. Ultrasound Obstet Gynecol 2001;18:583-586.

Miller AG, Aplin JD, Westwood M: Adenovirally mediated expression of insulin-like growth factors enhances the function of first trimester placental fibroblasts. J Clin Endocrinol Metab 2005;90:379-385.

Mittal P, Espinoza J, Hassan S, et al. Placental growth hormone is increased in the maternal and fetal serum of patients with preeclampsia. J Matern Fetal Neonatal Med 2007;20:651-9.

Modric T, Silha JV, Shi Z, Gui Y, Suwanichkul A, Durham SK, Powell DR, Murphy LJ. Phenotypic manifestations of insulin-like growth factor-binding protein-3 overexpression in transgenic mice. Endocrinology 2001;142:1958–1967.

Monzavi R, Cohen P. IGFs and IGFBPs: role in health and disease. Best practice and research clinical endocrinology and metabolism 2002;16:433-447.

Moy E, Kimzey LM, Nelson LM, Blithe DL. Glycoprotein hormone α-subunit functions synergistically with progesterone to stimulate differentiation of cultured human endometrial stromal cells to decidualized cells: a novel role for free subunit in reproduction. Endocrinology 1996;137:1332-1339.

Ning Y, Williams MA, Vadachkoria S, Muy-Rivera M, Frederick IO, Luthy DA. Maternal plasma concentrations of insulin-like growth factor-I and insulin-like growth factor-binding protein-1 in early pregnancy and subsequent risk of preeclampsia. Clinical Biochemistry 2004;37:968-973.

Olausson H, Lof M, Brismar K, Lewitt M, Forsum E, Sohlstrom A. Longitudinal study of the materanl insulin-like growth factor system before, during and after pregnancy in relation to fetal and infant weight. Horm Res 2008;69:99-106.

Osorio M, Torres J, Moya F, Pezzullo J, Salafia C, Baxter R, Schwander J, Fant M: Insulin-like growth factors (IGFs) and IGF binding proteins-1, -2, and -3 in newborn serum: relationships to fetoplacental growth at term. Early Hum Dev 1996; 46: 15–26.

Papadopoulou E, Sifakis S, Giahnakis E, Fragouli Y, Karkavitsas N, Koumantakis E, Kalmanti M. Increased human placental growth hormone at midtrimester pregnancies may be an index of intrauterine growth retardation related to preeclampsia. Growth Horm IGF Res 2006;16:290-296.

Poon LCY, Staboulidou I, Maiz N, Plascencia W, Nicolaides KH. Hypertesive disorders in pregnancy: screening by uterine artery Doppler at 11-13 weeks. Ultrasound Obstet Gynecol 2009a;34:142-148.

Poon LC, Maiz N, Valencia C, Plasencia W, Nicolaides KH. First-trimester maternal serum pregnancy-associated plasma protein-A and pre-eclampsia. Ultrasound Obstet Gynecol 2009b;33:23-33.

Powell DR, Allander SV, Scheimann AO, Wasserman RM, Durham SK, Suwanichkul A. Multiple proteins bind the insulin response element in the human IGFBP-1 promoter. Prog Growth Factor Res 1995;6:93-101.

Ritvos O, Ranta T, Jalkanen J, et al. Insulin-like growth factor (IGF) binding proteins from human decidua inhibits the binding and biological action of IGF-I in cultured choriocarcinoma cells. Endocrinology 1989;122:2150-2157.

Schiessl B, Strasburger CJ, Bidlingmaier M, et al. Role of placental growth hormone in the alteration of maternal arterial resistance in pregnancy. J Reprod Med 2007;52:313-316

Sheikh S, Satoskar P, Bhartiya D: Expression of insulin-like growth factor-I and placental growth hormone mRNA in placentae: a comparison between normal and intrauterine growth retardation pregnancies. Mol Hum Reprod 2001;7:287–292.

Shin JC, Lee JH, Yang DE, Moon HB, Rha JG, Kim SP. Expression of insulin-like frowth factor-II and insulin-like growth factor binding protein-1 in the placental basal plate from pre-eclamptic pregnancies. Int J Gynaecol Obstet 2003;81:273-280.

Sifakis S, Papadopoulou E, Konstantinidou A, Giahnakis E, Fragouli Y, Karkavitsas N, Koumantakis E, Kalmanti M. Increased levels of human placental growth hormone in the amniotic fluid of pregnancies affected by Down syndrome. Growth Horm IGF Res 2009;19:121-125.

Sifakis S, Akolekar R, Kappou D, Mantas N, Nicolaides KH. Maternal serum insulin like growth factor-I (IGF-I) at 11-13 weeks in preeclampsia. Prenat Diagn 2010;30:1026-1031

Sifakis S, Akolekar R, Mantas N, Kappou D, Nicolaides KH. Maternal serum human placental growth hormone (PGH) at 11 to 13 weeks of gestation in preeclampsia. Hypert Pregn 2011a;30:74-82

Sifakis S, Akolekar R, Kappou D, Mantas N, Nicolaides KH. Maternal serum insulin-like growth factor-binding protein-3 (IGFBP-3) at 11-13 weeks in preeclampsia. J Hum Hypertens. 2011b Mar 3. [Epub ahead of print]

Smith S, Francis R, Guilbert L, Baker PN: Growth factor rescue of cytokine mediated trophoblast apoptosis. Placenta 2002;23:322-330

Solomon CG, Graves SW, Green MF, Seely EW. Glucose intolerance as a predictor of hypertension in pregnancy. Hypertension 1994;23:717-721.

Suhonen L, Teramo K. Hypertension and preeclampsia in women with gestational glucose intolerance. Acta Obtet Gynecol Scand 1993;72:269-272.

Trollmann R, Klingmuller K, Schild RL, et al. Differential gene expression of somatotrophic and growth factors in response to in vivo hypoxia in human placenta. Am J Obstet Gynecol 2007;197:601.e1-601.e6.

Vatten LJ, Nilsen TIL, Juul A, Jeansson S, Jenum PA, Eskild A. Changes in circulting level of IGF-I and IGF-binding protein-1 from the first to second trimester as predictors of preeclampsia. European Journal of Endocrinology 2008;158:101-105.

Verhaeghe J, Van Bree R, Van Herck E, Laureys J, Bouillon R, Van Assche FA. C-peptide, insulin-like growth factor-I and factor-II, and insulin-like growth factor binding protein-1 in umbilical cord serum: correlations with birth weight. Am J Obstet Gynecol 1993;169:89-97.

Walenkamp MJ, van der Kamp HJ, Pereira AM, Kant SG, van Duyvenvoorde HA, Kruithof MF, Breuning MH, Romijn JA, Karperien M, Wit JM: A variable degree of intrauterine and postnatal growth retardation in a family with a missense mutation in the insulin-like growth factor I receptor. J Clin Endocrinol Metab 2006;91:3062-3070.

Wang HS, Lee JD, Cheng BJ, Soong YK. Insulin-like growth factor-binding protein 1 and insulin-like growth factor binding protein-3 in preeclampsia. Br J Obstet Gynaecol 1996;103:654-659.

Westwood M, Gibson JM, Davies AJ, Young RJ, White A: The phosphorylation pattern of insulin-like growth factor-binding protein-1 in normal plasma is different from that in amniotic fluid and changes during pregnancy. J Clin Endocrinol Metab 1994;79:1735-1741.

Yu J, Iwashita M, Kudo Y, Takeda Y: Phosphorylated insulin-like growth factor (IGF)-binding protein-1 (IGFBP-1) inhibits while non-phosphorylated IGFBP-1 stimulates IGF-I-induced amino acid uptake by cultured trophoblast cells. Growth Horm IGF Res 1998;8:65-70.

Zhou Y, Damsky CH, Chiu K, Roberts JM and Fisher SJ. Preeclampsia is associated with abnormal expression of adhesion molecules by invasive cytotrophoblasts. J Clin Invest 1993;91:950-960.

10

Placental Angiogenesis and Fetal Growth Restriction

Victor Gourvas[1], Efterpi Dalpa[2], Nikos Vrachnis[3] and Stavros Sifakis[4]
[1]Department of Pathology, General Hospital "G. Genimatas", Thessaloniki,
[2]Department of Pediatrics, General Hospital "G. Papageorgiou", Thessaloniki,
[3]2nd Department of Obstetrics & Gynecology, Aretaieion Hospital,
University of Athens, Athens,
[4]Department of Obstetrics & Gynecology, University Hospital of Heraklion, Crete,
Greece

1. Introduction

1.1 Vessel growth and angiogenesis

The process that involves vessel formation and growth has been described by the terms vasculogenesis and angiogenesis, as two distinct types [Demir et al., 2007]. Both of these processes are essential for normal uteroplacental development:

a. vasculogenesis, meaning new blood vessel formation from hemangiogenic stem cells (derived from mesenchymal cells) that differentiate to hemangioblastic stem cells, essentially occurring during fetal development. Vasculogenesis consists of three major steps: i. induction of hemangioblasts and angioblasts -mediated mainly through fibroblast growth factor (FGF), ii. assembly of primordial vessels -mediated mainly by vascular endothelial growth factor/vascular endothelial growth factor receptor system (VEGF/VEGFR) iii. transition from vasculogenesis to angiogenesis [Flamme et al., 1997];

b. angiogenesis, meaning new branches from pre-existing vessels, which is occurring in the female reproductive tract during the formation of the corpus luteum, during endometrial development and during embryo implantation and placentation. Two forms of angiogenesis have been described: sprouting and non-sprouting angiogenesis (intussusception) [Folkman et al., 1992]. The process of angiogenesis has three phases: initiation, proliferation-invasion and maturation-differentiation.

The vascularisation of placental villi starts at day 21 post conception (dpc), being the result of local de novo formation of capillaries rather than protrusion of embryonic vessels into the placenta [Demir et al., 1989]. Mesenchymal cells inside the villi transform into hemangiogenic precursor cells that migrate toward the periphery. In the latter, prior to the formation of the first vessels that are observed by about 28 dpc (erythrocytes are detected by 32 dpc), mesenchymal derived macrophages (Hofbauer cells) appear. Those macrophages will express angiogenic growth factors and, as they appear early, they suggest a paracrine role in the initiation of vasculogenesis. Angiogenic growth factors are also expressed by the maternal decidua and macrophages mediating the trohpoblast invasion [Ahmed et al., 1995]. In the meanwhile since the uterus and its contents demand an increased supply of blood during pregnancy, its vasculature undergoes three main adaptative changes: vasodilation, increased permeability, and growth and development of new vessels. So the villi mature and angiogenesis begins at around 32 dpc [Zygmunt et al., 2003].

Branching or sprouting angiogenesis (lateral ramification of pre-existing tubes) is first observed leading to the formation of a capillary network. During branching angiogenesis multistep processes are taking place including increased vascular permeability, degradation of basement membrane, increase in endothelial cell proliferation and migration, formation of endothelial cell tubes, and recruitment of pericytes to the outside of the capillary to form a stable vessel [Kaufmann et al., 2004]. From the 6th week a basal lamina begins to form around the capillaries that results to a web like arrangement of capillaries within the stroma of mesenchymal villi, and a superficially location of most of the capillaries in the immature intermediate villi (beneath the trophoblast, covering the villous surface). In the latter, from the 15th week onwards, fibrosal stromal core is being formed by the fusion of the adventicia of large central vessels, thus becoming a stem villus. In these larger villi a few central endothelial tubes (or early villous arteries and veins) have larger diameters, up to 100mm, and become surrounded by cells expressing alpha and gamma smooth muscles actins, vimentin and desmin. These contractile cells concentrate around the lumina, acquiring the full spectrum of cytoskeleton antigens. Following branching angiogenesis, non branching angiogenesis is observed from 24 weeks of gestation, due to the formation of mature intermediate villi, specialized in gas exchange. Those villi contain 1-2 long, poorly branched capillary loops, which coil and bulge through the trophoblastic surface, forming the terminal villi. These structures are the main site of diffusional gas exchange between the maternal and fetal circulations. This process includes decreased trophoblast proliferation and increased endothelial proliferation [Benirschke and Kaufmann, 1995].

As gestation increases, the terminal capillaries focally dilate and form large sinusoids, which counterbalance the effects of the long poorly branched capillaries on total fetoplacental vascular impedance. Increasing fetal blood pressure aids this dilation and fetoplacental blood flow rises throughout gestation to 40% of fetal cardiac output at term [Ahmed et al., 2000].

Pseudovasculogenesis is the process which remodelling of maternal uterine vessels occurs. Until 6 weeks post conception uterine arteries (spiral arteries) have high resistance and low capacity. After cytotrophoblast invasion they breakdown smooth muscle cells and replace maternal endothelial cells resulting to low resistance and high capacity vessels. Same process, but less extent occurs also in maternal veins. Pseudovasculogenesis is completed around 20 weeks of gestation.

1.2 Fetal growth restriction

Fetal growth restriction (FGR) is a complex condition in the field of current Obstetrics with an incidence rate of 4-7% of births and is associated with a 6- to 10-fold increased risk of perinatal morbidity and mortality [Jarvis et al., 2003]. FGR is not a disease entity with a unique pathophysiology. A variety of factors have been involved, including congenital abnormalities, drug abuse and infectious, immunological or anatomical factors. However, incomplete placentation (placental formation) is observed in most cases [Cetin et al., 2004].

Two types of FGR have been described: early onset, that the growth restriction is symmetrical and late onset that restriction of growth is asymmetrical. The first one is more severe and usually has its underline cause in a specific defect that acts from the beginning of conception such as chromosomal anomalies, infections or substance abuse. Second and more common is less severe with smaller impact on the fetus and the causes may vary. Many elements can be of greater or lesser importance in the progress of this entity. Incomplete placentation and factors controlled by hypoxia are the most common pathophysiologic mechanism.

A successful pregnancy outcome depends on the proper development of the fetoplacental vasculature in the villous core, which begins with the infiltration of cytotrophoblast in the endometrium and is completed in conjunction with the spiral arteries. It is widely accepted that shallow trophoblast invasion can lead to fetal hypoxia and impaired growth [Mayhew et al., 2004]. The proper and timely proliferation and differentiation of the villous cytotrophoblast stem cells, which are controlled by hypoxia, are crucial for adequate placentation [James et al., 2006]. Thus, the entire repertoire of hypoxia-associated growth factors is remarkably active during placental development.

1.3 Fetal growth restriction and angiogenesis

Angiogenesis is a placental factor playing an important role in the development of FGR. FGR occurs as a result of adequate vascular transformation and of terminal villous formation [Ahmed et al., 2000].

Based on the type of FGR (early or late onset) there are two models that may occur in the placental tissue. First is due to uteroplacental insufficiency and results to increased branching angiogenesis. Second and more common is due to placental failure and is accompanied by straight and unbranched capillaries, along with reduced cytotrophoblast proliferation, increased syncytial nuclei and erythrocyte congestion. All these suggest an increased rate of trophoblast proliferation. This situation has been interpreted as placental hyperoxia. Thus, fetoplacental blood flow is severely impaired and transplacental gas exchange is poor, placing the fetus at risk of hypoxia and acidosis [Macara et al., 1996].

Factors that are regulated by oxygen concentration are mainly important for the placental tissue to respond to hypoxic events. The most important known factors of this subgroup are hypoxia inducible factors (HIF).

2. Hypoxia inducible factors

Hypoxia Inducible Factors (HIF) are transcriptional factors that were discovered in mammalian cells under conditions of low oxygen, and appear to have a fundamental role in the cellular and systematic response to hypoxia, via the regulation of metabolism, cellular cycle, angiogenesis and apoptosis. HIFs are heterodimers constituted from the HIFa (1, 2 or 3) and HIFb or ARNT.

HIFa subunit is found in the cytoplasm and is transported in the nuclei in order to form HIF with the other subunit ARNT, which is expressed regularly in the nuclei, and achieve its transcriptional role. It has been found that transcriptional action of HIFa is achieved via bHLH (basic helix-loop-helix)-PAS domain in N-terminal. For this action the recruitment of co-activators p300 and CBP is needed. While HIF-1 and HIF-2 have similar structure and action, it appears that HIF-3 presents suspensive action in the hypoxia, which has not however been confirmed [Kiichi et al., 2006].

HIFa under normoxic conditions is hydroxylated in two Prolyl domains (Pro 402 and Pro 564) by their Prolyl Hydroxylation Domains (PHD-1,2 and 3), which induces the reaction with the von Hippel-Lindau (VHL) forming a dimmer that is proteosomical degradated. It appears that VHL is downregulated in hypoxia, consequently releasing the HIFa that at the same time is upregulated. PHD utilizes O_2 as a substrate with a Km that is slightly above atmospheric concentration. The enzymatic activity is modulated by changes in O_2 concentration under physiological conditions. This regulation appears to be common for all three HIFa factors [Min et al., 2002].

Deductively, the HIFa factors are upregulated by hypoxia, while the ARNT is stably expressed and in order to they carry out their transcriptional role, they should form a heterodimmer in the nuclei. Under normal conditions, while HIFs continue to be expressed, VHL and PHD-1, 2 and 3 are upregulated in order to complete protesomical degradation of HIFs. The existing data for HIF-1a and HIF-2a show a regulating role in angiogenesis, metabolism, cellular cycle and apoptosis; for HIF-3a however there is still lack of evidence regarding his precise role [Makino et al., 2001]. On the contrary, factors PHD-1, 2 and 3 appear to play all similar roles in the degradation of HIFa subunits [Salceda et al., 1997; Maxwell et al., 1999]. Important examples of factors that are regulated by HIF-1 are VEGF, PLGF, Flt-1 and Angiopoietin-2 regarding arterial destabilization and increased vascular permeability, MMPs, Angiopoietin-1, MCP-1 and PDGF regarding migration and proliferation of endothelial cells etc. Figure 1 represents the HIF pathway during normoxic and hypoxic conditions.

2.1 Hypoxia inducible factors in placenta

It is already known that one of the most important processes during gestation is the physiologic development of feto-placental unit that begins with the cytotrophoblast invasion in the endometrium and is completed with the creation of chorionic villi [Huppertz et al., 2007]. Initially the cytotrophoblast environment can be characterized as hypoxic, but after the completion of the conjunction with the spiral vessels there is a passage to physiologic oxygenation. During this process, structural changes are required for both the epithelium of endometrium and the endothelium and walls of the spiral arteries. The wall of vessels that is found to the side of fetus is replaced from trophoblasts. Cytotrophoblasts in this process turn from an expressive pattern of molecules of epithelial specification in an expressive pattern of adherence molecules that is more of endothelium cells differentiation. Many of these molecules are regulated by HIF. The cytotrophoblast tends to proliferate in hypoxia but to differentiate in physiological oxygenation, and these data show that cytotrophoblast activity depends on the presence of oxygen.

Results from studies in animal models have shown that at the initial stages of pregnancy where PO_2 is decreased, an increased action of regulating factors exists, mainly from HIF-1, HIF-2 and HIF-3. HIF-1 comprises a basic response of a cell to the hypoxic conditions. It is constituted by two subunits, HIF-1a and HIF-1b (ARNT). HIF-1a forms a heterodimmer with the HIF-1b and HIF-1, acts on the cell nucleus and regulates the expression of many genes that play role in angiogenesis, cellular cycle and metabolism [Semenza et al., 2000]. Similar function appears also for the HIF-2, while for HIF-3 the existing data is insufficient. The regulation of these factors is depending on the partial pressure of oxygen, a fact that makes them immediately connected with hypoxic conditions in the feto-placental circulation such as preeclampsia or FGR [Smith et al., 2001].

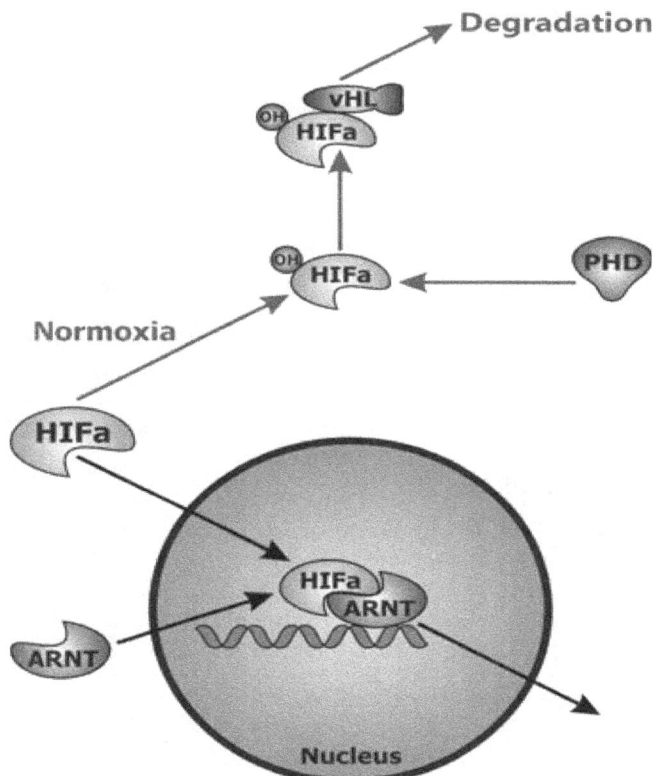

Fig. 1. Graphical representation of the HIF pathway during normoxic and hypoxic conditions. In normoxia (grey arrows) PHD hydroxylates HIF-a, which then binds to vHL, leading to its proteosomal degradation. In hypoxia (black arrows) HIF-a enters the nucleus, forms a dimer with ARNT, which then binds to DNA, leading to gene transcription activation [Gourvas et al., 2010].

Regulation of HIFs appears to relate not only with the induction/suspension of their expression, but also with their degradation. Thus, in physiologic conditions the a- subunits of HIF are degraded with a mechanism that includes factors PHD-1, 2 and 3 (prolyl hydroxylation domain) and VHL. They are responsible for the hydroxylation and degradation of HIFa, so that HIFa cannot activate ARNT in the nuclei. In a second phase one more hydroxylation can contribute in the suspension of HIF, which becomes in asn803 and suspends the interaction with co-activators p300/CBP, which is essential for the induction of transcription [Lando et al., 2002].

It is obvious that the regulation of HIF expression and function is achieved through a number of factors, such as PO_2, VHL and PHD-1, 2 and 3. Consequently, a measurement of expression only of HIF in conditions with decreased supply of oxygen may lead to false conclusions, especially by considering that their regulation is also posttranscriptional through the action of PHD and VHL. Later during gestation, when fetal-placental unit provides satisfactory quantities of O_2, HIFs are downregulated by decreased expression or degradation. In pathological situations, however, it is probable that this model is disturbed and the maintenance of decreased oxygenation affects the regulating action of these factors. Thus exists a change/imbalance in the expression of genes related with processes such as angiogenesis (VEGF, PLGF, PDGF, EPO, NOS2, FLT1 etc), metabolism (aldolase, hexokinase, pyrouvic kinase, lactic dehydrogonase etc) and cellular cycle (IGF, p21, p35srj etc). These changes may produce clinical signs and symptoms of FGR or preeclampsia or of both of them.

3. Angiogenetic growth factors in FGR

Numerous factors are thought to play a role in normal vascular adaptation to implantation. The VEGFs are specific stimulators of vascular permeability, as well as vascular endothelial cell protease production and migration, all of which are critical components of the angiogenic process [Folkman et al., 1987] Vascular endothelial growth factor also stimulate angiogenesis in a variety of in vivo and in vitro models [Klagsbrun et al., 1991]. The increased expression of VEGF-A, b-FGF, and eNOS that we have found in IUGR placentas may promote increased endothelial cell proliferation and migration and pathological angiogenesis [Kinzler et al., 2008].

VEGF, placental growth factor (PlGF), angiopoietins (Ang-1 and Ang-2) are involved not only in the regulation of vascular development and in remodeling during placentation, but also act as growth factors for driving growth and differentiation processes such as invasion. It has been hypothesized that an impairment of trophoblast invasion and a failure of spiral artery remodeling could have a role in the development of PE and FGR [Wulff et al., 2003].

Vascular endothelial growth factor-A (VEGF-A) and placental growth factor (PlGF) are probably the best-studied factors. VEGF interacts with VEGFR-1 (Flt-1) and VEGFR-2 (KDR) to promote endothelial cell proliferation, cell migration, and vascular permeability. PlGF shares biochemical and functional features with VEGF and interacts with VEGFR-1 (Flt-1). PlGF and VEGF-A have synergistic effects regarding angiogenesis, but vessels induced by PlGF are more mature and stable than vessels induced by VEGF-A [Chung et al., 2004]. PlGF is abundantly expressed in the human placenta. Both VEGF-A and PlGF may be important paracrine regulators of decidual angiogenesis and autocrine mediators of trophoblast function [Sherer et al., 2001].

A second family of growth factors, the angiopoietins, is also known for their regulating capacities regarding angiogenesis. Angiopoietin-1 (Ang-1) and angiopoietin-2 (Ang-2) bind with equal affinity to their receptor TIE-2, but have different functions. Ang-1 maintains vessel integrity and plays a role in the later stages of vascular remodeling [Geva et al., 2000]. Ang-2 is a functional antagonist of Ang-1 and leads to loosening of cell–cell interactions and allows access to angiogenic inducers like VEGF. Coexpression of VEGF and Ang-2 induces angiogenesis, but Ang-2 results in vascular regression in the absence of angiogenic signals. Ang-1 and Ang-2 have both been detected in decidual and placental tissues [Asahara et al., 1998].

Various decidual cell types are capable of producing angiogenic factors. We recently showed the production of PlGF, KDR, Flt-1, Ang-2, and TIE-2 by endothelial cells and extravillous trophoblasts. Decidual stromal cells, glandular epithelium, and perivascular smooth muscle cells were found to produce all studied angiogenic factors [Plaisier et al., 2007]. Uterine natural killer cells are also abundantly present in first-trimester decidua and are known to produce PlGF, VEGF, Ang-1, and Ang-2.

4. Conclusion

A successful pregnancy outcome depends on the proper development of the fetoplacental vasculature in the villous core, which begins with the infiltration of cytotrophoblast in the endometrium and is completed in conjunction with the spiral arteries. It is widely accepted that shallow trophoblast invasion can lead to fetal hypoxia and impaired growth. The proper and timely proliferation and differentiation of the villous cytotrophoblast stem cells, which are controlled by hypoxia, are crucial for adequate placentation and initiation of angiogenetic pathways. Numerous factors are thought to play a role in normal vascular adaptation to implantation. There is strong evidence that abnormal levels of angiogenic and antiangiogenic growth factors could in part be responsible for the pathophysiology associated with pregnancies complicated by FGR.

5. References

Ahmed AS, Li XF, Dunk CE, Whittle MJ, Rollason T. Colocalisation of vascular endothelial growth factor and its flt-1 receptor in human placenta. Growth Factors 1995;12:235-243.

Ahmed A, Dunk C, Ahmad S, Khaliq A. Regulation of placental vascular endothelial growth factor (VEGF) and placenta growth factor (PlGF) and soluble flt-1 by oxygen. A Review. Troph Res 2000;14:16-24.

Ahmed A, Perkins J: Angiogenesis and intrauterine growth restriction. Baillieres Best Pract Res Clin Obstet Gynaecol 2000;14:981-998.

Asahara T, Chen D, Takahashi T, et al. Tie2 receptor ligands, angiopoietin-1 and angiopoietin-2, modulate VEGF-induced postnatal neovascularization. *Circ Res.* 1998;83:233-240

Benirschke K, Kaufmann P (Eds). Pathology of Human Placenta. London: Springer-Verlag 1995

Cetin I, Foidart JM, Miozzo M, et al. Fetal growth restriction: a workshop report. Placenta 2004;25:753-757.

Chung J, Song Y, Wang Y, Magness RR, Zheng J. Differential expression of vascular endothelial growth factor (VEGF), endocrine gland derived-VEGF, and VEGF receptors in human placentas from normal and preeclamptic pregnancies. *J Clin Endocrinol Metab* 2004;89:2484-2490.

Demir R, Kaufmann P, Castellucci M, Erbengi T, Kotowski A. Fetal vasculogenesis and angiogenesis in human placental villi. Acta Anat (Basel) 1989;136:190–203

Demir R, Seval Y, Huppertz B. Vasculogenesis and angiogenesis in the early human placenta. Acta Histochem 2007;109:257-265.

Flamme I, Frolich T, Risau W. Molecular mechanisms of vasculogenesis and embryonic angiogenesis. J Cell Physiol 1997;173:206–210

Folkman J, Klagsbrun M. Angiogenic factors. Science 1987;233:442–447

Folkman J, Shing Y. Angiogenesis. J Biol Chem 1992;267:10931–10934

Geva E, Jaffe RB. Role of angiopoietins in reproductive tract angiogenesis. Obstet Gynecol Surv 2000;55:511-519.

Gourvas V, Sifakis S, Dalpa E, Soulitzis N, Koukoura O, Spandidos DA. Reduced placental prolyl hydroxylase 3 mRNA expression in pregnancies affected by fetal growth restriction. BJOG. 2010 ;117:1635-1642.

Huppertz B, Abe E, Murthi P, Nagamatsu T, Szukiewicz D, Salafia C. Placental Angiogenesis, Maternal and Fetal Vessels. A Workshop Report. Placenta 2007;28(supplement A):S94eS96

James JL, Stone PR, Chamley LW. The regulation of trophoblast differentiation by oxygen in the first trimester of pregnancy. Hum Reprod Update 2006;12:137-144.

Jarvis S, Glinianaia S, Torrioli M, et. al. Cerebral palsy and intrauterine growth in single births: European collaborative study. Lancet 2003;362:1106-1111.

Kaufmann P, Mayhew TM, Charnock-Jones DS. Aspects of human fetoplacental vasculogenesis and angiogenesis. II. Changes during normal pregnancy. Placenta 2004;25:114-126.

Hirota K, Semenza. GL Regulation of angiogenesis by hypoxia-inducible factor 1. Crit Rev Oncol Hematol 2006;59:15–26

Kinzler WL, Vintzileos AM. Fetal growth restriction. Curr Opin Obstet Gynecol 2008;2:125-131.

Klagsbrun M, D'Amore PA. Regulators of angiogenesis. Annu Rev Physiol 1991;53:217

Lando D, Peet, DJ, Whelan DA, Gorman JJ, Whitelaw ML. Asparagine hydroxylation of the HIF transactivation domain: a hypoxic switch. Science 295: 858-861, 2002

Macara LM, Kingdom JCP, Kaufmann P, Kohen G, Hair J, More IRA, Lyall F, Greer IA. Structural analysis of placental terminal villi from growth-restricted pregnancies with abnormal umbilical artery Doppler waveforms. Placenta 1996;17:37-48

Makino Y, Cao R, Svensson K, et al. Inhibitory PAS domain protein is a negative regulator of hypoxia-inducible gene expression. Nature 2001;414:550–554.

Maxwell PH, Wiesener MS, Chang GW, et al. The tumor suppressor protein VHL targets hypoxia-inducible factors for oxygendependent proteolysis. Nature 1999;399:271–275.

Mayhew TM, Charnock-Jones DS, Kaufmann P. Aspects of human fetoplacental vasculogenesis and angiogenesis. III. Changes in complicated pregnancies. Placenta 2004;25:127-139.

Min JH, Yang H, Ivan M. Gertler F, Kaelin WG Jr, Pavletich NP. Structure of an HIF-1-alpha-pVHL complex: hydroxyproline recognition in signaling. Science 2002;296:1886-1889.

Plaisier M, Rodrigues S, Willems F, et al. Different degree of vascularisation and its relation to the expression of VEGF, PlGF, angiopoietins and their receptors in 1st trimester decidua. Fertil Steril 2007;88:176-187.

Salceda S, Caro J. Hypoxia-inducible factor 1a (HIF-1a) protein is rapidly degraded by the ubiquitin-proteasome system under normoxic conditions. Its stabilization by hypoxia depends on redoxinduced changes. J Biol Chem 1997;272:22642–22647.

Semenza, G. L.HIF-1 and human disease: one highly involved factor. Genes Dev 2000;14:1983-1991.

Sherer DM, Abulafia O. Angiogenesis during implantation, and placental and early embryonic development. Placenta 2001;22:1-13

Smith SK. Angiogenesis and reproduction. BJOG 2001;108:777-783

Wulff C, Weigand M, Kreienberg R, Fraser HM. Angiogenesis during primate placentation in health and disease. Reproduction 2003;126:569–577.

Zygmunt M, Herr F, Munstedt K, et al: Angiogenesis and vasculogenesis in pregnancy. Eur J Obstet Gynecol Reprod Biol 2003;110(suppl):S10-S18.

11

The External Version in Modern Obstetrics

Esther Fandiño García[1] And Juan Carlos Delgado Herrero[2]
[1]Hospital de Jerez de la Frontera
[2]Hospital Juan Grande
Spain

1. Introduction

The incidence of breech presentation is 3-4% (Enkin et al 1995). It is still debated what is the best performance. In particular, both the role of the external cephalic version and the birth type have been extensively debated.

In contrast to cephalic presentations, breech presentations has a higher mortality and morbidity due to the associated incidence of prematurity, congenital malformations or intra-partum asphyxia. Thus, many efforts have been made in order to establish the best performance regarding the birth type: either vaginal delivery (in those women selected after evaluating different fetal and pelvic parameters) or the elective caesarian. On the other hand, the external version can be also considered. (American College Obstetricians and gynecologist [ACOG], 2001). It aims to avoid the vaginal delivery or caesarian complications by turning a breech presentation into a cephalic presentation.

Breech presentation is an independent factor associated with higher morbidity (Royal College of Obstetricians and Gynaecologists [RCOG], 2006). In fact, a high prevalence rate in children disabilities after breech presentation (16%) has been registered both in vaginal and caesarean delivery (Danielian et al, 1996).

Traditionally, there has always been a general agreement on the preference of caesarian delivery instead of a elective vaginal delivery in case of breech babies in the following circumstances: feet first, large fetus, intrapartum risk of loss of fetal well-being, congenital malformations (meaning a mechanical problem for a vaginal delivery) or in case of inexperienced obstetricians.

Some obstetricians advocate caesarean intervention in order to reduce the perinatal risks associated with breech presentation. Unfortunately this is based on their personal experience, medical legal aspects and non-randomized studies. Nevertheless, other obstetricians still advocate for vaginal delivery in selected cases, as it may reduce the maternal morbidity and the use of medical resources. In 2000, the results of a multicentric and randomized clinical study conducted by *Hannah* et al. in collaboration with *The Term Breech Trial* were published in *The Lancet* (Hannah et al, 2000). In this study, the caesarean delivery was highly recommended in breech babies at term. The Cochrane database also published a meta-analysis including *Hannah*'s project (Hofmeyr et Hannah, 2003). This analysis concluded that the elective caesarean reduces both the perinatal and neonatal morbidity and mortality at the expense of a moderate increase in maternal morbidity.

This study led to a worldwide change in medical practice. Several national recommended the caesarean delivery in term breech babies. In fact, in many American and European countries, this performance has become the only one to be considered.

In view of this opinion about avoiding the vaginal delivery in breech babies by using the caesarian delivery, there has been a growing interest in retaking the external version performances in order to reduce the caesarian delivery frequency.

Definitely, the external version has become more and more relevant as well as a controversial and a topical issue since this is a valid option against the elective caesarian. It has been shown that its use significantly reduces the vaginal delivery frequency as well as the caesarian delivery frequency in breech presentation in full term pregnancies. In spite of this fact, the external version is still not implemented in many countries.

This review article aims to discuss the complications in breech babies and the use of external version as an alternative (regarding the process itself, the conditions and the right moment to perform it, its contraindications, its adverse effects, etc.).

2. Material and methods

Articles have been searched in *Medline* and *Pubmed* database as well as in the *Cochrane Database of Systematic Reviews*. The search has been limited to those studies in human beings and articles in English or Spanish developed between 1995 and 2007. Current clinical practice guidelines (from the –American, British, Canadian and Spanish national associations of obstetricians and gynecologists on external version and breech presentation have also been reviewed. Key words: Breech, cephalic version, external version, adverse event "and" cephalic version.

3. Breech presentation

Breech presentation is defined as a fetus in a longitudinal lie with the buttocks or feet closest to the cervix and the head closest to the fundus of the uterus. There are three types of breeches.

The incidence of breech presentation in neonates before the 28th gestation-week is 20%. This percentage decreases to 3-4% with advancing gestational age. These data show that most babies turn around during the third trimester of pregnancy. Under normal circumstances, as the shape of the uterus changes, the fetus turns simultaneously to headfirst position between the 28th and the 32nd week of pregnancy. As of this moment, the uterus will expand more vertically than transversely. This situation facilitates the previous fetal position. Although the simultaneous turn is more common during the weeks of pregnancy mentioned above, this turn is also possible at delivery. However, this is more common in multiparous women rather than in primiparous women. Thus, it seems that the fetus plays an active role at adopting the best position in the uterus.

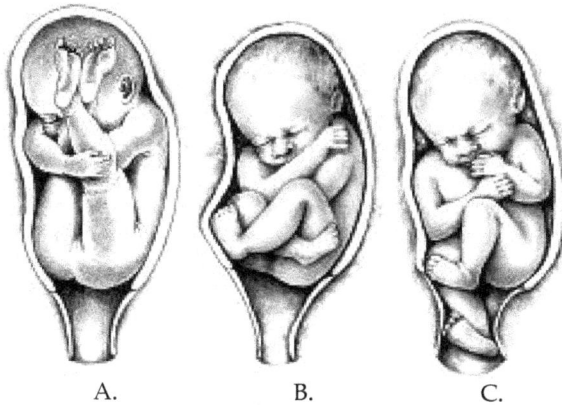

A.   B.   C.

Fig. 1. A. Frank breech (65-70%) The baby's legs are flexed at the hip, his or her knees are extended and feet next to the head. This is the most common type in pregnancies at term. **B.** Complete breech (5%) In this case, the baby's hips and knees are flexed. The fetus positions is the same as in the vertex presentation but, in this case, the polarity is reversed. **C.** Incomplete breech (-30%) The baby has one or both knees flexed so that baby's legs (not his or her bottom) are poised to deliver first. This type is common in preterm deliveries.

From the etiologic point of view, the breech presentation could be caused by situations avoiding or hampering the spontaneous cephalic version.

- Fetal factors: Prematurity, low weight, multiple pregnancy, structural anomalies, chromosomopathies, reduced fetal mobility.
- Maternal factors: Primiparous women, uterine malformations that change the uterus normal morphology, previous tumour, pelvic stenosis.
- Ovular factors: Anomalies of placental insertion (placenta previa), short umbilical cord and the changes in the amniotic fluid volume (both oligohydramnios and polyhydramnios).

The incidence of breech presentation is closely related to the gestational age. In the case of single-gestation pregnancies, the preterm delivery is probably the aspect that contributes the most to a breech presentation at delivery. Before the 28th week, the incidence is almost 10 times higher than at term, and almost 12% of preterm deliveries show breech presentation. However, 50%-80% of the cases do not show any etiologic factor responsible for the breech presentation (Sociedad Española de Ginecología y Obstetricia [SEGO], 2001).

4. The term breech trial: Clinical practice implications

The article: "Elective caesarean vs. vaginal delivery with breech presentation at term: The International Term Breech Trial", was a randomized trial published by Hannah et al. in The Lancet magazine in 2000. The conclusions of the study were immediately adopted by the medical society, leading to a great change in obstetric practice.

The purpose of the study was to create a clinical guideline based on the evidence regarding the best performance to follow with respect to breech presentation. The study was carried out in 121 centres of 26 different countries. It included a total of 2008 pregnant women at term with breech babies. Those women were randomly given the date of the planned caesarean or the planned vaginal delivery. After a three-month monitoring, it was performed a two-year monitoring.

There was a reduction in the neonatal mortality and morbidity in the elective caesarean delivery group when compared with the elective vaginal delivery group, without any significant increase of maternal morbidity or mortality. Furthermore, it was found that the adverse perinatal outcomes were less common when the caesarean had been planned before delivery, while they increased if the caesarean was performed intrapartum.

The subgroup analysis failed to demonstrate any independent association with deliveries performed after long delivery labor, those oxytocin or prostaglandin induced, those cases of incomplete breech presentation, those with unknown breech presentation and those breech presentation deliveries performed by inexperienced obstetricians.

Another subgroup analysis was carried out according to the national perinatal mortality rate (low versus high). In this case, the results showed some changes, obtaining a higher reduction of perinatal mortality in countries with lower national perinatal mortality rate than in those with higher mortality rates. Therefore, the benefits of the at term caesarean will be higher in countries with lower perinatal mortality rates, as it is the case of Spain. One reason for this difference could be that, in these countries, women were discharged at an early stage after the vaginal delivery. Therefore, the collection of neonatal complications has been less complete than the records concerning caesarean-born babies, as they need to stay longer in the hospital.

All subgroups analysis, except the already mentioned one, showed similar risk reductions when using an elective caesarean delivery, compared with the planned vaginal deliveries of the main study (Hannah et al, 2002).

Concerning maternal morbidity, the urinary incontinence occurring three months after delivery was lower in the planned caesarean group. Abdominal pain was more common in the planned caesarean group, while perineal pain was more common in the planned vaginal delivery. There were not statistically significant differences in low back pain, faecal incontinence, postpartum depression, maternal dissatisfaction with the method of care, breastfeeding, bonding with the newborn, bonding with the woman's partner or dyspareunia. However, neither the morbidity associated to uterine scars in subsequent pregnancies nor the ability to carry out everyday activities were evaluated.

As it has been mentioned, the results of the analysis of Hannah's three month after delivery study yield an significant impact for obstetrician practice and were adopted almost immediately by the medical societies. The Cochrane database also published a meta-analysis including *Hannah*'s project. This analysis concluded that the planned caesarean reduces both the perinatal and neonatal morbidity and mortality at the expense of a moderate increase in maternal morbility. These conclusions were included in the national associations of obstetrics and gynecology's clinical guidelines and protocols. Some of these societies are the Royal College of Obstetricians and Gynaecologists (RCOG), the Society of Obstetricians and Gynaecologists of Canada (SOGC) or the American College of Obstetricians and Gynaecologists (ACOG). Obviously, the Spanish Society of Obstetrics and Gynaecology

(SEGO, as per its Spanish initials) also included these conclusions and recommended in its breech presentation protocol the fact of informing the patient about the results from previous studies. This recommendation has caused an increase in breech presentation caesarians in pregnancies at term. Thus, a study published in 2003 and carried out in 80 centres and 23 countries stated that 92% of the centers studies had opted for the caesarean delivery in breech presentation instead of the vaginal delivery (Hogle et al, 2003).

The two year monitoring of this same project (published in 2004) did not show any difference between the groups concerning the following aspects: Breast feeding, bonding with the newborn or her partner; subsequent pregnancy; incontinence; depression; urinary, menstrual or sexual problems; fatigue; or distressing memories of the birth experience. The planned caesarean was related to a higher risk of constipation. It is remarkable the fact that the mothers from the planned caesarean group showed less concern about their babies' health than the ones from the planned vaginal delivery group (Hannah et al, 2004).

After two years, there were not any differences in the perinatal results between the elective caesarean and the elective vaginal delivery, regarding the risk of death or the developmental delay in two years old children. In other words, the lower number of neonatal deaths observed in the project after three months was compensated with a higher number of developmental delay in the elective caesarean delivery group (RCOG, 2006). This was a very surprising result, because three months after the project, performing a planned caesarean delivery proved a reduction both of risk of perinatal death and of severe neonatal morbidity. In conclusion, the planned caesarean delivery is not related to a risk of death reduction or to a developmental delay in two year old children, although this reduction is observed until six months after birth (whyte et al, 2003). Therefore, this new analysis two years after delivery revealed that the initial conclusion could not be maintained, as there were not any significant differences in neonatal morbidity and mortality between both groups. These new conclusions generated debated regarding the recommendations of The Term Breech Trial as the authors continued to reiterate the conclusions from the initial analysis in following papers despite the results obtained after the second year. Projects criticising the methodological reliability and setting out possible biases in Hannah's project. Even though, both the Cochrane and the different national obstetrics and gynaecology societies that adopted the initial results in its recommendations, have not gone into the question again since then. This is not surprising, as the breech presentation delivery is related to many risks from a medico-legal point of view, which makes the caesarean delivery option seem a more convenient option and with lower medico legal risk. Thus, for many obstetricians, Term Breech Trial has become an ideal excuse to adopt a type of delivery they already preferred over the other one.

All the aforementioned has resulted in a large increase of the caesarean delivery rates over the last few years. For instance, in the United Kingdom, caesarean delivery represented 2% of births in 1953, 18% in 1997 and 21% in 2001. In Norway, the rates has gone from 12,8% in 1999 to 13,0% in 2000 and 14% in 2001. The highest increase took place in the last few months of 2000, concurring with the publication of the Term Breech Trial. In the Netherlands, the caesarean delivery rate with breech presentation went from 50% to 80% in less than two months since the release of the Term Breech Trial (Rietberg et al, 2005).

This phenomenon must be analyzed, as we cannot obviate the non-negligible maternal risk related to caesarean, in spite of having notably decreased in the last few decades, thanks to the improvement of the surgical technique, the anesthesia, the infection control, thromboembolic prophylaxis, etc.

The caesarian is the most indendently associated factor with postpartum maternal mortality and morbidity (Minkoff et al, 2003). The mortality rate associated to elective caesarean almost tripled the vaginal delivery (Hall & Bewley, 1999). It is estimated that caesarean (both elective and urgent) quadruple the severe morbidity risks in comparison with vaginal delivery (Waterstone et al, 2001). Caesarean also increases the number of hospital readmissions. During 1995 and 1998, the Canadian hospital readmission rate during the three months after birth (attributable to complications following their birth) was 3,9% for caesarean delivery while for vaginal delivery was 2,6% (Health Canada, 2000). An American research also revealed higher hospitalization rates after a caesarean, with 1,8 relative risk compared with the vaginal delivery (Lydon-Rochelle, 2000).

Apart from this increase in postpartum morbidity after caesarean, there are also long-term risks and complications. The presence of uterine scars increases the risk of complications in subsequent pregnancies, such as ectopic pregnancy, placenta praevia, placenta accreta, premature placenta detachment and uterine rupture. It has been estimated that every caesarean performed to save a child will produce a uterine rupture in the subsequent pregnancy (Hodnett et al, 2005). In a project carried out in the Netherlands, it was calculated that the increase of 8.500 planned caesarean deliveries, which took place within four years of the Term Breech Trial would have avoided 19 perinatal deaths. However, it caused four avoidable maternal deaths. In subsequent pregnancies, it could cause 9 perinatal deaths caused by uterine rupture and 140 women could suffer complications related to the uterine scar (Palencia et al, 2006). The risk of intra-abdominal adhesions, endometriosis on implantation and adenomyosis. Caesareans have also been associated to emotional problems such as postpartum depression and distressing memories of the birth experience, as well as restrictions in everyday activities, and breastfeeding problems. However, it is not the case among those women electing the caesarian delivery. It has also been suggested that neonatal risks increase in caesarean delivery. Some of these risks are the following: increase in admissions to neonatal units (and mother-infant separations postbirth), iatrogenic prematurity, increase in neonatal respiratory problems and fetal deaths in the subsequent pregnancy.

In view of this situation, it is obvious the adequacy of the external version in pregnant women at term with breech presentation. This is the only performance able to turn a breech presentation into a cephalic presentation. Thus, the inherent risk of breech presentation delivery (both in vaginal or caesarean delivery) seems to disappear. A review of the strategies followed to reduce the caesarean risks identified the external cephalic version (ECV) as the only clinical performance gathering evidence (evidence level I) for the total reduction of primary caesarean rates. A Cochrane's review stated that the ECV implementation at term ($\geq$ 37th week) increases the probability of cephalic presentation at birth and reduces the necessity of a caesarean delivery. Thus, ECV should be recommended in the absence of contraindications for every woman with breech babies.

5. External cephalic version (ECV): Concept and history

The external cephalic version is an obstetrics performance aiming at turning a breech presentation into a cephalic one, more favourable to vaginal delivery. It can also be used to turn a transverse situation into a longitudinal (breech or cephalic) presentation. However, its current use is exclusively aimed at turning breech presentation into cephalic presentations.

This performance was widely used before 1970s, but it began to decline because it was considered an unsafe method. It has been performed from the time of Hippocrates (460-377 BC). Aristotle (384-322 BC) was the author of some texts describing that many doctors advised midwives to handle the baby's head so that it was presented at birth.

Over the last century, this performance gradually rose until the sixties, when it saw a boom caused by the increasing demand for a less medical intervention at birth. Before the seventies, the cephalic version was performed preterm because it was believed that this process could hardly be successful if it was performed at term. The external cephalic version was included in the daily obstetric practice due to the obvious and immediate effectiveness of the process as well as the results from non-randomized clinical projects. Its popularity began to decline in the mid-seventies due to the doubts raised about its effectiveness and safety. Reports about a considerable perinatal mortality associated to this performance were published (Bradley Watson, 1975) and the caesarian delivery was presented as the safest option against the external cephalic version or breech presentation. That is the reason why this practice was gradually abandoned until becoming an unusual performance. It must be considered that in those times there were neither ultrasound scans nor antenatal monitoring.

Subsequent projects proved that the external cephalic version in breech babies at term significantly reduced non cephalic presentation at birth as well as the rates of caesareans with no worse perinatal outcome. This situation, as well as the implantation of the Term Breech Trial's results made the external cephalic version be considered as the best option in order to avoid the caesarean in breech babies at term.

6. ECV impact on the reduction of caesarean deliveries and breech presentation at birth

The Cochrane, in a systematic review, assessed the external cephalic version at term effects. The results proved a clinically and statistically significant reduction of breech babies as well as of caesareans deliveries when the external cephalic version was used. No significant effects on perinatal mortality were observed. No significant differences in the incidence on Apgar score were observed (7 at the first minute or at the fifth minute, low umbilical artery PH level or perinatal death.

In fact, the Cochrane Foundation recommended offering the external version to every woman with normal pregnancies and breeching presentation at term (37th-42nd week) (level of recommendation A).

The cephalic version at term reduces the incidence of breech presentation (risk difference 52%, NNT 2) as well as the caesarean rate (risk difference 17%, NNT 6) at birth. In daily clinical practice, most of breech babies are born by elective caesarean, without considering the vaginal delivery possibility. That is why the number of caesarians has a further increase in daily clinical practice that in the projects. This reduction in the number of caesareans continues in spite of the increase of intrapartum caesareans (which has been observed in cephalic babies after a successful version in comparison to babies with spontaneous cephalic presentation). Furthermore, this increase is regardless of a higher induction rate and it is caused by both maternal and fetal indications.

Grade of recommendation	Description
A	Body of evidence can be trusted to guide practice
B	Body of evidence can be trusted to guide practice in most situations
C	Body of evidence provides some support for recommendation(s) but care should be taken in its application
D	Body of evidence is weak and recommendation must be applied with caution

Table 1. Definitions of Grade of Recommendation.

With respect to the external cephalic version effect on the perinatal outcome, the Cochrane data base indicates that, even though no statistically significant differences on perinatal mortality were observed, there is not enough evidence to precisely evaluate the risks related to the process. More projects must be carried out to determine the adverse effects as well as on the external version practice at birth or on the foetuses in non-longitudinal situation.

7. ECV procedure

Before starting the version, the woman must be informed about the importance of keeping calm. She must also know that the procedure can be uncomfortable, although it is not painful. The external version cannot be performed without her consent or when the abdominal wall shows resistance. For this reason, the woman must be aware of the importance of her cooperation.

Before the performance, the abdomen is liberally coated with ultrasonic gel in order to decrease friction and lessen the chances of an over vigorous manipulation

First of all, the baby must be moved up and away from the pelvis in the right direction in order to increase the fetal flexion. If this manoeuvre is not successful, the next version trial must not be carried out. With both hands on the surface of the baby's buttocks, they must be gently elevated. It can also be possible to try to move the baby's head towards one of both sides, but this must never be done before the buttocks have been moved. Sometimes, you may need help to handle one of the fetal poles. The relaxation of the uterus, abdomen and legs and the Trendelenburg position will facilitate the maneuver.

Secondly, the baby's must be move by palpating the backbone. This can be achieved by using both hands simultaneously. While with one hand, the babies feet are moved upwards, with the other hand the baby's head must be moved to the opposite side and towards the pelvis. The rotation must continue until achieving the optimal vertex position (SEGO, 2001).

It must not be performed any sudden manoeuvres, but moderate and sustained pressure, trying that the fetus make the rest of the movement. Basically, the purpose is that the fetus itself finds a more comfortable position than the one that it has under pressure.

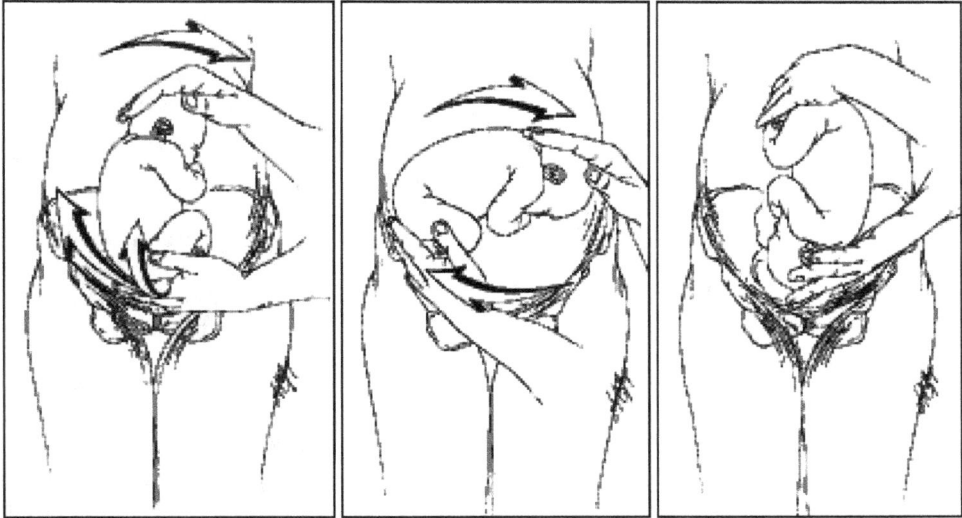

Fig. 2. Maneuvers to secure the cephalic presentation in fetuses with breech presentation.

During the maneuver the fetal presentation must be monitored with the ultrasound scan and the fetal cardiac frequency with continuous cardiotocography. Transitional fetal bradycardia commonly occurs. It is spontaneously solved in most of cases. However, the version must be stopped if it is sustained and still continues after relieving the pressure. It will also be stopped if it does not succeed after a short period of time or in case of severe pain. The benefit of performing the version without anesthesia is that the pain suffered is an indicator of the limit of pressure in the maneuver. Furthermore, the use of epidural analgesia has not proved neither a greater success in the maneuver, nor a reduction in subsequent caesarean rate (Hofmeyr, 2003). After the procedure, the tocolytics perfusion will be stopped and the success of the manoeuvre will be confirmed by ultrasound scanning.

Regardless of the success or the failure of the version, the fetal status must be evaluated again after performing the procedure. The fetus must be monitored for at least 45 minutes. If the cardiotocographic record is normal and there is no vaginal bleeding or pain, the patient can be discharged, although a 24 hour relative rest will be recommended.

If this technique does not succeed and the fetus returns to breech presentation, the version can be repeated after 5-7 days. It is estimated that 5-10% of the fetus return to the presentation previous to the version, as the cause that generated the abnormal presentation continues. This spontaneous reversion is more common in multiparous than in nulliparous mothers. However, there is no scientific evidence recommending the immediate labor induction in order to reduce the possibility of reversion (American College of Obstetricians and Gynecologist [ACOG], 2001).

Rh (-) patients will be given anti-D gamma globulin after the version, as it is estimated that the risk of fetomaternal hemorrhage is approximately 1%.

8. ECV: Prerequisites

The following prerequisites are necessary before performing an external version:

- Informed consent signed by the pregnant.
- Absence of contraindications.
- Previous checking of fetal wellbeing (reactive NST [Non Stressing Test]).
- Ultrasound scanning to reveal any contraindications in order to perform the method instead of a vaginal delivery. It will also be useful to know: the fetal estimated weight, the fetus presentation, position and situation, the amniotic fluid index, and the location of the placenta and of the umbilical cord. Using an ultrasound scan while performing the maneuver is very advantageous.
- Performance of the procedure near a operating theatre equipped for an emergency caesarean, in case of potential severe complications.
- The pregnant woman must be placed in the supine position, in semi-Fowler and with a light Trendelenburg in order to facilitate the buttocks move.
- Insertion of an intravenous (IV) to perfuse uterine relaxants (a ritodrine dose of 200 µg/min).

9. ECV: Contraindications

The Spanish, British and Canadian obstetrics and gynaecology association agree that there is not enough evidence to draw up a contraindication list. Nevertheless, they do take into account some situations that seem to be related to an increase in morbidity and mortality. Among them, the following can be considered:

- Fetal compromise or suspected fetal compromise (abnormal RGTC)
- Placenta praevia
- Abruptio placentae
- Vaginal bleeding in the previous seven days.
- Oligohydramnios
- Intrauterine fetal demise.
- Severe malformations.
- Rupture of membranes.
- Multiple gestation.
- RH isoimmunization.

- Severe uterine anomaly.
- Alterations of coagulation.
- Existence of some caesarean delivery indicators.

Determining which situations could be considered as relative contraindications is more difficult, but the following are some of them:

- Hypertensive disorders during pregnancy (preeclampsia with proteinuria).
- Delayed fetal growth with alteration in uteroplacental Doppler flow.
- Deflexed fetal head.
- Estimated weight >3800-4000 grams.
- Anterior placenta.
- Already initiated labour.
- Unstable fetal position.
- Regarding the previous caesarean, there are not any randomised projects yet, so there are not enough data to advise for or against performing it in this situation.

10. ECV: Predictors and success rate

The spontaneous version rate in nulliparous women, as of the 36th week, is 8%. However, if the version is not successful, this rate is only 5%. The probability of reversion after a successful version is only 5%.

Depending on the series, the external version success oscillates between 30-80%. This success also depends on the race, parity, uterine tone, amniotic fluid volume, cephalic engagement, possibility of palpation of cephalic pole and use of tocolytics. The highest success rates have been observed in multiparous nonwhite women with relaxed uterus, when the breech presentation is not fixed and the cephalic pole can be easily palpated (Lau et al, 1997). This would be the optimal condition in order to obtain a successful version.

Many authors have been looking for patterns aiming at predicting the cephalic version success or failure (Newman et al, 1993). Those factors considered as the most significant tones in a failed external version are the following: the cephalic pole palpation, the engagement presentation level and a tense uterus when palpated. When these factors are missing, the probability of a failed external version is only 6%. However, the failure probability increases over 80% if more than one of these three factors occurs. Thus, in a group composed of 243 pregnant women subject to an external cephalic version, the ECV was successful in 94% of the cases when none of these factors occurred, as well as in at least 20% of the cases if two of those factors occurred and 0% of the cases if the three factors took place.

Nevertheless, other factors considered as significant independent predictors in the past, as the placental location, the backbone position, the breech type, the maternal body mass index and the fetal weight seem to be less significant if the three factors mentioned above are controlled (they are not independent factors). However, it must be taken into account that the usefulness of these indicators is still awaiting confirmation by further research.

Even though some projects reveal that the higher amniotic fluid volume is, the more successful ECV can be. This statement has not been proved yet and it can also imply a higher number of spontaneous revisions.

Pregnant women should be informed that approximately 50% of those external versions performed by an experienced professional are successful, even though the results must be separately identified for each patient (level of recommendation B) (RCOG, 2006).

11. Making the ECV easier

The procedures that have proved their usefulness in randomized studies are only the tocolytics aiming at relaxing the uterus at the version.

In a 2005 *Cochrane*'s review, tocolytics were related to a reduction of the failure risk in external cephalic version both with nulliparous and multiparous women, as well as to a reduction in the caesarean rate. In the "tocolytic groups" the achievement of the external cephalic version in a minute and the fetal bradycardia was less common. These results are valid for tocolytics such as ritodrine, salbutamol and terbutaline (both by an intravenous or subcutaneous injection). However, no evidence has been proved in order to use other tocolytics suggested in other projects (such as the intravenous nitroglycerin, sublingual glyceryl trinitrate or nifidipine). Thus, pregnant women should be warned about the tocolytics adverse effects (evidence level Ia and recommendation level A).

In the same revision it was concluded that despite the fact that many multiple studies have been carried out, there is not enough scientific evidence proving the use of epidural analgesia, vibroacoustic stimulation or amnioinfusion in order to facilitate the version.

A small prospective study published in 2010 concluded that the factors increasing the probability of success and reducing the rate of adverse effects in ECV are a single attempt at the maneuver, total duration of the maneuver of less than 5minutes, and use of salbutamol as a uterine relaxant (Delgado et al, 2010).

There were contradictory results regarding the outcomes using the epidural or spinal analgesia to facilitate the version maneuvers. Therefore, the use of regional analgesia in order to facilitate the external cephalic version cannot be recommended.

In the case of the acoustic stimulation of the fetus, there is a small project which proved a significant reduction in the external cephalic version failure rate in midline fetal spine positions. Nevertheless, as this project is small, the confirmation of the results by other projects is necessary before including this procedure into the clinical practice.

No randomized clinical studies on the amnioinfusion practices as a method to facilitate the external version were found.

12. ECV: The right moment for its performance

The external version should be performed as of the 37th week (at term). The reasons for this recommendation are the following: the fetus is mature and, in case any problem takes place, the labour can be induced easily. Moreover, the spontaneous cephalic versions without trying the external cephalic version or the reversion after a successful external cephalic version are less common at term.

The *Cochrane*'s meta-analysis on cephalic versions in fetus at term (at least 37 weeks) evidently prove that the possibility of breech presentation and the caesarean practice can be substantially reduced without significantly increasing the perinatal mortality. As a result, there are many reasons for the clinical use of the external cephalic version at term (with the suitable precautions) in any pregnant woman where the cephalic vaginal delivery probability overcomes the version risk.

However, another *Cochrane*'s meta-analysis in pregnancies at term indicated that the early external cephalic version (from the 32nd to the 37th week) has not proved any significant effect on the position of the fetus at term (from the 38th to the 40th week) or on the caesareans incidence or perinatal results. In view of the absence of evidence on the effectiveness of the early external cephalic version and the existence of (observational) studies which relate it to higher risks, no procedure can be currently recommended.

Controlled and randomized studies have established that external cephalic version at term increases the probability of cephalic presentation at delivery and that, therefore, the necessity of a caesarian is reduced. However, the success rates are low (particularly in North America and Europe). The ECV studies at term carried out in Africa expressed high success rates. However, these results were not repeated in the studies from North America and Europe. It was suggested that this situation could be caused by the pelvic structure differences in white women, making the fetus prematurely engage and, thus, hampering the ECV.

In order to solve this problem and with the purpose of increasing the success rates, the University of Toronto carried out a pilot study to determinate if the ECV at preterm (at th 34th or 35th week) could be more effective than when started at term (≥ the 37th-38th week). This study was aimed at reducing the breech presentation rates at delivery if the procedure was previously performed. If the breech presentation rate was finally reduced, an wider study to consider the caesarean rates, fetal results and neonatal adverse results should be carried out. It was observed an significant reduction both in the cephalic presentation rates at delivery (9,5%) and in the caesareans (7%). However, these results were not relevant enough since the sample was very small. No differences in the neonatal results from both groups were shown. Apart from that, the reversion rate in breech presentation was low in both groups. Besides, most of women stated that they could consider the ECV in prospective pregnancies. That shows an increase of the acceptance level (Hutton et al, 2003).

These results show that the ECV at the 34th-35th week could be more effective than ECV at term. Taking into account that the caesarian rate decreased 9% (~10%) with ECV at the 34th week, 10 patients should be treated (NNT) in order to prevent 1 caesarian. This means that only 10 women would need a preterm ECV (instead of receiving a ECV at term) in order to avoid 1 caesarean. However, these results must be reconfirmed by a wider study. The fetal safety and the preterm version must also be verified before recommending a change in the clinical practice. The *Early External Cephalic Version 2 Trial* project has been recently approved (in May, 2007). This project will indicate if early ECV is better than ECV at term in order to avoid the caesarean delivery (University of Toronto, 2007).

13. ECV: Adverse effects

The external version is a procedure that is not exempt from potential problems. Nonetheless, if it is properly performed, the risk of complications is low. The Cochrane's systematic review on the external cephalic version in babies at term concluded that the ECV reduced breech presentations and caesareans, without expressing statistically significant differences on perinatal mortality. However, there is not enough evidence to specifically assess the risks related to the procedure.

The available information from the isolated observational studies and classical obstetrics books describe many complications such as hemorrhage, rupture of membranes, umbilical cord arround the fetal neck, placental abruption, start of labour, fetomaternal transfusion, uterine rupture and fetal demise. The most common complication among the described complications is the fetal bradycardia which, as it has already been said, is spontaneously solved in most of the cases when the manoeuvre is stopped. It seems to be due to a temporary fetal hypoxia caused by an increased pressure generated by the uteroplacental blood flow alteration during the version manoeuvres. After the version, the nonreactive CTGR (Cardiotocography Registry), which are temporary as well, are less common. If the bradycardia continues, a caesarean must be urgently performed. For all these reasons, it is recommended to perform the technique in an appropriate room for the immediate care of the aforementioned complications. However, given the low rate of described complications, specifically incomparison with the vaginal delivery, it is not necessary to perform a patient's presurgical preparation (previous absolute diet, premedication prior to general anesthesia or peripheral venous cannulation).

Some temporary Doppler alterations in the umbilical and middle cerebral arteries, as well as an increase in the amniotic fluid volume after the version have also been described The reasons for these alterations are currently unknown. Studies about the posible ECV effects over the fetal blood circulation revealed a reduction in the pulsatility of the middle cerebral artery. However, there were not any modifications in the umbilical artery. Therefore, it does not seem to change the placental blood flow. Furthermore, the reduction in the rate of pulsatility of the middle cerebral artery was more common in multiparous, in posterior placenta or if the procedure was difficult. However, it was not related to the fact that the version was successful (Lau et al, 2000). A recently released article associates the changes in the pulsatility rate with the pressure on the uterine wall during the manoeuvre and also reveals variations in the middle cerebral artery in cases of posterior placenta, as well as in the umbilical artery when it is lateral (Leun et al, 2004). In any case, it seems to be a physiological response and it has never been related to a negative perinatal result.

Once the cephalic version has been completed, many complications have been proved at delivery, such as greater frequency of labor dystocia, risk of fetal suffering, caesarean caused by birth anomalies and induction failure. The reasons for these complications are unknown and they are not clearly related to the version procedure itself. After having analyzed 169 successful versions in a project, it was observed a caesarean rate at delivery 2,25 times higher in comparison with the control group (fetus with spontaneous cephalic presentation). This increase was due to the higher fetal suffering rate and dystocias. It was also proved an increase in the instrumental vaginal birth (Lau et al, 1997). A higher risk of dystocia and fetal suffering in cephalic presentation after version may require a more careful intrapartum monitoring.

Given the absence of clinical evidence available about the possible adverse effects and their real consequences two meta-analyses have been recently released. The purpose of these analyses was to analyse the adverse effects related to the extreme version procedure, as well as to know its frequency. The most common adverse effects found were the CTGR alterations (between 1% and 47%, depending on the series), specially fetal bradycardia. Most of these alterations are temporary, as they are solved between the first 5 and 60 minutes. The prolonged decelerations that required an emergency caesarean only represented 1,1%, and in all cases the fetuses were born in good condition. There was no increase in the significant risk of nuchal cord in pregnant women subject to external version in comparison with the pregnant women with breech presentation where the version was not performed. The projects describe only 0,054% of cord prolapse cases (Nassar et al, 2006), which is a really low risk compared with the risk in breech or transverse presentation fetus with premature rupture of membranes. The vaginal bleeding after the version occured in approximately three in a thousand pregnants. The incidence of placenta abruption occurred in 0,12%, which is lower than the 0,34%, which represents the at term pregnant overall population. Other reviews, however, did not find any case in its series. Concerning the fetal adverse effects, the femoral fracture also has to be mentioned, occurring one only case among all of them.

The incidence of fetal demise after the procedure was 1,64 in a thousand versions performed. Thus, it was not clearly related to the external version and none of the cases occurred during the first 24h after the procedure. Anyway, this figure is not higher than antepartum fetal demise (between the 36th and the 40th week) rate (6,2 in a thousand newborns).

Concerning the maternal adverse effects found, the external version can be painful for the patient. Approximately 35% of the pregnants suffer mild discomfort during the version and 5% severe pain. The procedure may be stopped for this reason, and it has been observed that when the version fails the pain is higher than when it succeeds. The available data about the use of analgesia during the manoeuvre are still few. 4% suffered tachycardia or palpitations, which were solved one hour later without the use of medication. In less than 2% of the cases, it occurred fetomaternal transfusion. The results did not show any significant differences concerning the start of labour during the 24h after the version compared with the breech presentations where the version was not performed.

Basically, the data released in the two only meta-analyses reveal a low complication rate and show the external cephalic version as a safe procedure. Nevertheless, new projects supporting the aforementioned results are strongly needed.

Pregnant women should be informed of the possible (although in a low rate) complications of the external version (recommendation level B).

14. ECV: Quality indicators

The auditable standards for the external version are:

- Detection of antepartum breech presentation.
- Percentage of patients with breech presentation who are offered the external version.
- Version success figures.
- Complications occurring during or after the maneuver.
- Maternal experience of the version.

15. ECV: Associated costs

A 2001 British project analyses the hospital costs derived from the external version. The purpose was to determine the difference of costs between performing an external version, a vaginal delivery or a caesarean delivery for the breech presentations. The costs were calculated for the "accepted ECV" vs. "non-accepted ECV" option. Both options included the probable emergence of adverse effects, as well as the different deliveries (breech presentation, cephalic, planned caesarean, emergency caesarean, etc.) The results proved £248-£376 saving per patient. Therefore, offering ECV implies lower hospital costs than if it was not offered. An obstetrics service offering daily ECV will be cheaper than a service which does not offer it (James et al, 2001).

A cost-benefit analysis was also carried out including the *The Term Breech Trial* data. Surprisingly, it demonstrated that healthcare costs in the caesarean group were less than those produced in the vaginal delivery group. It also proved that there were not any differences regarding parity. Even though the caesarean intrapartum costs were higher, the vaginal delivery patients need more antepartum and intrapartum care as well as the babies, who need more intensive and intermediate cares, apart from the costs related to the epidural analgesia. Many studies expressing higher healthcare costs in induced labor or oxytocin stimulation have been published (Bost, 2003). These results show that the caesarean in breech presentation at term, despite being safer, it is also cheaper than vaginal labour (Palencia et al, 2006). However, this statement cannot be taken for granted, since the analysis did not take into account the long term costs (in prospective pregnancies, for instance) as well as the maternal risks.

16. ECV: Alternatives

Other methods used to correct the fetal position are acupuncture, homeopathy and postural methods. There is an awakening interest in exploring alternative medicines during pregnancy and labour. This interest is especially important in the case of external version alternatives since this is considered as s "dangerous" manoeuvre by pregnant women. The alternative medicine has become so important that *Cochrane* has carried out some reviews on the effectiveness of these methods, in particular, those referring to postural methods and the moxibustion use in cephalic version.

Throughout the history, midwives and doctors have used many different techniques referring to the best position to facilitate the cephalic version. However, few articles have been published about this topic in the medical literature. The knee-chest position and the supine position with the pelvis elevated with a wedge-shaped cushion are the most common techniques. The available evidence from the controlled clinical trials is so far insufficient to uphold the use of postural methods (Hofmeyr et Kulier, 2000).

Moxibustion is a type of Chinese medicine which involves burning a herb close to the skin in order to cause a heating sensation. It has also been stated that the acupuncture point called Bladder 67 (BL67) (or *Zhiyin*, according to its Chinese name) placed on the top of the fifth toe can correct breech presentations. How it works is totally unknown, but it seems to stimulate the production of maternal hormones (placental estrogens and prostaglandin) and the uterine contractions, as well as the fetal activity. In spite of not having found any adverse effects, Cochrane did not find enough evidence to prove that the moxibustion might be useful for correcting a breech presentation. The results suggest that moxibustion may be effective to reduce the external cephalic version need and caused a reduction in the use of oxytocin. However, some additional evidence is needed to confirm (or to reject) a benefit with respect to the breech presentation correction (Coyle et al, 2005; Hutton & Hofmeyr, 2006).

Therefore, there is not enough scientific evidence to recommend neither postural methods nor moxibustion to facilitate the spontaneous cephalic version (recommendation level A).

17. Conclusions

The ECV is safe and useful for reducing caesarean rates. The external version success goes from 30% to 80%. The experience of the obstetrician who performed the technique plays a key role in ensuring success (Fandino et al, 2010). An obstetrics service offering daily ECV will be cheaper than a service which does not offer it (James et al, 2001). Tocolycs are recommended to be used during the manoeuvre to reduce adverse effects and increase the success rate.

18. References

American College of Obstetricians and Gynecologist. Clinical Management Guidelines for Obstetricians-Gynecologists. External cephalic version. Int J Gynecol Obstet 2001; 72: 198-204.

Bost BW. Caesarean delivery on demand: what will it cost? Am J Obstet Gynecol 2003; 188:1418-23.

Coyle ME, Smith CA, Peat B. Cephalic version by moxibustion for breech presentation. Cochrane Database Syst Rev. 2005 Apr 18;(2):CD003928.

Danielian PJ, Wang J, Hall MH. Long term outcome by method of delivery of fetuses in breech presentation at term: population based follow up. BMJ 1996; 312:1.451-3.

Delgado JC, Fandino E, Duenas JL, Carrasco A. Analysis of factors influencing the development of adverse effects in the external cephalic version. Prog Obstet Ginecol. 2011;54:60-4.

Enkin M, Keirse JN, Renfrew M, Neilson J, A Guide to Effective Care in Pregnancy and Childbirth, Second Edition, Oxford University Press (1995)

Fandino E, Duenas JL, Delgado JC; Carrasco A, Bedoya C. Obstetrics and perinatal results on the introduction of an external cephalic version program. Prog Obstet Ginecol. 2010; 53(02): 41-5 - vol.53 núm 02.

Hall MH, Bewley S. Maternal mortality and mode of delivery. Lancet 1999; 354:776.

Hannah ME, Hannah WJ, Hewson SA, Hodnett ED, Saigal S, et al. Planned caesarean section versus planned vaginal birth for breech presentation at term: a randomised multicentre trial. Term Breech Trial Collaborative Group. Lancet 2000; 356:1375-83.

Hannah ME, Hannah WJ, Hodnett ED, Chalmers B, Kung R, William A. Outcomes at 3 months after planned cesarean vs planned vaginal delivery for breech presentation at term. JAMA 2002; 287(14):1822-31.

Hannah ME, Whyte H, Hannah WJ. Maternal outcomes at 2 years after planned caesarean section versus planned vaginal birth for breech presentation at term: The international randomized Term Breech Trial. American Journal of Obstetrics and Gynecology 2004;191, 917-27.

Health Canada. Canadian Perinatal Surveillance System: Canadian perinatal health report, 2000.Ottawa: Minister of Public Works and Government Services Canada, 2000.

Hodnett ED, Hannah ME, Hewson S, Whyte H, Amankwah K, Cheng M, Gafni A, Guselle P, Helewa M .Mothers' views of their childbirth experiences 2 years after planned Caesarean versus planned vaginal birth for breech presentation at term, in the international randomized Term Breech Trial. J Obstet Gynaecol Can. 2005 Mar;27(3):224-31

Hofmeyr GJ, Hannah ME. Review Planned caesarean section for term breech delivery. [Cochrane Database Syst Rev. 2003]

Hofmeyr GJ, Kulier R. Review Cephalic version by postural management for breech presentation. Cochrane Database Syst Rev. 2000 (2): CD000051.

Hofmeyr GJ. Interventions to help external cephalic version for breech presentation at term (Cochrane Review). The Cochrane Library, Issue 1, 2003. Oxford: Update Software.

Hogle KL, Kilburn L, Hewson S, Gafni A, Wall R, Hannah ME. Impact of the international term breech trial on clinical practice and concerns: a survey of centre collaborators. J Obstet GynaecolCan 2003; 25:14-6.

Hutton EK, Hofmeyr GJ. External cephalic version for breech presentation before term. Cochrane Database Syst Rev. 2006 Jan 25; (1):CD000084. Epub 2006 Jan 25.

Hutton EK, Kaufman K, Hodnett E, Amankwah K, Hewson SA, McKay D, Szalai JP, Hannah ME for the Early External Cephalic Version Trial Group. External cephalic version beginning at 34 weeks gestation versus 37 weeks gestation: a randomized multicenter trial. Am J Obstet Gynecol 2003;189:245-54.

James M, Hunt K, Burr R. A decision analytical cost analysis of offering ECV in a UK district general hospital BMC Health Services Research 2001, 1:6. This article is available from: http://www.biomedcentral.com/1472-6963/1/6

Lau TK, Lo KWK, Chan LYS, Leung TY, Lo YMD. Cell-free fetal DNA in maternal circulation as a marker of feto-maternal haemorrhage in patients undergoing external cephalic version near term. Am J Obstet Gynecol 2000;183: 712–716

Lau TK, Lo KWK, Dan W et al. Predictors of succeful external cephalic version at term: a prospective study. Br J Obstet Gynaecol 1997;104: 798-802.

Lau TK, Lo KWK, Rogers M. Pregnancy outcome after successful external cephalic version for breech presentation at term. Am J Obstet Gynecol 1997;176: 218–223.

Leung TY, Sahota DS, Fok WY, Chan LW, Lau TK. External cephalic version induced fetal cerebral and umbilical blood flow changes are related to the amount of pressure exerted BJOG: An International Journal of Obstetrics and Gynaecology 2004; 111 (5), 430–435.

Lydon-Rochelle M, Holt VL, Martin DP, Easterling TR. Association between method of delivery and maternal rehospitalization. JAMA 2000;283:2411-6.

Maternal, Infant and Reproductive Health Research Unit. Trial protocol; Early External Cephalic version 2. University of Toronto. February 2007.

Minkoff H, Chervenak FA. Elective primary cesarean delivery. N Engl J Med 2003; 384(10):946-50.

Nassar N, Roberts CL, Barratt A, Bell JC, Olive EC, Peat B. Systematic review of adverse outcomes of external cephalic version and persisting breech presentation at term Paediatric and Perinatal Epidemiology 2006; 20 (2), 163–171.

Newman RB, Peacock BS, VanDorsten JP, Hunt HH. Predicting success of external cephalic version. Am J Obstet Gynecol 1993;169:245-50.

Palencia R, Gafni A, Hannah ME, et al. The costs of planned cesarean versus planned vaginal birth in the Term Breech Trial. CMAJ 2006;174(8):1109-13.

Palencia R, Gafni A, Hannah ME, Ross S, Willan AR, Hewson S, McKay D, Hannah W, Whyte H, Amankwah K, Cheng M, Guselle P, Helewa M, Hodnett ED, Hutton EK, Kung R, Saigal S; Term Breech Trial Collaborative Group. The costs of planned cesarean versus planned vaginal birth in the Term Breech Trial. CMAJ. 2006 Apr 11;174(8):1109-13.

Rietberg, C. C. T. Elferink-Stinkens, P. M. Visser, G. H. A. The effect of the Term Breech Trial on medical intervention behaviour and neonatal outcome in The Netherland: an analysis of 35 453 term breech infants. BJOG: An International Journal of Obstetrics and Gynaecology 2005; 112: 205-209.

Royal College of Obstetricians and Gynaecologists. External cephalic version and reducing the incidence of breech presentation. Guideline N°20, December 2006

Royal College of Obstetricians and Gynaecologists. The Management of Breech Presentation. Guideline N° 20, June 2006.

Sociedad Española de Ginecología y Obstetricia. Parto en presentación de nalgas. Protocolos de Procedimientos Diagnósticos y Terapéuticos en Obstetricia N° 34, Octubre 2001.

Sociedad Española de Ginecología y Obstetricia. Versión externa en presentación de nalgas. Protocolos de Procedimientos Diagnósticos y Terapéuticos en Obstetricia N° 18, Octubre 2001.

Waterstone M, Bewley S, Wolfe C. Incidence and predictors of severe obstetric morbidity: casecontrol study. BMJ 2001;322:1089-94.

Whyte H, Hannah M, Saigal S, Term Breech Trial Collaborative Group. Outcomes of children at 2 years of age in the Term Breech Trial. American Journal of Obstetrics and Gynecology 2003;189:S57.

12

Blood Parameters in Human Fetuses with Congenital Malformations and Normal Karyotype

Chantal Bon[1], Daniel Raudrant[2], Françoise Poloce[1],
Fabienne Champion[2], François Golfier[2], Jean Pichot[1] and André Revol[3]
[1]Department of Biochemistry, Hospital Croix-Rousse, Lyon
[2]Department of Gynecology – Obstetrics, Hospital Lyon-Sud, Pierre-Bénite Cedex
[3]Department of Biochemistry, Hospital Lyon-Sud, Pierre-Bénite Cedex
France

1. Introduction

Congenital malformations can be defined as structural anomalies arising during the periods of embryogenesis and organogenesis (Roux, 2001).

However, during the fetal period, various external factors of infectious, vascular or toxic origin can also interfere with the development of previously formed structures (Gallot, 2002).

The causes of malformations are either endogenous (genetic) or exogenous, and there are probably interactions between the genetic and the exogenous factors (Roux, 2001). The precise cause of the malformation process, however, is most often unknown and the underlying physiopathological mechanisms are not elucidated (Brent, 1986).

The biology of fetal blood has been widely described in cases of isolated intra-uterine growth restriction (Cox et al., 1988; Economides et al., 1989; Weiner et al., 1989; Pardi et al., 1989; Roberts et al., 1999) but few studies have been conducted in fetuses with morphological anomalies (Bocconi, 1997; Lallata, 1998), and their biochemical profile remains little known.

We present the results of a study on 53 pregnancies with the complication of congenital malformations of variable expression and severity, and during which a fetal blood sampling was performed for fetal karyotyping. The gestational age ranged from 21 to 38 weeks of amenorrhea (average age: 28.5 ±4.45 WA). The karyotype proved to be normal for all the fetuses in this group.

The acid-base balance (pH, pCO_2, bicarbonate concentration) and the oxygenation level of the fetuses (pO_2, SaO_2) were evaluated on umbilical venous blood (UVB), taken by cordocentesis. At the same time, the glucose, lactate, free fatty acid, aceto-acetate, beta-hydroxybutyrate and cholesterol concentrations were measured, being essential biochemical constituents in relation to the nutritional status.

The aim of the work was to identify cases of fetal suffering and / or malnutrition, and to define the blood chemistry profile of this fetal population.

The results were compared with those of a control group of 73 healthy fetuses, with an average gestational age of 26 ± 5.7 weeks of amenorrhea, the results of which have already been published (Bon et al., 1997, 2007).

2. Materials and methods

2.1 Population studied

The pregnant women had consulted the Obstetrics department of the Hôtel-Dieu Hospital in Lyon, France (Professor D Raudrant). They were informed of the risks of fetal blood sampling and gave their consent.

The study was conducted in accordance with the recommendations of the Helsinki Declaration, paragraph II-6, and was approved by the hospital's Ethics Committee.

The gestational age at the time of blood sampling was calculated from the date of the last menstrual period, and confirmed by early ultrasound examination, carried out between 8 and 12 weeks of gestation.

2.1.1 Pathological group

This comprised 53 fetuses, with an average gestational age of 28.5 ±4.45 weeks of amenorrhea, for which the ultrasound examination had revealed one or more congenital malformations.

The various fetal anomalies found are described in table 1; in all cases, they were confirmed at birth or the end of pregnancy. The fetal blood sampling allowed a karyotype analysis which proved normal for all the fetuses in this group, so a chromosomic anomaly could be ruled out. Fetal growth was assessed in successive ultrasound examinations, by the measurement of three characteristic parameters: the transversal abdominal diameter, the biparietal diameter and the femoral length, the values being compared to those of the department's reference tables based on gestational age. Some fetuses presented growth restriction, associated with the morphological anomaly.

2.1.2 Control group

It is composed of 73 fetuses, with an average gestational age of 26.3 ±5.7 weeks of amenorrhea, in which cordocenteses were carried out for the prenatal diagnosis, due to a risk incurred by the fetus: suspicion of infection (30 cases of toxoplasmosis, 2 cases of rubella, 13 cases of varicella), fetal karyotype check (18 cases), and risk of fetal thrombopenia (10 cases). These fetuses were not affected by the suspected pathologies and had a normal karyotype; they had a normal morphology, growth and vitality for their gestational age.

All the babies were born at full term, had a birth weight above the 10th percentile of the reference curves in the department; their good health was confirmed by pediatric examination. The group studied could be regarded as similar to a reference population.

• Renal malformations	14 cases
• Obstructive uropathy, Prune Belly syndrome	1 case
• Unilateral obstructive uropathy	4 cases
• Bilateral obstructive uropathy	3 cases
• Cystic dysplasia (just 1 cyst)	1 case
• Unilateral multi-cystic renal dysplasia	3 cases
• Bilateral multi-cystic renal dysplasia	2 cases
• Digestive malformations	8 cases
• Stenosis of the small intestine with hydramnios	4 cases
• Stenosis of the oesophagus with hydramnios	2 cases
• Other digestive malformations	2 cases
• Cardiac malformations	5 cases
• Complete atrioventricular canal	1 case
• Interventricular communication	1 case
• Transposition of the major vessels	1 case
• Transposition of the large vessels, interventricular communication, interauricular communication	1 case
• Abnormal pulmonary venous return	1 case
• Malformations of the central nervous system	11 cases
• Hydrocephaly	4 cases
• Hydrocephaly and microcephaly	1 case
• Hydrocephaly and agenesis of the corpus callosum	1 case
• Microcephaly	2 cases
• Porencephalic cyst	1 case
• Spina bifida	2 cases
• Pulmonary malformations	3 cases
• Type 1 cystic adenomatoid malformation	1 case
• Type 2 cystic adenomatoid malformation	1 case
• Pulmonary hypoplasia with amniotic band syndrome	1 case
• Ascites	4 cases
• Isolated fetal ascites	3 cases
• Ascites with fetoplacental anasarca	1 case
• Multicystic hepatic tumour	1 case
• Limb reduction anomaly	1 case
• Anomaly of the extremities (club foot, club hand)	2 cases
• Genital anomaly (left ovarian cyst)	1 case
• Polymalformative syndrome	1 case
• Familial recurrent chylothorax	1 case
• Microphthalmia	1 case

Table 1. Pathological group. Fetal anomalies observed.

2.2 Sampling procedures

Fetal blood was obtained by cordocentesis from the umbilical vein, a technique carried out without maternal premedication, and only under local anesthesia at the puncture site (Daffos, 1983).

Five hundred microlitres of umbilical venous blood were collected in a heparinised syringe for gasometric and acid-base analyses, pH, partial CO_2 pressure (pCO_2), bicarbonate concentration, partial oxygen pressure (pO_2) and oxygen saturation (SaO_2).

The concentrations of ketone bodies (aceto-acetate and beta-hydroxybutyrate), free fatty acids (FFA) and cholesterol were evaluated on the same sample.

Two hundred microlitres of umbilical venous blood were collected on sodium fluoride to measure glucose and lactate, and 200 µl were collected without anticoagulant to measure hCG.

The good quality of the sample was verified, in particular the absence of contamination by maternal blood or amniotic fluid (Forestier, 1988). An immediate check was made by determining the erythrocyte group iI, and then a Kleihauer test, red and white cell count and a leukocyte differential count were carried out.

The serum hCG concentration of fetal blood was also measured, this test being proposed as a sensitive contamination marker due to the low hCG content of fetal serum, compared with that of the maternal blood and / or amniotic fluid (Dommergues et al., 1993).

Fetal blood samples were stored in ice at +4°C and transported to the laboratory immediately. The blood pH and gas measurement and the deproteinisation of the whole blood with perchloric acid for the ketone bodies determination were carried out upon receipt of the samples; the deproteinisation supernatants were decanted and kept at -20°C.

The blood was centrifuged at +4°C for the other analyses. The plasma glucose, lactate, cholesterol and hCG concentrations were determined immediately; the free fatty acid contents were determined subsequently on the plasma kept at -20°C.

The sample storage conditions were verified for the quantitative analysis carried out after freezing.

2.3 Analytical methods

The gasometric and acid-base analyses (pH, pO_2, pCO_2, bicarbonate, SaO_2) were carried out using the ABL 300 analyser (Radiometer, Copenhagen, Denmark).

The glucose and lactate concentrations were determined with the Ektachem 500 automated analyser (Kodak, New York, United States) by an enzymatic method using glucose oxidase (EC 1.1.3.4) and lactate oxidase (EC 1.13.12.4) and a measurement by reflectometry (reference interval in adult blood: 3.6 – 5.8 mmol/l for glucose and 0.7 – 2.1 mmol/l for lactate).

The total free fatty acid concentration was measured by a manual colorimetric enzymatic assay (Okabe et al., 1980), using an acyl-coenzyme A synthetase (EC 6.2.1.3), an acyl-coenzyme A oxidase (EC 1.3.3.6) and a peroxidase (EC 1.11.1.7) (Biomérieux, Marcy l'Etoile, France).

The ketone bodies content was determined by a fluorimetric enzymatic micromethod based on the measurement of NADH fluorescence (Olsen, 1971). Fluorescence was quantified on a spectrofluorimeter, the Kontron SFM (Kontron, Zurich, Switzerland), the excitation and emission wavelengths being 350 and 460 nm respectively. The reagents (lactate dehydrogenase, beta-hydroxybutyrate dehydrogenase, NADH, NAD) were supplied by Boehringer (Mannheim, Germany).

The adult blood reference values with the techniques used are from 0.018 to 0.078 mmol/l for aceto-acetate and 0.050 to 0.100 mmol/l for beta-hydroxybutyrate.

The cholesterol concentrations were measured by an enzymatic assay using a cholesterol esterase (EC 3.1.1.13) and a cholesterol oxidase (EC 1.1.3.6.) (Biomérieux, Marcy l'Etoile, France); the reference interval in adult blood is 3.6 – 7 mmol/l.

The hCG content was determined using the IMx automated analyser (Abbott Diagnostics, Abbott Park, United States), by a microparticle enzyme immunoassay.

2.4 Statistical analysis

The comparative study between the results of the control group and the pathological group was carried out using the Student's t-test (unpaired series) and the Mann-Whitney U test (non-parametric test). The search for a possible relation between different constituents measured in the umbilical venous blood was carried out by calculating the linear correlation coefficient r and the Spearman coefficient rs. The significance of the correlations was evaluated with Fisher's exact test.

In the control group, an analysis by linear regression was used to study any changes in the parameters according to gestational age (expressed as weeks of amenorrhea).

A p value below 0.05 was considered to be statistically significant.

3. Results

The results obtained from fetuses with malformations were compared with those from control fetuses, with normal growth and morphology.

The means and standard deviations were calculated for all 53 fetuses and per sub-group, with a minimum of 3 cases per category of malformation. When a type of anomaly is presented only by one or two fetuses, the results are given individually.

3.1 Gasometric and acid-base parameters in the umbilical venous blood (tables 2 and 3, figure 1)

The results were compared with norms established in the control population for the gestational age considered, as the pH, pO_2 and SaO_2 decrease physiologically in the UVB during gestation, whereas the pCO_2 and the bicarbonate concentration rise (Bon et al., 1997).

The acidemia and hypoxemia statuses were defined by pH and pO_2 values beyond a standard deviation below the mean, and the hypercapnia statuses by pCO_2 values higher by more than one standard deviation to the mean.

Only the pO_2 and the SaO_2 of the entire group (n=53) are significantly reduced when compared to the norms of the control group, whereas the other parameters have not significantly changed.

However, the results are scattered and were analysed by sub-group.

	Controls	Malformations (entire group)	Renal malformations	Digestive malformations	Cardiac malformations	Malformations of the central nervous system	Pulmonary malformations	Ascites
n	73	53	14	8	5	11	3	4
pH	7.31 0.054	7.28 0.090	7.31 0.033	7.31 0.023	7.22** 0.130	7.24** 0.125	7.23 0.049	7.28 0.107
pCO_2 (kPa)	5.99 0.85	6.17 1.27	5.79 0.67	6.02 0.58	7.62** 2.05	6.52 1.60	6.47 0.65	5.65 0.45
HCO_3^- (mmol/l)	22.16 1.90	21.46 2.45	21.73 1.86	22.77 1.44	22.92 3.73	20.04** 2.66	20.23 1.72	19.97 3.42
pO_2 (kPa)	6.02 1.69	4.89*** 1.60	5.53 1.61	4.35** 1.16	4.01** 1.27	4.38** 1.20	5.30 1.92	4.47 2.38
SaO_2	0.71 0.18	0.58*** 0.23	0.67 0.19	0.54** 0.16	0.43** 0.22	0.53** 0.24	0.61 0.24	0.54 0.35

The results are expressed as means and standard deviations.
n = number of samples
** $p < 0.01$
*** $p < 0.001$

Table 2. Gasometric and acid-base parameters in the umbilical venous blood (number of cases $\geq$ 3).

3.1.1 Renal malformations (n=14)

Four cases of moderate hypoxemia (pO_2 between 3.1 and 4.04 kPa) were found in the following pathologies: one case of Prune Belly syndrome, two cases of bilateral obstructive uropathy, and one case of multicystic renal dysplasia.

The pH is still within normal limits, whereas the pCO_2 is elevated in one case, associated with an increase in the plasma bicarbonate concentration.

The bicarbonate level is reduced in 3 cases, lying between 18 and 20 mmol/l.

3.1.2 Digestive malformations (n=8)

The pO_2 value is low for 3 fetuses, including 2 cases of duodenal stenosis and one case of oesophagus stenosis with hydramnios.

The pH and the pCO_2 remain within normal limits, while the plasma bicarbonate concentration was found to be raised in 2 cases.

3.1.3 Cardiac malformations (n=5)

This sub-group is characterised by a state of acidemia, hypoxemia and hypercapnia in 3 cases out of 5.

The mean pH and pO_2 are significantly decreased and the mean pCO_2 significantly increased, when compared with the control group values.

One case in particular of severe acidosis (pH of 6.99), both gaseous and metabolic, was observed in a fetus presenting a complex cardiopathy, with a complete atrioventricular canal.

The gasometric and acid-base balance was however found to be normal in two fetuses, one of which presented a transposition of the main vessels and the other an abnormal pulmonary venous return.

3.1.4 Malformations of the central nervous system (n=11)

The pH, pO_2, SaO_2, and bicarbonate concentration are on average significantly lower than those of the control group.

A state of acidemia, often gaseous and metabolic, is present in 5 cases, and a state of hypoxemia in 6 cases.

These anomalies are found in fetuses with hydrocephaly or spina bifida.

Also noted is one case of acidemia (pH of 7.18), associated with hypercapnia (pCO_2 of 7.99 kPa), in the presence of microcephaly linked to a cytomegalovirus (CMV) infection.

3.1.5 Pulmonary malformations (n=3)

The pH and the pO_2, and likewise the bicarbonate concentration of the UVB, are lower in a fetus presenting a major cystic adenomatoid malformation of the left lung, type 2, with the start of hydrops and hydramnios.

In the case of type 1 adenomatoid malformation, the biological balance is normal.

The third clinical case (pulmonary hypoplasia with amniotic band syndrome) is associated with acidosis (pH of 7.20) with hypercapnia (pCO_2 of 7.22 kPa); at birth, the infant presented generalised cyanosis and acute respiratory distress.

3.1.6 Ascites (n=4)

This subgroup is characterized by scattered results.

The gasometric and acid-base balance is normal in 3 cases. However, in the presence of ascites with the complication of fetoplacental anasarca, we found acidosis (pH 7.10), which was essentially metabolic (bicarbonate concentration of 14.9 mmol/l), and severe hypoxemia (pO_2 of 1.20 kPa).

3.1.7 Other malformations (isolated cases, n=8)

The gasometric balance shows acidemia, hypoxemia and hypercapnia, in the presence of a multicystic hepatic tumour.

A decrease in pO_2 is observed in the fetus presenting a genital anomaly, whereas the pH, pCO_2, and bicarbonate concentration are within the normal range.

One state of probably gaseous alcalosis, in the presence of a polymalformative syndrome, is found.

The case of chylothorax, with pleural effusion, is complicated by gaseous acidosis with moderate hypoxemia.

	Hepatic tumour	Reductional anomaly of the limbs	Anomaly of the extremities	Genital anomaly	Polymalformative syndrome	Familial recurrent chylothorax	Microphthalmia
n	1	1	2	1	1	1	1
pH	7.19*↘	7.33	7.32 7.36	7.31	7.49*↗	7.25*↘	7.36
pCO_2 (kPa)	8.56*↗	5.33	5.25 6.08	5.57	3.75*↘	7.24*↗	5.01
HCO_3^- (mmol/I)	23.9	21.1	19.9 25.6	20.9	21.5	23	21.3
pO_2 (kPa)	2.74*↘	7.28	7.01 5.91	2.97*↘	5.07	3.79*↘	7.08
SaO_2	0.23*↘	0.85	0.82 0.79	0.33*↘	0.77	0.43*↘	0.86

n = number of samples
* value outside the normality interval for the gestational age
↗ value increased
↘ value decreased

Table 3. Gasometric and acid-base parameters in the umbilical venous blood (number of cases ≤ 2).

3.2 Metabolic parameters in the umbilical venous blood (tables 4 and 5, figure 1)

The results were analysed by type of pathology and compared with the norms established for the gestational age considered.

In the reference population, the umbilical venous concentrations of the parameters studied were found to be stable during gestation, with the exception of lactate which rises physiologically (Bon et al., 2007).

The limit of normal values was set at one standard deviation more or less on either side of the mean value of the control group, except for free fatty acids and ketone bodies for which the limits were set at the 10th and 90th percentiles of the values of this group.

	Controls	Malformations (entire group)	Renal malformations	Digestive malformations	Cardiac malformations	Malformations of the central nervous system	Pulmonary malformations	Ascites
n	73	53	14	8	5	11	3	4
Glucose (mmol/l)	3.48 0.36	3.57 0.90	3.48 0.53	3.57 0.44	3.68 0.44	3.48 0.45	2.36 0.70	3.02 0.96
Lactate (mmol/l)	1.48 0.45	2.15*** 1.12	1.87* 0.64	1.86* 0.59	2.42*** 0.80	2.44*** 1.27	2.6 2.34	2.42 2.35
Free fatty acids (mmol/l)	0.125 0.046	0.138 0.049	0.177*** 0.030	0.124 0.022	0.188** 0.045	0.091* 0.045	0.130 0.032	0.142 0.044
Aceto-acetate (mmol/l)	0.111 0.059	0.126 0.084	0.128 0.093	0.178** 0.120	0.072 0.037	0.139 0.074	0.136 0.073	0.091 0.015
Beta-hydroxy-butyrate (mmol/l)	0.321 0.149	0.345 0.240	0.350 0.296	0.394 0.278	0.173 0.054	0.398 0.272	0.370 0.242	0.350 0.070
Cholesterol (mmol/l)	1.67 0.35	1.59 0.44	1.72 0.40	1.69 0.35	1.76 0.29	1.23** 0.38	1.27 0.47	1.49 0.50

The results are expressed as means and standard deviations.
n = number of samples
* $p < 0.05$
** $p < 0.01$
*** $p < 0.001$

Table 4. Metabolic parameters in the umbilical venous blood (number of cases ≥ 3).

3.2.1 Renal malformations (n=14)

Lactatemia is moderately increased in 4 cases, in relation with a fall in the pO_2.

Glycemia is no different, on average, from that of the control group; however, a low umbilical venous glucose concentration, at 2.8 mmol/l, is found in one case of multicystic renal dysplasia.

An increase in UVB free fatty acids level is also observed.

3.2.2 Digestive malformations (n=8)

Few metabolic anomalies are found, with the exception of an increase in lactatemia in 3 cases, and an increase in ketone bodies, in particular aceto-acetate, in 2 cases.

3.2.3 Cardiac malformations (n=5)

The metabolic balance shows a significant increase in lactatemia, with umbilical venous concentrations lying between 1.4 and 3.1 mmol/l; a small increase in the serum concentration of free fatty acids is also found.

3.2.4 Malformations of the central nervous system (n=11)

Hyperlactatemia is present in 6 cases, associated with a diminution in the pO_2, with lactate concentrations being between 3 and 5.4 mmol/l.

This sub-group is also characterised by a decrease in the average free fatty acid concentration, and by a significant fall in cholesterolemia. UVB cholesterol is found at a lower level than that of the control group in over 50% of cases, the lowest concentration being 0.93 mmol/l.

3.2.5 Pulmonary malformations (n=3)

Umbilical venous glucose and cholesterol concentrations are found to be reduced in the 2 cases of cystic adenomatoid malformations of the lung.

3.2.6 Ascites (n=4)

The results are within the normal range in the three cases of isolated fetal ascites.

The case of ascites with the complication of fetoplacental anasarca shows severe metabolic changes: hyperlactatemia of 5.9 mmol/l, hypoglycemia of 1.7 mmol/l, and hypocholesterolemia of 1.05 mmol/l.

3.2.7 Other malformations (isolated cases, n=8)

Hypoglycemia, hyperlactatemia, and a fall in the venous umbilical ketone bodies concentration are found in the case of multicystic hepatic tumour.

Likewise, in the two fetuses presenting anomalies of the extremities, the following are noted: elevated umbilical venous glycemia of 6.8 and 7.1 mmol/l, with maternal glycemia being 7.0 and 7.8 mmol/l respectively.

Lactatemia is significantly increased in the presence of a genital anomaly (left ovarian cyst).

A moderate rise in the lactate and ketone bodies UVB concentrations is observed in the case of familial recurrent chylothorax.

	Hepatic tumour	Reductional anomaly of the limbs	Anomaly of the extremities	Genital anomaly	Polymalformative syndrome	Familial recurrent chylothorax	Microphthalmia
n	1	1	2	1	1	1	1
Glucose (mmol/l)	2.5*↘	3.5	6.8*↗ 7.1*↗	3.6	3.7	4.0	4.6
Lactate (mmol/l)	2.9*↗	1.2	1.6 1.7	4.3*↗	1.8	2.3*↗	1.5
Free fatty acids (mmol/l)	0.076	0.179	0.068 0.135	0.087	0.117	0.113	0.134
Aceto-acetate (mmol/l)	0.020*↘	0.101	0.090 0.098	/	0.105	0.195*↗	0.110
Beta-hydroxy-butyrate (mmol/l)	0.105*↘	0.236	0.230 0.284	/	0.294	0.640*↗	0.470
Cholesterol (mmol/l)	1.20	1.45	1.92 2.34	1.43	1.82	2.17	2.43

n = number of samples
* value outside the normality interval for the gestational age
↗ value increased
↘ value decreased

Table 5. Metabolic parameters in the umbilical venous blood (n ≤ 2).

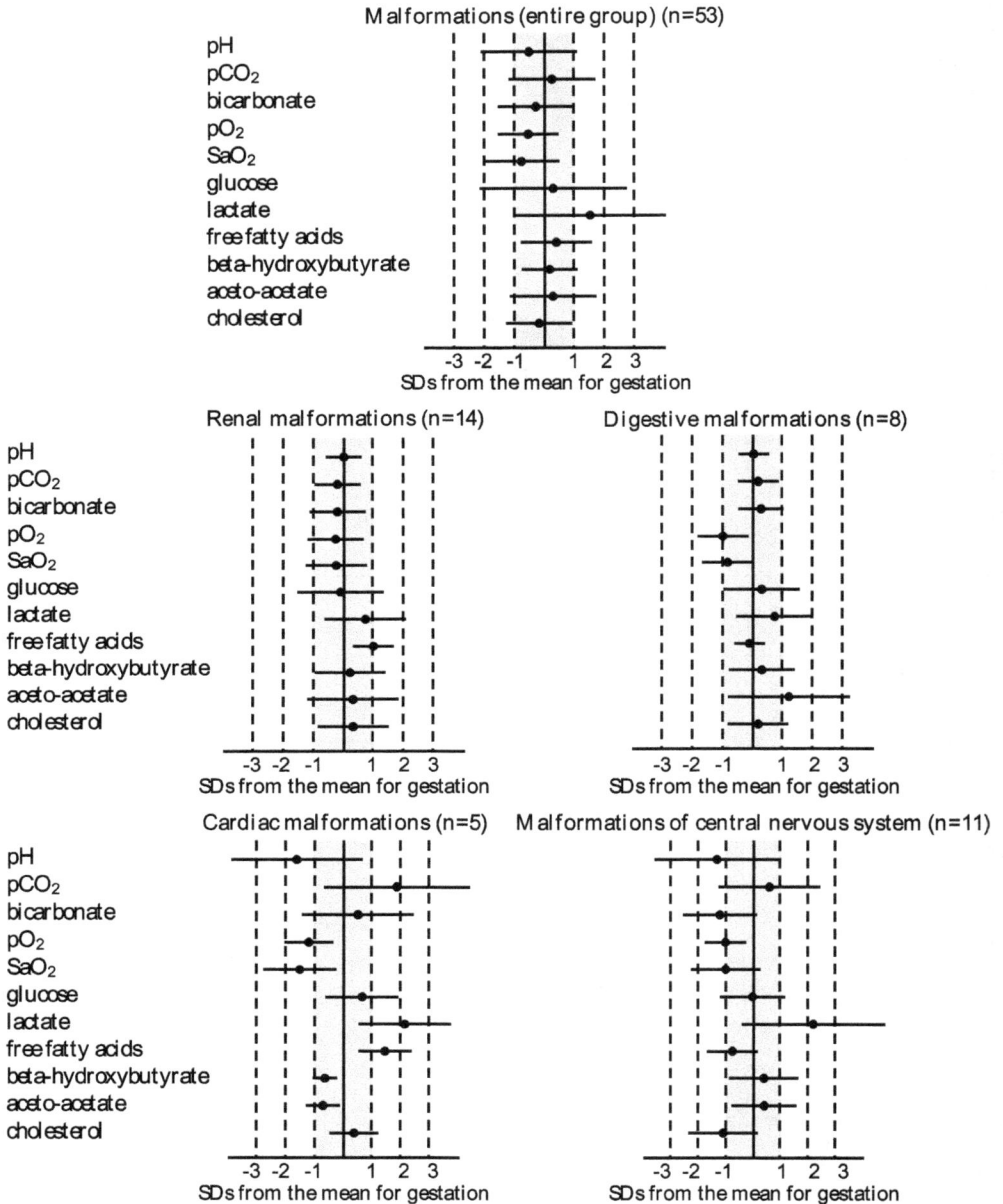

Fig. 1. Means (circles) and standard deviations (bars) of UVB constituents in pathological group and sub-groups (number of samples ≥ 5). Values are expressed as number of standard deviations (SDs) from the mean of control group. Shaded area indicates extent of reference range for the different variables.

4. Discussion

During its intra-uterine life, the conceptus can be exposed to various agents (physical, chemical and infectious) which may interfere with its development. However, they are responsible for only 5% of the congenital malformations observed, as around 5% are attributable to chromosome anomalies, 10 to 20% to hereditary diseases, and 70% due to indeterminate causes (Gallot, 2002). The fetus' response to an aggression depends mainly on its level of maturity.

We have studied 53 pathological pregnancies, for which a fetal blood sampling was performed following confirmation by ultrasound of one or more fetal malformation(s), or a risk of malformation; the population studied is characterised by its heterogeneity, as previously described.

The fetal karyotype was found to be normal in all cases.

In this context, the obstetrical decision as to whether or not to continue the pregnancy, depends principally on the prognosis associated with the malformation.

The acid-base parameters measured allow a state of fetal distress to be diagnosed, the metabolic parameters assessed characterise the level of energy supply to fetus affected by morphological anomalies, some 20% of which also presented growth restriction.

The fetal origin of the umbilical venous blood taken was carefully checked in our study protocol, in particular with the measurement of hCG serum concentration; reference values in the fetal blood were established previously for this parameter (Bon et al., 1999).

4.1 Acid-base balance and gasometric data

The pH is not significantly different, on average, from that of the control group; however, the analysis of results showed a state of acidemia to be present in 12 fetuses, i.e. 22% of the group; this relates mainly to cases of cardiac malformation, central nervous system malformations, pulmonary malformations, one case of effusion with anasarca, and one case of hepatic tumour.

The plot on a Davenport diagram of the pH and total CO_2 shows that acidosis is usually mixed: gaseous and metabolic. However, gaseous acidosis is predominant as the pH is significantly correlated with the pCO_2 ($r = -0.866$, $p < 0.001$), while the correlation between pH and plasma bicarbonate concentration is less significant ($r = 0.402$, $p = 0.003$). The pCO_2 is significantly increased in the event of cardiac malformations.

In the presence of effusion with fetoplacental anasarca and flooding with amniotic fluid, acidosis is of essentially metabolic origin, due to the high level of lactic acid in the amniotic fluid.

The most frequent gasometric anomaly is the fall in the partial oxygen pressure, present in over 40% of observations. The state of hypoxemia is not specific to any pathology; it is found in all types of malformation, with the exception of anomalies of the limbs and extremities.

Strictly fetal causes - anemia or cardiovascular failure - can be the cause of fetal hypoxia, responsible for a deviation in the metabolism towards anaerobia.

Cerebral hypoxia is often associated with a poor neurological prognosis, and depending on its severity, can be the cause of an apoptotic process. A state of hypoxemia frequently accompanies malformations of the central nervous system.

The fall in the umbilical venous pO_2 is associated in 15% of cases, with a rise in the pCO_2, leading to a state of gaseous acidosis. An impaired transplacental diffusion of respiratory gases may be the cause; indeed, placental lesions (infarct and thromboses of the villositary vessels) were indicated in some observations.

The episode of acidosis may be secondary to anomalies in development, as a fetus with malformations probably has limited regulation abilities and insufficient resources to fight against acidosis.

Conversely, a state of hypoxemia and then acidemia was able to favour the occurrence of malformations, due to a greater sensitivity of the fetus to an external, infectious, toxic aggression. An episode of acidosis may facilitate a toxic drug being passed on to the fetus, with the pH gradient between maternal blood and fetal blood influencing the transfer of certain drugs, such as weak acids (Fontaine, 2001).

4.2 Metabolic parameters

Nutritional and metabolic anomalies are less frequent and often less severe than acid-base anomalies.

The umbilical venous glucose concentration, an essential energetic substrate for the fetus, does not differ, on average, from that of the control group, which means that the hormonal factors of glycemic regulation are functional in the pathological group, with the neoglucogenesis abilities being maintained.

However, ten cases of hypoglycemia are noted, often associated with hypoxemia. A fall in blood glucose may be secondary to a fall in the transplacental passage of glucose, in parallel to the reduced diffusion of oxygen, or alternatively to a fetal or placental over-consumption of glucose, associated with an acceleration of anaerobic glycolysis; these mechanisms were mentioned with regard to severe growth retardation (Economides et al., 1989, Nicolini et al., 1989).

Fetal glycemia is low in the presence of a multicystic hepatic tumour; it is accompanied by a fall in ketone bodies and cholesterol concentrations in the umbilical venous blood; these biological results are the consequence of hepatic dysfunction. In the case of effusion with fetoplacental anasarca, the fall in the umbilical venous glycemia is probably the result of dilution by amniotic fluid.

Umbilical venous glucose was found to be elevated in some cases, in particular concentrations of 6.8 and 7.1 mmol/l are associated with maternal venous concentrations of 7.2 and 7.8 mmol/l. At these conditions, these values are the expression of a pre-diabetic or diabetic state in the mother, and this can be implicated in the occurrence of the malformation (Boivin et al., 2002, Gabbe et al., 2003).

Umbilical venous lactatemia is, on average, significantly higher in the pathological group than in the control group. Hyperlactatemia, present in 34% of observations, is secondary to hypoxia, with a significant negative correlation between pO_2 and lactate in the UVB ($r = -0.420$, $p < 0.02$). The rise in lactate may also be associated with poor lactate clearance by the placenta and is one of the components of metabolic acidosis.

Umbilical venous concentrations of free fatty acids were found to be significantly lowered in the group of fetuses with malformations of the central nervous system.

Few data are available on the maternal-fetal metabolism of free fatty acids during pathological pregnancies.

In a group of 24 patients with a pregnancy complicated by intra-uterine growth restriction (Ortega - Senovilla, 2010), an increase in free fatty acid and retinol concentrations was found in the maternal plasma, in comparison with the results of the control group; the authors put forward the hypothesis of a limitation in the transplacental transfer of retinol and free fatty acids, lower concentrations of which are found in the fetal plasma. A similar mechanism can be mentioned in the case of pregnancies complicated by fetal malformations, or alternatively an accelerated turnover of free fatty acids in the fetal compartment could be implicated.

Umbilical venous concentrations of ketone bodies and in particular beta-hydroxybutyrate are very scattered in the pathological group and do not differ, on average, from those of the control group. However, in some pregnancies, namely around 15% of cases, a moderate increase in ketone bodies concentration was found in the umbilical venous blood: in three cases of renal malformations, two cases of digestive malformations, three cases of malformations of the central nervous system and one case of pulmonary malformation.

Fetal ketone bodies can be supplied by transplacental transfer from the maternal blood (Pere et al., 2003), and there is also probably an intrinsic fetal production (Tannirandorm et al., 1999). The teratogenic action of beta-hydroxybutyrate has been suspected in certain diabetic pregnancies (Jovanovic et al., 1998).

Cholesterol, an essential constituent for embryo development and growth, is found at a reduced umbilical venous concentration in some pathological pregnancies: in the presence of renal malformations (2 cases out of 14), pulmonary malformations (2 cases out of 3), ascites with anasarca (1 case), hepatic tumour (1 case), and malformations of the central nervous system (7 cases out of 11); in this final sub-group, umbilical venous cholesterolemia is, on average, significantly lower than that of the control group.

It should be borne in mind that cholesterol is essential for the development of the central nervous system and cerebral growth (Roux et al., 1997, 2000).

Cholesterol is mainly synthesised in the fetal compartment as maternal cholesterol does not readily pass through the placenta (Carr et al., 1982).

In the pathological pregnancies, the inadequate production of cholesterol by the fetal liver may be associated with hepatic immaturity, or alternatively with defective oxygenation conditions in the fetus; we noted the frequency of cases of hypoxemia in the group of fetuses studied.

The possibility of a fetal liver disorder was reported by Roberts et al. in growth-restricted fetuses.

The decrease in cholesterolemia may be related to growth problems which are often associated with morphological anomalies. The fundamental role of cholesterol in embryo development is well established, and anomalies in cholesterol synthesis are involved in a number of human malformation syndromes (Porter et al., 2003; Guizzetti et al., 2005).

5. Conclusion

We studied a group of 53 fetuses with malformations of varying clinical expression and severity, and measured in the fetal blood essential biochemical parameters which may be associated with fetal well-being; the results obtained were compared with those from a group of 73 fetuses with normal growth and morphology.

The disparity in the populations studied make the interpretation of the results difficult. Around 20% of the pathological pregnancies are accompanied by a state of fetal distress with acid-base balance alterations. Gaseous acidosis is present in the cardiac malformations; acidosis is mixed in the malformations of the central nervous system and pulmonary malformations, and is essentially metabolic in the case of fetoplacental anasarca.

The gasometric anomaly most frequently encountered is hypoxemia, present in around 40% of observations and in almost all types of pathology.

The reduction in the umbilical venous pO_2 probably reflects an impaired transplacental transfer of respiratory gases and placental dysfunction; it may also be related to a maternal cause (such as an episode of hypoxemia), or a properly fetal cause such as fetal anemia.

Metabolic anomalies, often less common, are associated with acid-base anomalies. The decrease in umbilical venous glucose, found in 18% of the pathologies studied, leads to a suspicion of a reduced transplacental passage of glucose, in parallel to the reduced diffusion of oxygen.

Conversely, the umbilical venous hyperglycemia present in some cases, is secondary to a maternal hyperglycemia and probably associated with a diabetic or pre-diabetic state in the mother.

Changes to concentrations of lactate, free fatty acids, ketone bodies and cholesterol are markers of a disrupted fetal metabolism. Hyperlactatemia is associated with impaired oxygenation conditions and inadequate placental clearance.

The reduction in umbilical venous cholesterolemia found in some pregnancies reflects defective metabolic conditions in the fetus. It has possible consequences on fetal growth and is possibly linked to the morphological anomalies found, with cholesterol being an essential constituent for the development of the embryo.

The results obtained are however a reflection of an instantaneous measurement and the biochemical anomalies found may be a consequence of the malformations.

Moreover, in nearly 50% of cases, the blood chemistry and the in utero living conditions of the fetus with congenital malformations are not very disrupted compared with those of the normally constituted fetus.

6. Acknowledgment

We express our sincere thanks to physicians who performed fetal blood samplings and allowed us to realize this work (Department of Obstetrics and Gynecology, Hôtel-Dieu Hospital, Lyon, France).

7. References

Bocconi, L., Nava, S., Fogliani, R., Rizzuli, T. & Nicolini, U. (1997). Trisomy 21 is associated with hypercholesterolemia during intrauterine life. *Am J Obstet Gynecol*, Vol.176, No.3, pp. 540-543, ISSN 0002-9378

Boivin, S., Derdour-Gury, H., Perpetue, J., Jeandidier, N. & Pinget, M. (2002). Diabetes and pregnancy. *Ann Endocrinol* (Paris), Vol.63, No.5, pp. 480-487, ISSN 0003-4266

Bon, C., Raudrant, D., Poloce, F., Champion, F., Thoulon, JM., Pichot, J. & Revol, A. (1997). Acid-base equilibrium and oxygenation of human fetus. Study of 73 samples obtained by cordocentesis. *Ann Biol Clin*, Vol.55, No.5, pp. 455-459, ISSN 0003-3898

Bon, C., Gelineau, MC., Raudrant, D., Pichot, J. & Revol, A. (1999). Fœtal blood human chorionic gonadotropin concentrations in normal and abnormal pregnancy. *Immunoanal Biol Spec*, Vol.14, pp. 37-46, ISSN 0923-2532

Bon, C., Raudrant, D., Golfier, F., Poloce, F., Champion, F., Pichot, J. & Revol, A. (2007). Feto-maternal metabolism in human normal pregnancies: study of 73 cases. *Ann Biol Clin*, Vol.65, No.6, pp. 609-619, ISSN 0003-3898

Brent, RL. (1986). The complexities of solving the problem of human malformations. *Clin Perinatol*, Vol.13, pp. 491-503, ISSN 0095-5108

Carr, BR. & Simpson, ER. (1982). Cholesterol synthesis in human fetal tissues. *Clin Endocrinol Metab*, Vol.55, pp. 447-452, ISSN 0021-972X

Cox, WL., Daffos, F., Forestier, F., Descombay, D., Aufrant, C., Auger, MC. & Gaschard, JC. (1988). Physiology and management of intrauterine growth retardation: a biologic approach with fetal blood sampling. *Am J Obstet Gynecol*, Vol.159, No.1, pp. 36-41, ISSN 0002-9378

Daffos, F., Capella-Pavlovsky, M. & Forestier, F. (1983). Fetal blood sampling via the umbilical cord using a needle guided by ultrasound. *Prenat Diagn*, Vol.3, pp. 271-277, ISSN 0197-3851

Dommergues, M., Bunduki, V., Muller, F., Mandelbrot, L., Morichon-Delvallez, N. & Dumez, Y. (1993). Serum hCG assay: a method for detection of contamination of fetal blood samples. *Prenat Diagn*, Vol.13, pp. 1043-1046, ISSN 0197-3851

Economides, DL. & Nicolaides, KH. (1989). Blood glucose and oxygen tension levels in small for gestational age fetuses. *Am J Obstet Gynecol*, Vol.160, pp. 385-389, ISSN 0002-9378

Fontaine, P. (2001). Comment et pourquoi l'équilibre métabolique de la mère affecte-t-il l'embryon. *Diabetes Metab*, Vol.27, pp. 3S13-3S18, ISSN 1262-3636

Forestier, F., Cox, WL. & Daffos, F. (1988). The assessment of fetal blood samples. *Am J Obstet Gynecol*, Vol.158, pp. 1184-1188, ISSN 0002-9378

Gabbe, SG. & Graves, CR. (2003). Management of diabetes mellitus complicating pregnancy. *Obstet Gynecol*, Vol.102, No.4, pp. 857-868, ISSN 0029-7844

Gallot, D., Laurichesse, H. & Lemery, D. (2002). Prévention des risques fœtaux: infection, médicaments toxiques, irradiation. *La Rev du Prat*, Vol.52, pp. 751-764, ISSN 0035-2640

Guizetti, M. & Costa, LG. (2005). Disruption of cholesterol homeostasis in the developing brain as a potential mechanism contributing to the developmental neurotoxicity of ethanol: an hypothesis. *Med Hypotheses*, Vol.64, pp. 563-567, ISSN 0306-9877

Jovanovic, L., Metzger, BE., Knopp, RH., Conley, MR., Park, E. & Jack Lee, Y. (1998). The diabetes in early pregnancy study. *Diabetes Care*, Vol.21, No.11, pp. 1978-1984, ISSN 0149-5992

Lallata, F., Salmona, S., Fogliani, R., Rizzuli, T. & Nicolini, U. (1998). Prenatal diagnosis of genetic syndromes may be facilitated by serendipitous findings at fetal blood sampling. *Prenat Diagn*, Vol.18, pp. 834-837, ISSN 0197-3851

Nicolini, U., Hubinont, C., Santolaya, J., Fisk, NM., Coe, AM. & Rodeck, CH. (1989). Maternal-fetal glucose gradient in normal pregnancies and in pregnancies complicated by alloimmunization and fetal growth retardation. *Am J Obstet Gynecol*, Vol.161, pp. 924-927, ISSN 0002-9378

Okabe, H., Ujil, Y., Nagashima, K. & Noma, A. (1980). Enzymic determination of free fatty acids in serum. *Clin Chem*, Vol.26, No.11, pp. 1540-1543, ISSN 0009-9147

Olsen, C. (1971). An enzymatic fluorimetric micromethod for the determination of aceto-acetate, beta-hydroxybutyrate, pyruvate and lactate. *Clin Chim Acta*, Vol.33, pp. 293-300, ISSN 0009-8981

Ortega-Senovilla, H., Alvino, G., Taricco, E., Cetin, I. & Herrera, E. (2010). Enhanced circulating retinol and non-esterified fatty acids in pregnancies complicated with intrauterine growth retardation. *Clinical Science*, Vol.118, No.5, pp. 351-358, ISSN 0143-5221

Pardi, G., Cetin, I., Marconi, AM., Lanfranchi, A., Bozetti, S., Ferrazzi, E., Buscaglia, M. & Battaglia, FC. (1993). Diagnostic value of blood sampling in fetuses with growth retardation. *N Engl J Med*, Vol.328, No.10, pp. 692-696, ISSN 0028-4793

Pere, MC. (2003). Materno-foetal exchanges and utilisation of nutrients by the fetus: comparison between species. *Reprod Nutr Dev*, Vol.43, pp. 1-15, ISSN 0926-5287

Porter, FD. (2003). Human malformation syndromes due to inborn errors of cholesterol synthesis. *Curr Opin Pediatr*, Vol.15, No.6, pp. 607-613, ISSN 1040-8703

Roberts, A., Nava, S., Bocconi, L., Salmona, S. & Nicolini, U. (1999). Liver function tests and glucose and lipid metabolism in growth-restricted fetuses. *Obstet Gynecol*, Vol.94, No.2, pp. 290-294, ISSN 0029-7844

Roux, C., Wolf, C., Llirbat, B., Kolf, M., Mulliez, N., Taillemite, JL., Cormier, V., Le Merrer, M., Chery, F. & Citadelle, D. (1997). Cholestérol et développement. *CR Soc Biol*, Vol.191, No.1, pp. 113-123, ISSN 0037-9026

Roux, C., Wolf, C., Mulliez, N., Gaoua, W., Cormier, V., Chery, F. & Citadelle, D. (2000). Role of cholesterol in embryonic development. *Am J Clin Nutr*, Vol.71 (5 suppl), pp. 1270S-1279S, ISSN 0002-9165

Roux, C. (2001). Tératogénèse, In: *Médecine et biologie du développement*, Saliba, E., Hamamah, S., Gold, F., Benhamed, M., (108-122), Masson (ed), Paris, ISBN 2-225-83168-8

Tannirandorm, Y., Phaosavasdi, S., Numchaisrika, P., Wongwathanavikrom, R. & Leepipathpaiboon, S. (1999). Fetal metabolism. *J Med Assoc Thai*, Vol.82, No.4, pp. 383-387, ISSN 0025-7036

Weiner, CP. & Williamson, RA. (1989). Evaluation of severe growth retardation using cordocentesis - hematologic and metabolic alterations by etiology. *Obstet Gynecol*, Vol.73, pp. 225-229, ISSN 0029-7844

13

Reduced Fetal Movements

Julia Unterscheider[1] and Keelin O'Donoghue[2]
[1]*Royal College of Surgeons in Ireland, Rotunda Hospital Dublin,*
[2]*Anu Research Centre, University College Cork, Cork University Maternity Hospital,*
Ireland

1. Introduction

Maternal awareness of fetal movements serves as an indicator of fetal wellbeing and its reduction alerts clinicians to pregnancies at risk of complications. A reduction of fetal movements (FM) causes concern and anxiety, both for the mother and obstetrician, and is a common reason for referral to hospital. Decreased fetal movements affect up to 15% of pregnancies (Sergent *et al.*, 2005; Heazell *et al.*, 2008). Of those women, 85% are concerned about fetal wellbeing and 53% are afraid that the baby might die (Tveit *et al.*, 2006). The perception of reduced movements is highly subjective to the mother and has clinical significance as a predictor of adverse pregnancy outcome - therefore any concerns should be taken seriously and assessed appropriately.

Conditions associated with diminished fetal movements are summarised in Table 1 and may vary from serious clinical diagnoses such as intrauterine fetal death, intrauterine fetal growth restriction and oligohydramnios, hydrops fetalis and polyhydramnios to other causes such as fetal sleep, anterior placental location, increased body mass index, maternal smoking, metabolic and endocrine disorders or a busy mother who is simply not concentrating on fetal movements. The most common single cause of stillbirth is intrauterine fetal growth restriction (IUGR). Some reports suggest 11-29% of women presenting with reduced FM carry a small for gestational age (SGA) fetus under the 10th centile (Heazell *et al.*, 2005; Sinha *et al.*, 2007). Sergent *et al* retrospectively reviewed 160 patients complaining of reduced FM and reported 4.3% of fetuses with severe growth restriction in their cohort (Sergent *et al.*, 2005). The clinical significance of reduced FM may be unclear until pathological underlying causes have been excluded. Placental dysfunction has been identified as a key factor in pregnancies affected by diminished FM (Warrander *et al.*, 2011). There are a wide variety of investigations available, some of which are not proven to be useful in the detection of a fetus at risk or to promote timely intervention. This can lead to unnecessary investigation of otherwise uncomplicated pregnancies, which results in maternal anxiety, inconvenience and increased obstetric intervention.

The Confidential Enquiry into Stillbirths and Deaths in Infancy (CESDI) under the umbrella of the National Institute for Clinical Excellence (NICE) collected and analysed data of deaths between 20 weeks gestation and one year of life. In their 8th annual report they reviewed 422 stillbirths and found that 45% of them were associated with suboptimal care; 69 cases (16.4%) were related to altered or reduced fetal movements. Concerns were raised over the failure of (a) the mother to report reduced FM, (b) the clinician explaining the importance of changes in FM to the woman and (c) professionals to act appropriately when decreased FM occur.

Intrauterine fetal death (IUD)
Fetal sleep
Fetal position
Fetal congenital malformation (i.e. neurological, musculo-skeletal)
Fetal anaemia or hydrops
Acute or chronic hypoxia from placental insufficiency leading to
i. Reduced amniotic fluid volume (oligohydramnios) or
ii. Small for gestational age fetus (SGA)/ intrauterine growth restriction (IUGR)
Polyhydramnios
Increased maternal weight
Anterior placental localisation
Maternal sedating drugs which cross the placenta (alcohol, benzodiazepines, barbiturates, methadone, narcotics)
Smoking
Administration of corticosteroids for promotion of fetal lung maturity
A busy mother who is not concentrating on fetal activity
Maternal anaemia, metabolic disorders, hypothyroidism
Acute or chronic feto-maternal haemorrhage

Table 1. Conditions associated with maternal perception of reduced fetal movements (Unterscheider *et al.*, 2009)

In February 2011, the Royal College of Obstetricians & Gynaecologists has issued a clinical practice guideline (Green-top Guideline 57) on the management of reduced fetal movements which summarises the current evidence of how to best manage these complicated pregnancies.

This chapter provides a comprehensive overview of the clinical significance, investigation and management of reduced fetal movements in the low risk pregnant population over 24 weeks gestation. It will further provide guidance to the clinician in the critical assessment of these pregnancies to ensure high quality antepartum and intrapartum care, safe delivery and improved perinatal outcomes.

2. Physiology

Mothers usually report fetal movements from around 20 weeks gestation with a peak at 28-34 weeks gestation (Mangesi & Hofmeyr, 2007). Fetal movements have been defined as any discrete kick, flutter swish or roll (Neldam, 1983). Multiparous women may notice movements earlier (16-20 weeks gestation) than primiparous women (20-22 weeks gestation) (Grant *et al.*, 1989). FM follow a circadian pattern and are an expression of fetal wellbeing. Fetal movements are usually absent during fetal sleep, periods which usually last 20-40 minutes and rarely exceed 90 minutes (Patrick *et al.*, 1982). A recent study confirmed that fetal movements are significantly better in the evening than in the morning (Ozkaya *et al.*, 2011). A gradual decline during the third trimester is suggested to be due to improved fetal coordination and reduced amniotic fluid volume, coupled with increased fetal size (Grant *et al.*, 1989). Some ultrasound studies on fetal behaviour show that fetal movements do not become less frequent in the third trimester but that the movements change as coordination improves and a pattern of cycling becomes established.

Decreased FM are regarded as a marker for suboptimal intrauterine conditions, possibly of placental dysfunction and intrauterine stress and should alert the clinician to pregnancies at risk. The fetus responds to chronic hypoxia by conserving energy and the subsequent reduction of FM is an adaptive mechanism to reduce oxygen consumption. It is recognised that an IUD is preceeded by cessation of FM for at least 24 hours (Sadovsky & Yaffe, 1973). Over 55% of women experiencing a stillbirth perceive a reduction in fetal movements prior to diagnosis (Efkarpidis *et al.*, 2004).

3. Definition

There is a lack of consensus on how many movements are regarded as normal or abnormal. FM in a healthy fetus vary from 4 to 100 per hour (Mangesi & Hofmeyr, 2007). Maternal perception of fetal movements range from 4-94% of actual movements seen on concurrent ultrasound scanning (Heazell *et al.*, 2008). The positive predictive value of the maternal perception of reduced FM for fetal compromise is low, 2% to 7% (Macones & Depp, 1996).

Haezell *et al* recently confirmed that there is little agreement amongst midwives and obstetricians on the definition of reduced FM. Definitions ranged from less than 10 movements in 2 hours (Whitty *et al.*, 1991) to 12 and 24 hours. In this study, the maternal perception of decreased movements for 24 hours gained the greatest acceptance and the authors suggest this is currently the most appropriate method to identify reduced FM (Heazell *et al.*, 2008; Heazell & Frøen, 2008). Reports on published definitions found most midwives and obstetricians favoured the definition of less than 10 movements in 12 hours (Heazell *et al.*, 2008). This concurs with the 1976 definition of Pearson and Weaver who developed the 'count-to-ten kickchart'. Using this kickchart, women record their first 10 movements of each day, and if this is not reached after 12 hours, are advised to seek further assessment (Grant *et al.*, 1989; Heazell *et al*, 2008; Person & Weaver, 1976). A recent prospective cohort study showed that the mean time to perceive 10 movements is approximately 10 minutes in normal third trimester pregnancies (Winje *et al.*, 2011). Other studies showed that the mean time to perceive 10 movements varied between 21 minutes for focused counting to 162 minutes with unfocused perception of fetal movements (Grant et al., 1989; Moore & Piacquadio, 1989).

There is no evidence that any formal definition of reduced FM is of greater value than subjective maternal perception in the detection of fetal compromise. Therefore maternal perception of reduction or sudden alteration of fetal movements should be considered clinically important. There is currently no universally agreed definition of reduced FM.

4. Current practice

A wide range of investigations are performed for the complaint of reduced FM. Investigations considered include symphyseal fundal height measurement (SFH), cardiotocography (CTG), biophysical score (BPP), fetal weight estimation (EFW), liquor assessment, umbilical artery (UA) Doppler velocimetry, formal fetal movement counting (kickcharts) and vaginal examination. These investigations may lead to interventions such as a membrane sweep or induction of labour.

An anonymous structured web-based questionnaire recently performed amongst 96 Irish obstetricians (Unterscheider *et al.*, 2010) found that there was a lack of guidance in the management of reduced FM with only one third of clinicians having a clinical practice guideline in their institution. Table 2 summarizes the management and assessment methods. Results of this study demonstrated that CTG was the most favoured method of assessing fetal wellbeing (93%) followed by the use of kickcharts (64%), while 54% of obstetricians assessed the fetus with a biophysical score and 52% performed an ultrasound scan to assess liquor volume. Only 34% applied simple SFH measurement and 23% assessed umbilical artery Doppler velocimetry. In the same study, fetal biometry was performed by 20% of obstetricians and the same percentage offered vaginal examination to assess favourability. The minority recommended admission (2%) or induction of labour (4%). The study confirmed that clinicians apply multiple combinations of assessment methods with 98% of doctors performing more than one investigation. This highlights the uncertainty over optimal assessment methods in this common clinical scenario.

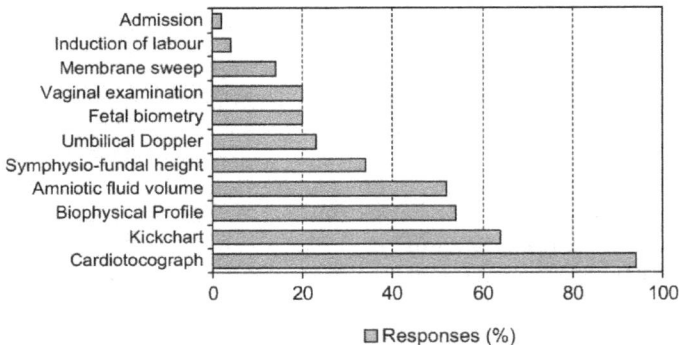

Table 2. Management and assessment methods of reduced fetal movements employed by Obstetricians in Ireland (Unterscheider *et al.*, 2010)

Haezell *et al* recently reviewed the current practice in the United Kingdom where most obstetricians (70%) had institutional guidelines available. In contrast to the Irish study they found that only 3% of midwives and 5% of obstetricians were using kickcharts in their routine antenatal care. The majority of respondents in this questionnaire performed CTG and SFH measurement. Further evaluation including fetal biometry, umbilical artery Doppler or full biophysical profile was based on results of CTG, SFH measurement and clinical situation. The most frequently reported management option for both midwives and obstetricians was to consider admission and delivery.

There are no randomised controlled trials addressing the optimal management of reduced FM. All published studies are limited by the variation in definition and outcomes. The main outcome measure of interest, stillbirth, is relatively uncommon with an incidence of 1 in 200 births in developed countries (Stanton *et al.*, 2006), therefore large scale studies would be required to answer the question of optimal management.

5. Assessment methods

5.1 Which investigations are beneficial?

5.1.1 Basic Assessment

Every patient who presents with reduced FM over 24 weeks gestation should have the following assessed:

- Detailed history/ duration of the presenting complaint.
- Risk factors in this or the previous pregnancy.
- Maternal blood pressure, pulse rate, temperature and urinalysis.
- Auscultation of the fetal heart or a CTG over 15-20 minutes (Preboth, 2000)
- Clinical examination including abdominal palpation and SFH measurement

5.1.2 Symphyseal fundal height measurement (SFH)

A clinical opinion about the size of the baby including abdominal palpation and the measurement of SFH should be part of every assessment and is helpful in the management of reduced FM. Despite the fact that abdominal palpation only detects 30% of small for gestational age fetuses (RCOG, 2002), SFH measurement has a positive predictive value of 60% and a negative predictive value of 76.8% (Heazell et al., 2005). This implies that if the SFH is within normal limits, fetal growth restriction or placental insufficiency is unlikely to be present. Serial SFH measurements have an increased specificity and sensitivity (Heazell et al, 2005; Pearce & Campbell, 1987) as the trend in growth is of more value than a single measurement in predicting poor fetal outcome. As 50-70% of fetuses with a birthweight below the 10th centile are constitutionally small (RCOG, 2002), Gardosi et al suggested that plotting measurements on customised SFH charts adjusted for maternal weight, height, parity and ethnic group results in increased detection of growth restriction and fewer hospital referrals (Gardosi & Francis, 1999). The SFH mean at 36 weeks gestation on drawn charts is 34-34.8cm (Calvert, Quaranta, Nottingham) which implies that using 'SFH in cm equals gestational age in weeks' would lead to significant over-diagnosis of SGA fetuses.

We conclude that, in the absence of anything better, the measurement of SFH and its plotting on customised charts is recommended in selecting which patients should undergo further investigation (Unterscheider et al., 2009).

5.1.3 Non stress test – Cardiotocography (CTG)

CTG it is widely accepted as the primary method of antenatal fetal monitoring to assess the current status of the fetus (Pattison & McCowan, 2000) but its use is particularly difficult and cannot be recommended before 28 weeks gestation (Preboth, 2000). Between 24 and 28 weeks gestation auscultation of the fetal heart may be sufficient and CTG can be performed. A reactive CTG is defined by two accelerations exceeding 15bpm, sustained for at least 15 seconds in a 20 minute period (Devoe, 1990). Loss of variability is associated with fetal sleep, sedation or central nervous system depression, including fetal acidosis. The absence of accelerations or appearance of decelerations along with a history of reduced FM may indicate fetal hypoxia (Lee & Drukker, 1979) and is associated with fetal demise and Caesarean section delivery (ACOG, 2000). CTG is useful in the detection of acute hypoxia but is a poor test for chronic hypoxia (Heazell *et al.*, 2005). Large scale studies show that CTG does not reduce stillbirth or perinatal morbidity (Pattison & McCowan, 2000). Nevertheless a reactive CTG is significantly more likely to be followed by a normal delivery and a normal perinatal condition than non-reactive tests (Neldam, 1986).

Computerised CTGs are in use in many units in the United Kingdom and suggested to be more reliable, objective and accurate than visual inspection (Dawes *et al.*, 1996). Fetal heart rate measurements are automatically calculated by a computer, and compared to reference values (centiles) according to gestation. The use of computerised CTG improves discrimination between normal and questionable records in gestations ranging from 24-42 weeks.

5.1.4 Amniotic fluid index (AFI) or deepest vertical pool (DVP)

There are three ways to assess liquor volume; these include AFI, DVP and subjective assessment. In 1980 Manning & Platt proposed the measurement of the DVP for assessment of fetal wellbeing. This was revised by Phelan in 1987 who suggested that four pockets are better than one. Some studies show that AFI has poor correlation with actual fluid volume and suggest that measuring the DVP is slightly more reliable in assessing liquor volume (Chauhan *et al.*, 1997). This finding agrees with a recent Cochrane review on the use of AFI versus DVP which concluded that the DVP measurement in the assessment of amniotic fluid volume during fetal surveillance seems a better choice since the use of the amniotic fluid index increases the rate of diagnosis of oligohydramnios and the rate of induction of labour without improvement in peripartum outcomes (Nabhan & Abdelmoula, 2008). Table 3 shows the reference values for AFI and DVP according to gestation. An AFI less than 5cm is associated with adverse outcome.

Mean at term:	AFI 12cm
Polyhydramnios:	DVP ≥ 8cm, AFI ≥ 20cm
Oligohydramnios:	DVP ≤ 2cm, AFI ≤ 5cm
Borderline:	AFI 5-8cm (5% chance of oligohydramnios in 4 days)
Normal:	AFI 8-18cm (0.5% chance of oligohydramnios in 1 week)

Table 3. Reference values for Amniotic fluid index (AFI) and deepest vertical pocket (DVP)

In general, if reduced liquor volume is detected, further evaluation of the fetus is recommended, given the association of oligohydramnios with placental insufficiency, premature rupture of membranes and fetal renal abnormality. Lin *et al* found that oligohydramnios was present in 29% of growth restricted fetuses. An AFI or DVP measurement is also recommended in postdates pregnancies. The 5th centile for AFI at 37 weeks is 8.8cm (Moore) or 6.9cm (Magann).

5.1.5 Fetal biometry

A Cochrane review showed that routine ultrasound after 24 weeks gestation in low-risk pregnancy does not improve perinatal outcome (Bricker & Neilson, 2007). Nevertheless, if reduced FMs are reported, fetal ultrasound assessment for abdominal circumference (AC) or EFW is indicated in cases where SFH measurement suggests SGA. More than 40 formulas to estimate fetal weight exist, and numerous growth curves have been designed to plot these serial measurements. In late gestation, a single AC measurement is more accurate than head measurement. AC measurements have reported sensitivities of 72.9-94.5% and specificities of 50.6-83.3% and EFW has sensitivities between 33.3-89.2% and specificities of 53.7-90.9% (RCOG, 2002). AC and EFW measurements are better to predict a small for gestational age fetus under the 10th centile than large for gestational age fetuses (RCOG, 2002). Similar to SFH, serial measurements, ideally two weeks apart, are more accurate than single estimates in the prediction of growth restriction. As with SFH measurements they can be plotted on customised centile charts to increase sensitivity and specificity.

In conclusion, fetal biometry assessment should be performed if SFH suggests SGA and if there is suspected oligohydramnios. The most common single cause of stillbirth is intrauterine growth restrition, therefore sonographic assessment is recommended if small fetal size is suspected or if the clinical assessment is limited, i.e. in case of increased maternal body mass index. It should also be considered in second and subsequent presentations or if neither pregnant woman nor clinician are reassured by the initial assessment (Unterscheider et al., 2009).

The correlation with placenta derived factors such as reduced first trimester pregnancy associated plasma protein-A (PAPP-A) or placental protein-13 (PP-13) may suggest underlying placental dysfunction in patients with reduced FM. Fetal biometry is recommended in such cases (Warrander et al., 2011).

5.2 Which investigations are of limited value in the management of reduced FM in the low risk population?

5.2.1 Umbilical artery (UA) Doppler velocimetry

There is little evidence for the use of UA Doppler velocimetry in the assessment of reduced FM. UA Doppler is of benefit in high-risk pregnancies including the assessment of IUGR pregnancies in order to reduce perinatal mortality (Neilson & Alfirevic, 2000) but has not been shown to be of value as a screening test for detecting fetal compromise in the general obstetric population. Korszun et al suggested that adding UA and uterine artery (Ut.A) Doppler velocimetries to conventional CTG in the assessment of reduced FM might be reassuring for the managing clinician. Dubiel et al compared CTG with UA Doppler in the assessment of 599 women with low risk pregnancies complaining of reduced FM; CTG and UA Doppler were normal in 93% of patients. The overall perinatal mortality in their study was 3.8%. They found that CTG seemed to be a better predictor of mortality and infant handicap than Doppler velocimetry. Sergent et al reported only one highly pathological UA Doppler in their retrospective review of 160 pregnancies affected by reduced FM.

We conclude that UA Doppler is of limited use in the assessment of reduced fetal movements (Unterscheider et al., 2009). It is useful in the assessment of the IUGR fetus.

5.2.2 Fetal vibroacoustic stimulation test

A fetal vibroacoustic stimulation test may elicit fetal heart rate accelerations and increased fetal body movements, and may reduce the incidence of non-reassuring CTG and subsequent obstetric intervention (Pearson & Weaver, 1976). A Cochrane review by Tan &

Smyth examining 4,838 participants confirmed that fetal vibroacoustic stimulation reduced the incidence of non-reactive CTGs (RR 0.62, 95% CI, 0.52-0.74) and also reduced the overall mean testing time. The authors concluded that further randomised trials were needed to determine the optimal intensity, frequency, duration and position of vibroacoustic stimulation and also to evaluate the efficacy, predictive reliability, safety and perinatal outcome.

5.3 Which investigations are of no value in the management of reduced FM in the low risk population?

5.3.1 Fetal movement counting (count-to-ten kickcharts)

Formal fetal movement counting was first suggested in 1973 by Sadovsky & Yaffe. Sadovsky instructed women to count movements three times a day after meals. Counting movements using kickchart (Cardiff "count to ten" chart) is now more frequently employed. We have recently shown that 64% of obstetricians working in Ireland handed out kickcharts to patients presenting with reduced FM (Unterscheider et al., 2010) The use of kickcharts is easy, simple and can be done at home. However, in a large study of 68,000 women, Grant et al were unable to demonstrate a reduction in the incidence of antepartum fetal death using formal movement counting. They reported that formal FM counting by 1,250 women prevented, at best, one unexplained antepartum late fetal death and that a random adverse effect was just as likely (Grant et al., 1989). The use of kickcharts increased attendences for assessment of fetal wellbeing (15.5% vs 9.8%) and was associated with a 2.6 fold increased obstetric intervention rate (Heazell et al., 2005; Whitty et al., 1991). Another report demonstrated higher intervention rates (32% vs 21%) and caesarean section rates (24% vs 14%) (Sinha et al., 2007).

In October 2003 NICE and the National Collaborating Centre for Women's and Children's Health published their guideline on the routine antenatal care of healthy pregnant women. They came to the conclusion that routine formal FM counting should not be offered. This statement has been renewed in their 2008 guideline. In contrast, the American College of Obstetricians and Gynaecologists supports formal movement counting. In their bulletin on antepartum fetal surveillance they instruct the woman to count 10 movements, preferably after a meal, and to write down the hours this takes (ACOG, 2000). They do not provide a definition of reduced fetal movements or advise a timeframe in which these movements should be achieved, which reflects the dilemma and controversy of the definition and management of reduced FM.

Although formal fetal movement counting is not recommended, women should be educated about the physiology of fetal movements and the need to seek assessment if movements change, decrease or cease given the association with stillbirth and the identification of these concerns in the recent CESDI report.

5.3.2 Biophysical profile (BPP)

The biophysical profile (BPP) combines a CTG with ultrasound assessment of fetal movements, fetal tone, fetal breathing movements and liquor volume. A score of 8-10 confirms fetal well-being. Lalor et al recently published their Cochrane review on the use of BPP in high risk pregnancies and report that the available evidence from randomised controlled trials does not support the use of BPP as a test of fetal wellbeing (Lalor *et al.*, 2008). There was no significant difference between the groups in perinatal deaths (RR 1.33, 95% CI 0.60 to 2.98). Combined data from two high-quality trials suggest an increased risk of caesarean section in the BPP group (RR 1.60, 95% CI 1.05 to 2.44, n = 280, interaction test P = 0.03) (Tuffnell *et al.*, 1991). Observational studies however suggest that BPP has a good negative predictive value, meaning that fetal death is rare in women in the presence of a normal BPP (Dayal *et al.*, 1999).

6. Optimal management of reduced fetal movements prior to and beyond 24 weeks' gestation

Reduced fetal movements prior to 24 weeks gestation should be managed with auscultation of the fetal heart and clinical examination (basic assessment). Between 24 and 28 weeks gestation evidence suggests that fetal heart auscultation is sufficient for assessment, however CTG can be performed. The evaluation of a CTG can be difficult at this early gestation and its interpretation can be improved by computerised CTG applying the Dawson & Redmond criteria. It is essential to carry out a basic assessment including comprehensive stillbirth risk evaluation. If clinical examination is suggestive of small fetal size, ultrasound for fetal biometry, liquor volume and congenital structural abnormalities is recommended.

Beyond 28 weeks gestation, CTG should be part of the assessment of women presenting with reduced FM (refer to section 5.1.3). Figure 1 summarizes the recommended management approach to women presenting with reduced FM after 28 weeks gestation.

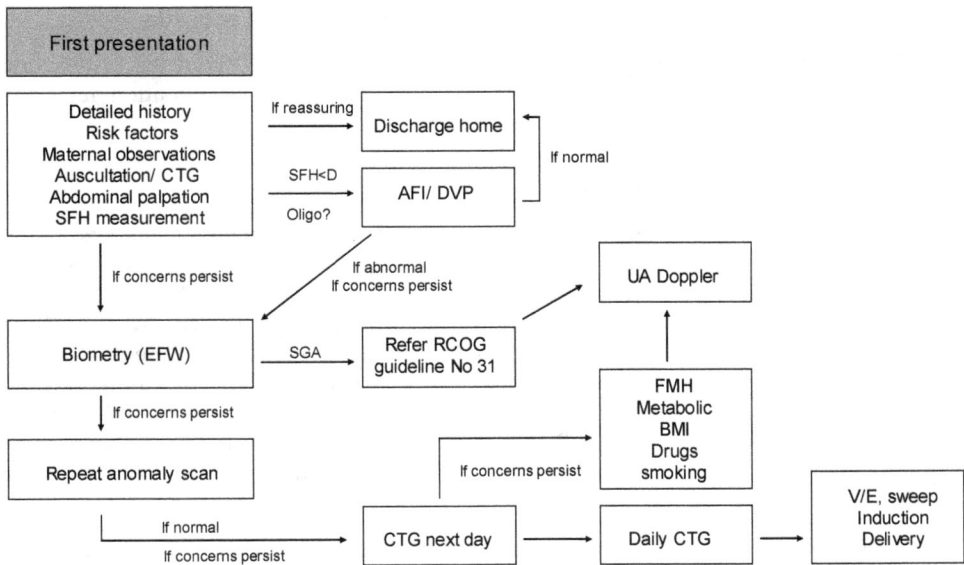

Fig. 1. Reduced fetal movement assessment flowchart (Unterscheider *et al.*, 2009)

7. Management of second and subsequent presentations

Up to 5% of women will re-present with reduced FM (Sinha *et al.*, 2007). If the perception of reduced FM persists, consideration should be given to other causes such as fetal structural anomalies (4.3%), anaemia or feto-maternal haemorrhage. There is little evidence how to manage these pregnancies, however women who present on two or more occasions with reduced FM are at increased risk of poor perinatal outcome compared with those who attend only once (OR 1.92; 95% CI 1.21 – 2.02) (O'Sullivan *et al.*, 2009). A practical approach would be to perform ultrasound assessment to rule out SGA, structural anomalies and oligo- or polyhydramnios and invite the woman for daily CTGs until mother and clinician are reassured. A blood test should ultimately be considered looking for maternal metabolic disorders or feto-maternal haemorrhage. Smoking should be discouraged. If concerns persist in later gestation, induction of labour or delivery can be considered.

8. Reduced fetal movements in multiple gestations

There is little guidance on the assessment and management of reduced FM in multiple gestations but a practical approach would incorporate clinical assessment and CTG followed by sonographic evaluation of chorionicity, biometry, liquor volume and umbilical artery Doppler. Given that fetal biometries are concordant and appropriate for gestational age, there are no structural abnormalities, signs of selective IUGR or twin-to-twin transfusion syndrome (TTTS), the mother can be reassured but careful follow-up should be arranged. Serial sonographic assessment for multiple gestations, more frequently in monochorionic gestations, is recommended.

9. Documentation of reduced fetal movements in maternal records

As in all areas of good clinical practice, meticulous documentation about the history and duration of the presenting complaint, stillbirth risk assessment, examination methods, recommendation for follow-up and advice is essential.

10. Summary and recommendation

Every mother who presents with the concern of reduced or altered fetal movements should be taken seriously. The initial assessment should include a detailed history of the presenting complaint, maternal observations, abdominal palpation, SFH measurement and CTG. If this is reassuring for the mother and clinician, no further evaluation is needed. Amniotic fluid assessment should be added in postdates pregnancies. If the mother re-presents or initial assessment is non-reassuring further tests should be performed; these include amniotic fluid assessment and estimation of fetal weight. Kickcharts are of no value and should therefore not be given out to pregnant women. Biophysical profile scoring has not been shown to be of benefit either, and UA Doppler velocimetry and vibroacoustic stimulation are of limited use in the assessment of reduced FM.

This review describes significant variation in clinical routines reported in the management of reduced FM, which do not correlate well with current information given to pregnant women, the available literature, or expert guidelines. This leads to clinical uncertainty for both pregnant women and healthcare professionals.

This comprehensive review is based on current evidence and experience from expert groups and reflects good clinical practice. For the development of evidence-based guidelines the authors suggest further randomised controlled trials to assess the different suggested management plans. This is likely to be difficult given current established clinical practice and ethical difficulties surrounding trials in pregnancy. Therefore, a sensible approach to the management of reduced FM based on good clinical practice as set out in this chapter seems reasonable.

11. References

American College of Obstetricians and Gynecologists Practice bulletin. (2000). Antepartum fetal surveillance. Clinical management guidelines for obstetrician-gynecologists. *Int J Gynaecol Obstet* 68:175-185.

Bricker L & Neilson JP. (2007). Routine ultrasound in late pregnancy (after 24 weeks gestation). *Cochrane Database Syst Rev.* CD001451.

Chauhan SP, Magann EF, Morrison JC, Whitworth NS, Hendrix NW & Devoe LD. (1997). Ultrasonic assessment of amniotic fluid does not reflect actual amniotic fluid volume. *Am J Obstet Gynecol.* 177(2):291-296.

Chauhan SP, Sanderson M, Hendrix NW, Magann EF & Devoe LD. (1999). Perinatal outcome and amniotic fluid index in the antepartum and intrapartum periods: A meta-analysis. *Am J Obstet Gynecol.* 181(6):1473-1478.

Confidential Enquiry into Stillbirths and Deaths in Infancy (CESDI). 8th Annual Report. (2001). Maternal and Child Health Research Consortium. London.

Dawes GS, Moulden M & Redman CW. (1996). Improvements in computerized fetal heart rate analysis antepartum. *J Perinat Med.* 24(1):25-36.

Dayel AK, Manning FA, Berck DJ, Mussalli GM, Avila C & Harman CR. (1999). Fetal death after normal biophysical profile score: an eighteen year experience. *Am J Obstet Gynecol* 181: 1231-1236.

Dubiel M, Gudmundsson S, Thuring-Jönsson A, Maesel A & Marsal K. (1997). Doppler velocimetry and nonstress test for predicting outcome of pregnancies with decreased fetal movements. *Am J Perinatol.* 14(3):139-144.

Efkarpidis S, Alexopoloulos E, Kean L, Liu D & Fay T. (2004). Case-control study of factors associated with intrauterine fetal deaths. *Med Gen Med* 6:53.

Gardosi J & Francis A. (1999). Controlled trial of fundal height measurement plotted on customised antenatal growth charts. *BJOG* 106(4):309-317.

Grant E, Elbourne D, Valentin L & Alexander S. (1989). Routine formal fetal movement counting and risk of antepartum late death in normally formed singletons. *Lancet.* 12;2(8659):345-349.

Haezell AE, Sumathi GM & Bhatti NR. (2005). What investigation is appropriate following maternal perception of reduced fetal movements? *J Obstet Gynaecol.* 25(7):648-650.

Haezell AE, Green M, Wright C, Flenady V & Frøen JF. (2008). Midwives and obstetricians knowledge and management of women presenting with decreased fetal movements. *Acta Obstet Gynecol Scand.* 87(3):331-339.

Heazell AE & Frøen JF. (2008). Methods of fetal movement counting and the detection of fetal compromise. *J Obstet Gynaecol.* 28(2):147-154.

Korszun P, Dubiel M, Kudla M & Gudmundsson S. (2002). Doppler velocimetry for predicting outcome of pregnancies with decreased fetal movements. *Acta Obstet Gynecol Scand.* 81(10):926-930.

Lalor JG, Fawole B, Alfirevic Z & Devane D. (2008). Biophysical profile for fetal assessment in high risk pregnancies. *Cochrane Database Syst Rev.* CD000038.

Lee CY & Drukker B. (1979). The nonstress test for antepartum assessment of fetal reserve. *Am J Obstet Gynecol.* 15;134(4):460-470.

Lin CC, Sheikh Z & Lopata R. (1990). The association between oligohydramnios and intrauterine growth retardation. *Obstet Gynecol.* 76(6):1100-1104.

Macones, GA & Depp, R. Fetal monitoring. (1996). In: Wildschut HIJ, Weiner CP, Peters TJ. (editors). When to screen in obstetrics and gynaecology. London: WB Saunders; pp. 202–218.

Mangesi L & Hofmeyr GJ. (2007). Fetal movement counting for assessment of fetal wellbeing. *Cochrane Database Syst Rev.* 24;(1):CD004909.

Manning FA, Platt LD & Sipos L. (1980). Antepartum fetal evaluation: development of a fetal biophysical profile. *Am J Obstet Gynecol.* 15;136(6):787-795.

Moore TR & Piacquadio K. (1989). A prospective evaluation of fetal movement screening to reduce the incidence of antepartum fetal death. *Am J Obstet Gynecol* 160:1075-1080.

National Institute for Clinical Excellence and National Collaborating Centre for Women's and Children's Health. (2003). Clinical Guideline CG6 Antenatal care: routine care for the healthy pregnant woman.

Nabhan AF, Abdelmoula YA. (2008). Amniotic fluid index versus single deepest vertical pocket as a screening test for preventing adverse pregnancy outcome. *Cochrane Database Syst Rev.* CD006593.

Neilson JP & Alfirevic Z. (2000). Doppler ultrasound for fetal assessment in high risk pregnancies. *Cochrane Database Syst Rev.* CD000073.

Neldam S. (1986). Fetal movements as an indicator of fetal well-being. *Dan Med Bull* 33:213-321.

O'Sullivan O, Stephen G, Martindale E & HeazellAE. (2009). Predicting poor perinatal outcome in women who present with decreased fetal movements. *J Obstet Gynecol* 29:705-710.

Ozkaya E, Baser E, Cinar M, Korkmaz V & Kucukozkan T. (2011). Does diurnal rhythm have impact on fetal biophysical profile. *J Matern Fetal Neonatal Med.* 23. [Epub ahead of print]

Patrick J, Campbell K, Carmichael I, Natale R & Richardson B. (1982). Patterns of gross fetal body movements over 24-hour observation intervals during the last 10 weeks of pregnancy. *Am J Obstet Gynecol* 142:363-371.

Pattison N & McCowan L. (2000). Cardiotocography for antepartum fetal assessment. *Cochrane Database Syst Rev.* CD001068.

Pearce JM & Campbell S. (1987). A comparison of symphysis-fundal height and ultrasound as screening tests of light-for-gestational age infants. *BJOG.* 94(2):100-104.

Pearson JF & Weaver JB. (1976). Fetal activity and fetal well-being: an evaluation. *BMJ.* 29;1(6021):1305-1307.

Phelan JP, Smith CV, Broussard P & Small M. (1987). Amniotic fluid volume assessment with the four-quadrant technique at 36-42 weeks' gestation. *J Reprod Med.* 32(7):540-542.

Preboth M. (2000). ACOG guidelines on antepartum fetal surveillance. *Am Fam Physician* 62:1187-1188.

Royal College of Obstetricians and Gynaecologists. (2002). The investigation and management of the small-for-gestational-age fetus. RCOG Green-top Guideline No 31.

Royal College of Obstetricians and Gynaecologists. (2011). Reduced Fetal Movements. RCOG Green-top Guideline 57.

Saastad E, Tveit JVH, Bordahl PE, Stray-Pederson B & Frøen JF. (2006). Information and maternal concerns for decreased fetal movements. Proceedings of the Norwegian Perinatal Society Conference.

Sadovsky E & Yaffe H. (1973). Daily fetal movement recording and fetal prognosis. *Obstet Gynecol.* 41(6):845-850.

Sergent F, Lefevre A, Verspyck E & Marpeau L. (2005). Decreased fetal movements in the third trimester: what to do? *Gynecol Obstet Fertil.* 33(11):861-869.

Sinha D, Sharma A, Nallaswamy V, Jayagopal N & Bhatti N. (2007). Obstetric outcome in women complaining of reduced fetal movements. *J Obstet Gynaecol.* 27(1):41-43.

Stanton C, Lawn JE, Rahman H, Wilczynska-Ketende K & Hill K. (2006). Stillbirth rates: delivering estimates in 190 countries. *Lancet.* 6;367(9521):1487-1494.

Tan KH & Smyth R. (2001). Fetal vibroacoustic stimulation for facilitation of tests of fetal wellbeing. *Cochrane Database Syst Rev.* CD002963.

Tuffnell DJ, Cartmill RS & Lilford RJ. (1991). Fetal movements; factors effecting their perception. *Eur J Obstet Gynecol Reprod Biol.* 10;39(3):165-167.

Tveit JV, Saastad E, Børdahl PE, Stray-Pederson B & Frøen JF. (2006). The epidemiology of decreased fetal movements. *Proceedings of the Norwegian Perinatal Society Conference.*

Unterscheider J, Horgan R, O'Donoghue K & Greene R. (2009). Reduced fetal movements. *The Obstetrician & Gynaecologist* 11:245-251.

Unterscheider J, Horgan R, Greene R & Higgins J. (2010). How do Irish Obstetricians manage reduced fetal movements in an uncomplicated pregnancy at term. Results from an anonymous online survey. *J Obstet Gynaecol* 30(6):578-582.

Warrander LK & Heazell AEP. (2011). Identifying placental dysfunction in women with reduced fetal movements can be used to predict patients at risk of pregnancy complications. *Med Hypotheses.* 76(1):17-20.

Whitty JE, Garfinkel DA & Divon MY. (1991). Maternal perception of decreased fetal movements as an indication for antepartum testing in a low-risk population. *Am J Obstet Gynecol.* 165:1084-1088.

Winje B, Saastad E, Gunnes N, Tveit J, Stray-Pedersen B, Flenady V & Frøen J. (2011). Analysis of 'count-to-ten' fetal movement charts: a prospective cohort study. *BJOG*. doi: 10.1111/j.1471-0528.2011.02993.x. [Epub ahead of print]

14

Oxytocin and Myometrial Contractility in Labor

N. Vrachnis[1], F.M. Malamas[2], S. Sifakis[3],
A. Parashaki[4], Z. Iliodromiti[1], D. Botsis[1] and G. Creatsas[1]

[1]*2nd Department of Obstetrics and Gynecology,*
University of Athens Medical School, Aretaieio Hospital, Athens,
[2]*1st Department of Obstetrics and Gynecology,*
University of Athens Medical School, Alexandra Hospital, Athens,
[3]*Department of Obstetrics and Gynaecology, University Hospital of Heraklion, Crete,*
[4]*Health Center of Thira, Thira,*
Greece

1. Introduction

Oxytocin (OT), a hormone exerting central and peripheral actions, plays an essential role in the mechanisms of parturition and lactation. It acts through its receptors, the number of which increases in the uterus towards labor, thus augmenting the uterotonic effect. Activated oxytocin receptors (OTR) by oxytocin, signal via a large number of intracellular pathways causing increased myometrial contractions by means of increased intracellular Ca^{+2} ion, increased myosin light chain phosphorylation and increased production of prostaglandins.

Molecules that antagonize the action of oxytocin have been developed for use as tocolytic agents in the treatment of preterm labor. One presently available tocolytic, the oxytocin receptor antagonist atosiban, acts on both myometrial and decidual OTRs. However, research is in progress aimed at the development and clinical application of new oxytocin receptor antagonists with an enhanced pharmacological profile translating as higher affinity for the receptor as well as better bioavailability and improved safety. In this chapter we describe the function of oxytocin in labor and review the use of atosiban for the treatment of preterm labor, while also evaluating the current development of other OTR antagonists that are potential candidates as tocolytic drugs in the future.

2. Oxytocin synthesis and function

Oxytocin (OT) is a nine amino acid neuropeptide synthesized by the magnocellular neurons of the supraoptic and paraventricular nuclei of the hypothalamus. It is released into the circulation by exocytosis from the posterior pituitary and nerve terminals in response to various stimuli. The amino acids sequence in the OT molecule is: Cysteine-Tyrosine-Isoleukine-Glutamine-Asparagine-Cysteine-Proline-Leukine-Glycinamide, and with a sulfur bridge between the two cysteines. The structure of OT is very similar to that of the nonapeptide vasopressin, which differs from oxytocin by two amino acids. Oxytocin is also synthesized in such peripheral tissues as the uterus, corpus luteum, placenta, amnion, and testis (Gimpl and Fahrenholz, 2001).

Oxytocin, involved in numerous physiological and pathological processes, exerts a variety of actions, including the regulation of the hypothalamo-pituitary-adrenal axis in response to stress, cell proliferation, pregnancy, luteal function, maternal behavior, erectile function, and ejaculation (Viero et al., 2010).

3. The oxytocin receptor signaling

Oxytocin has only one receptor, which belongs to the rhodopsin-type class I G-protein coupled receptor (GPCR) superfamily. The gene of the oxytocin receptor is present in a single copy on chromosome 3p25 and contains 3 introns and 4 exons. Oxytocin and other molecules of similar structure, such as arginine vasopressin (AVP) and oxytocin agonists or antagonists, can bind to the receptor. The affinity for OT is about 10-fold higher than for AVP. The cell surface transmembrane OTR is activated after binding of OT molecule, and the receptor subsequently causes activation of the various intracellular signal pathways, this finally resulting in the numerous effects of the hormone, including contraction. OTR is coupled to the $G_{q/11}$ a- class guanosine triphosphate (GTP) binding proteins. Binding of OT activates, via $G\alpha_{q/11}$, phospholipase C (PLC) which hydrolyzes phosphatidylinositol 4,5-bisphosphate (PIP2) to inositol 1,4,5- triphosphate (InsP3) and diacylglycerol (DAG). InsP3 results in the release of Ca^{2+} ions from intracellular stores, while DAG activates protein kinases type C (PKC), which further phosphorylates other proteins, thus bringing about a trophic effect on myometrial cells via the eukaryotic translation elongation factor 2 (eEF2). Release of Ca^{2+} ions initiates smooth muscle contractions as Ca^{2+} binds to calmodulin and the Ca^{2+}-calmodulin system activates myosin light-chain kinase. This mechanism causes myometrial contractions, as well as contraction of mammary myoepithelial cells leading to milk ejection (Gimpl and Fahrenholz, 2001). The major pathway that mediates the signal of OTR after binding of OT is the Gq/PLC/InsP3 pathway. The OTR is, however, also coupled with other G proteins, Gs and Gi, which give rise to various other cellular effects, e.g. inhibition of cellular growth (Viero et al., 2010).

OTR additionally acts on voltage-gated or receptor coupled channels; this activation, which leads to membrane depolarization and the entry of extracellular Ca^{2+} into the cells, eventually triggers various cellular responses and further promotes smooth muscle contractility.

OTR also activates the mitogen-activated protein kinase (MAPK) and the Rho kinase pathways. Rho associated protein kinases are involved in many cellular phenomena, among them cell migration, cell cycle control and cell contractility. Activation of OTR and MAPK results, in both cases, in elevated cytosolic phospholipase A2 (cPLA2) activity. cPLA2 hydrolyzes phospholipids while liberating arachidonic acid, that results in increased production of prostaglandins via cyclooxygenase-2 (COX-2), an enzyme up-regulated by MAPK (Molnar and Hertelendy, 1995; Soloff et al., 2000). RhoA kinase increases phoshporylated myosin light chains. The increase in intracellular Ca^{2+} ions, the activation of the Rho and MAP kinase pathways, and the increased production and secretion of prostaglandins all together result in the contractile effects of OT-OTR activation.

4. Changes in circulating oxytocin and oxytocin receptor levels in labor

In humans, circulating oxytocin is not necessary for the initiation and completion of parturition, since normal labor can be achieved in cases of pituitary dysfunction (Phelan et al., 1978). Additionally, oxytocin circulation levels do not increase significantly in pregnancy or at the beginning of labor but are increased at the expulsive stage, while oxytocin pulsatile changes occur in pregnant women at term. Apart from in the pituitary, OT is also produced locally, and, in fact, placental OT acting in a paracrine fashion may be more important than circulating OT for the mechanism of labor. OTR is also up-regulated at the end of gestation and sensitivity to oxytocin-induced contractions is greatly increased compared to the non-pregnant uterus. A significant increase in the number of oxytocin receptors in the myometrium and decidua is observed in women with both term and preterm labor (Petraglia et al., 1996). Although steroid hormones are also thought to influence the number of OTR, the mechanisms of regulation are complex and not yet fully elucidated (Mirando et al., 1990, Wathes et al., 1996; Zingg et al., 1995). After parturition the binding sites of OT in uterus decline rapidly, while OTR expression in mammary glands remains high during the period of lactation (Petraglia et al., 2010).

However, continuous exposure to high doses of oxytocin leads to desensitization and down-regulation of OTR (Plested and Bernal, 2001). Desensitization is a phenomenon that prevents overstimulation of cells after prolonged agonist stimulation. This phenomenon is observed in GPCR receptors and is brought about by means of different mechanisms at many levels, such as phosphorylation, internalization or changes at the receptor mRNA levels. Rapid desensitization of GPCR receptors, taking place within seconds or minutes, occurs in two steps: 1. phosphorylation of the receptor, causing inhibition of G-protein activation; 2. binding of proteins, called arrestins, preventing G-protein activation and promoting receptor internalization. Internalization of the receptor after continuous OT stimulation is yet another mechanism of desensitization. Though it has been suggested that once internalized, the receptor does not return to the cell surface, recent data suggest that intracellular trafficking and recycling of the OTR to the cell surface does indeed take place (Conti et al., 2009). OTR desensitization is a phenomenon that occurs after prolonged agonist stimulation, i.e. lasting for several hours (Terzidou, 2007). Continuous OT treatment reduces the mRNA of the OTR, this possibly due to suppression of OTR transcription or destabilization of the mRNA molecule. In cultured human myometrial cells, treatment with OT for up to 20 hours causes OTR desensitization which effects in a reduction of the OT binding sites from 210×10^3 sites/cell to only 20.1×10^3 sites/cell, without receptor internalization. However, while the total amount of OTR protein is not diminished, treatment reduces OTR mRNA levels (Phaneuf et al., 1998). In vivo, in women with oxytocin-induced or oxytocin-augmented labor there is also a reduction in myometrial oxytocin binding sites and in OTR mRNA levels. Compared to women not in labor, in cases of oxytocin-augmented or oxytocin-induced labor, the median number of binding sites was reduced from to 477 fmol/mg^{-1} protein to 140 fmol/mg^{-1} protein and 118 fmol/mg^{-1} protein, respectively, both differences being statistically significant. Compared to women not in labor, in cases of labor augmentation and induction OTR mRNA levels were reduced by 60- and 300-fold, respectively (Phaneuf et al., 2000). Oxytocin receptor down-regulation has great significance in clinical practice. Long-term oxytocin infusion may fail to augment labor or may lead to postpartum uterine atony which cannot be managed with additional oxytocin infusion. However, oxytocin is normally secreted in pulses, this pulsatile secretion likely being a mechanism that prevents desensitization from occurring. This might explain why in women in labor, induction of labor requires significantly lower doses of oxytocin when oxytocin is administered in pulses, compared with continuous oxytocin infusion (Dawood, 1995).

5. Experimental or clinical use of oxytocin agonists

The widespread distribution of OTR has led to the development of OTR agonist molecules that could be used as pharmacological tools (agents used experimentally to study the functions of oxytocin and its receptor) or as potential drugs for the management of obstetric disorders and neuropsychiatric diseases, including anxiety-related disorders, autism and schizophrenia. OTR agonists may be peptide (such as [Thr⁴]OT, [HO¹][Thr⁴]OT, [Thr⁴,Gly⁷]OT and [HO¹][Thr⁴,Gly⁷]OT) or non-peptide molecules (such as WAY-267464 and other compounds) (Borthwick, 2006; Manning et al., 2008). WAY-267464 exerts oxytocinergic actions, such as anxiolytic effects, in mice (Ring et al., 2010).

Clinically, synthetic oxytocin is used for labor induction and augmentation and the treatment of postpartum hemorrhage. Carbetocin, a synthetic oxytocin analog, is also indicated for prevention of uterine atony after delivery by cesarean section in spinal or epidural anesthesia. It also has the advantage of longer half life than oxytocin (4-10 times) and it is administered in a single dose, intramuscularly or intravenously, compared to oxytocin continuous infusion (Rath, 2009).

6. Tocolytic action of oxytocin antagonists

Since the most recognized signs of preterm labor are uterine contractions, the main method for postponement of preterm labor is currently the pharmacological inhibition of uterine contractions. The inhibition of myometrial contractions is called tocolysis, and a drug administered to that end is referred to as a tocolytic agent. The aim of tocolytic agents is to maintain pregnancy for 24-48 hours, to allow the beneficial effects of corticosteroids administration to take place (reduced risk of perinatal death, neonatal respiratory distress syndrome, etc), usually after 18 hours, and also to permit safe transfer of the mother to a center with neonatal intensive care facilities. There are several tocolytics agents, such as ritodrine (a beta-receptor agonist), calcium-channel blockers, nitric oxide donors (as glyceryl trinitrate), and COX-2 inhibitors such as indomethacin (Simhan and Caritis, 2007).

Selective human oxytocin receptor antagonists, such as atosiban and barusiban have also been synthesized as tocolytic agents for the management of preterm labor. Atosiban, an oxytocin analog (1-Deamino-2-D-Tyr-(O-ethyl)-4-Thr-8-ornoxytocin), is based on modification of amino acids in the structure of oxytocin at positions 1, 2, 4 and 8, thus being a competitive inhibitor of the OTR that blocks OT binding. It is also a mixed vasopressin V1a/OT antagonist that results in the incidence of related unwanted effects. Vasopressin V1a receptors (V1aR) expression are also present in myometrium.

The onset of uterine relaxation after atosiban administration is fast. Atosiban is given intravenously as shown in Table 1 and the total dose should preferably not exceed 330 mg.

Dose and administration		
Step 1	6.75 mg	i.v. bolus, in one minute
Step 2	18 mg/h i.v.	i.v. infusion for 3 hours
Step 3	6 mg/h i.v.	i.v. infusion for up to 45 hours

Side effects: Nausea, vomiting, hyperglycemia, headaches, dizziness, tachycardia, hot flushes, hypotension, injection site reactions, pruritis, rush, pyrexia, insomnia

Table 1. Dose, method of administration, and side effects of atosiban.

Clinically, atosiban, which requires continuous intravenous administration, is as effective as β2-adrenergic agonists, but without producing their adverse effects. Subcutaneously administered after a period of preterm labor, atosiban given as maintenance therapy was not shown to be associated with a reduction of the incidence of preterm birth nor with any improvement of neonatal outcome. In a study in which a total of 513 women were randomized to receive either atosiban or placebo administered with a subcutaneous infusion pump in order to prevent recurrence of preterm birth, atosiban compared to placebo did not reduce the incidence of preterm birth before 37 weeks (RR 0.89; 95% CI 0.71 to 1.12), 32 weeks (RR 0.85; 95% CI 0.47 to 1.55), or 28 weeks (RR 0.75; 95% CI 0.28 to 2.01). Outcomes were also similar for both groups with respect to birth weight, respiratory distress syndrome, patent ductus arteriosus, necrotizing enterocolitis, and intraventricular hemorrhage (Papatsonis et al., 2009).

In Europe and other countries atosiban is the only oxytocin/vasopressin antagonist used today for preterm delivery. However, this does not apply to the USA where the Food and Drug Administration has not granted approval of the drug as a tocolytic because of sufficient lack of evidence as to its efficacy and improvement of neonatal outcomes.

Clinical studies have determined that atosiban is safer than beta-receptor agonists. A large study (Worldwide Atosiban versus Beta-agonists Study Group, 2001) demonstrated that atosiban was comparable in clinical effectiveness to conventional beta-agonist therapy (ritodrine, salbutamol or terbutaline), but was better tolerated and was associated with fewer maternal cardiovascular side effects (ClinicalTrials.gov, 2001). Atosiban is also safer than calcium channel blockers. Meanwhile, clinical studies have shown nifedipine to be equally effective as atosiban, although the maternal side effects were significantly more common among women allocated to nifedipine rather than atosiban (Al-Omari et al., 2006). Cyclooxygenase inhibitors act as tocolytics by inhibiting prostaglandins production but also present significant side effects (King et al., 2005). Conversely, evidence is as yet not strong enough for recommendation of the use of nitric oxide donors as inhibitors of preterm delivery (Duckitt and Thornton, 2002). Nevertheless, atosiban has not been proven to be superior in terms of neonatal outcome, concerns having been expressed in other studies (Papatsonis et al., 2005).

Atosiban's limited bioavailability—which necessitates parenteral administration and hospitalization—together with its low affinity for OTR and the binding to V1a receptors that causes side effects, have led to endeavors for the identification of new peptide and non-peptide oxytocin antagonists for the management of preterm labor. While many such substances have been discovered, these drugs are still being evaluated at the experimental level and clinical studies in most cases have ceased or have been completed unsuccessfully (Manning et al., 2008). These compounds are either peptide or non-peptide molecules.

The OT antagonists shown in Table 2 bind for both oxytocin and AVP receptors. However, limitations exist, these being: a) there are major differences among them with regard to their selectivity for a specific OT receptor; b) selectivity also varies according to the AVP receptor (V1a, V1b, V2); c) there are striking differences among species as to both receptors' affinity for a given antagonist; and d) specification as to receptors' affinity varies in the literature according to the experimental method used.

	Oxytocin antagonists	OT and AVP receptor binding
I. Peptide	Atosiban	Yes
	FE 200 400 (Barusiban)	Yes
II. Non-peptide	GSK221149A (Retosiban)	Yes
	SSR-126768A	Yes
	L-368,899	Yes

Table 2. OT antagonists with tocolytic action and AVP receptor binding

The V2 and V1a peptide antagonist d(CH$_2$)$_5$[Tyr(Me)^2]AVP (known as Manning compound) is a potent OT antagonist in vitro and in vivo (Chan et al., 1996). d(CH$_2$)$_5$[Tyr(Me)^2]AVP is also a mixed V1a/OT antagonist for human VP and OT receptors.

Several others highly selective OT peptidic antagonists have been designed and synthesized. These include d(CH$_2$)$_5$[Tyr(Me)^2]OVT, desGly-NH$_2$,d(CH$_2$)$_5$[Tyr(Me)^2,Thr^4]OVT (which is about 18 times more potent as an OT antagonist in the rat than as a V1a antagonist) and desGly-NH2,d(CH$_2$)$_5$[D-Tyr^2,Thr^4]OVT (which is 95 times more potent as an OT antagonist in the rat than as a V1a antagonist). Moreover, the peptide d(CH$_2$)^5,[D-Thi^2,Thr^4,Tyr-NH$_2$^{9}]OVT is a very selective oxytocin antagonist while being a very weak V1a antagonist, as is also desGly-NH$_2$,d(CH$_2$)$_5$ [D-Trp^2, Thr^4, Dap^5]OVT in the rat. On the other hand, there are between species striking differences in the affinity of most antagonists for OT and AVP receptors. The first peptide above, d(CH$_2$)$_5$[Tyr(Me)^2]OVT, is 5 times more potent as an V1a antagonist than as a OT antagonist in the rat, whereas in humans it is about 9 times more potent as an OT antagonist than as a V1a antagonist.

Some of the new peptide OT/VP antagonists have higher affinity for human receptor than the peptide atosiban, which, as noted, is the only antagonist used today in Europe. These new peptides are desGly-NH$_2$,d(CH$_2$)$_5$[D-2-Nal^2,Thr^4]OVT, desGly-NH$_2$,d(CH$_2$)$_5$[2-Nal^2,Thr^4]OVT, d(CH$_2$)$_5$[D-2-Nal^2,Thr^4,Tyr-NH$_2$^{9}]OVT, and d(CH$_2$)$_5$[2-Nal^2, Thr^4, Tyr-NH$_2$^{9}]OVT. These four peptides may be candidates as potential tocolytic agents for the prevention of preterm labor (Manning et al., 2008).

Barusiban is a selective peptide oxytocin antagonist that exerts a high affinity for the human oxytocin receptor On the contrary, it displays low affinity for the vasopressin (V1a) receptor. It possesses greater potency and a longer duration of action than atosiban. Contractility studies with isolated human myometrium have revealed that barusiban inhibits oxytocin-induced myometrial contractions of both preterm and term myometrium, this action being at least as potent as that of atosiban (Pierzynski et al., 2004). In a study with eight pregnant monkeys, following induction of stable contractions by OT, barusiban or atosiban were administered. Barusiban's duration of action was generally longer than 13–15 hours, while atosiban's effect ceased within 1.5–3 hours. For long-term treatment, continuous high-dose infusions of barusiban (150 µg/kg/h) or the beta-2 agonist fenoterol (3 µg/kg/h) were administered. Barusiban reduced uterine activity in response to daily OT challenge and prolonged pregnancy more effectively than fenoterol (Reinheimer, 2007).

Although barusiban suppresses oxytocin-induced preterm labor in non-human primates, in a recent study it was no more effective than placebo in terminating preterm labor in pregnant women at between 34[+0]-35[+6] weeks of gestation. This study was conducted at 21 participating centers with subjects from six different European countries. Participants were randomly assigned to receive a single intravenous bolus dose of 0.3, 1, 3, or 10 mg barusiban or placebo (acetate buffer). The percentage of women who did not deliver within 48 hours was not significantly different between the placebo group and any of the barusiban groups (P = 0.21-0.84). No significant decreases in the number of uterine contractions compared with placebo were registered. All doses of barusiban were well tolerated and there were no adverse events that would lead to withdrawal from the study. Finally, there was no statistically significant difference in maternal or neonatal adverse effect between the placebo and barusiban groups (Thornton et al., 2009).

The lack of peptide antagonists characterized by oral bioavailability have led researchers to seek an effective non-peptide oxytocin antagonist. The non-peptide oxytocin antagonist 2'-methyl-1',3'-oxazol-4'-yl morpholine amide derivative 74 (GSK221149A or retosiban) when administered orally or intravenously produced a dose-dependent decrease in oxytocin-induced uterine contractions in rats, after either single or multiple dosing for 4 days. In addition, spontaneous uterine contractions in late-term pregnant rats (at 19–21 days gestation) were significantly reduced by intravenous administration of GSK221149A at a dose of 0.3 mg/kg. In vitro experiments using Chinese hamster ovary (CHO) cell membranes expressing human OT receptors or human V1a, V1b, or V2 receptors, and human endothelial kidney (HEK) cells expressing rat oxytocin receptors showed that GSK221149A also has a higher affinity for human and rat oxytocin receptors than for V1a and V2 receptors (McCafferty et al., 2007). GSK221149A is over 15-fold more potent compared to atosiban for the OTR (Borthwick and Liddle, 2011). GSK221149A is on a Phase ll Clinical trial described as "A randomized, double-blind, placebo-controlled, dose ranging study to investigate the safety, tolerability, pharmacokinetics and pharmacodynamics of GSK221149A administered intravenously and to investigate the pharmacokinetics of GSK221149A administered orally to healthy, pregnant females with uncomplicated pre-term labor between 30[+0] and 35[6] weeks' gestation" . The estimated date for study completion was June 2011 and no results have so far been published.

Another non-peptide molecule, 1-((7,7-Dimethyl-2(S)-(2(S)-amino-4-(methylsulfonyl) butyramido) bicyclo[2.2.1]-heptan-1(S)-yl)methyl)sulfonyl)-4(2methylphenyl) piperazine, known as L-368,899, was shown to be a potent OT antagonist that inhibits spontaneous nocturnal uterine contractions in pregnant rhesus monkeys. L-368,899 also blocked OT-stimulated uterine activity in postpartum women with a potency similar to that in the pregnant rhesus monkey (Pettibone et al., 1995). The pharmacokinetics and oral bioavailability, however, were suboptimal, and further clinical evaluation was not undertaken (Freidinger and Pettibone, 1997). L-368,899 is moreover brain penetrant. In a study, the non-peptide OT antagonist L-368,899 was accumulated when injected intravenously in four male monkeys in limbic brain areas. This antagonist when injected iv in one adult female monkey altered maternal and sexual behavior (Boccia et al., 2007).

WAY-162720 is another high-affinity, potent, and selective non-peptide antagonist of the OTR. WAY-162720 also penetrates the brain and is a tool for studies of OT on the CNS effects. In one study, the effects of OT on both the behavioral and autonomic parameters of the anxiety response in male mice were examined. Oxytocin showed an anxiolytic-like effect comparable to those observed with the reference anxiolytic alprazolam. The administration of WAY-162720 fully reversed the effects of centrally administered OT (Ring et al., 2006).

The non-peptide SSR-126768A (4-Chloro-3-[(3R)-(+)-5-chloro-1-(2,4-dimethoxybenzyl) -3-methyl-2-oxo-2,3-dihydro-1H-indol-3-yl]-N-ethyl-N-(3-pyridylmethyl)-benzamide, hydrochloride) produced a competitive antagonistic effect against OT in rat myometrial strips, while after oral administration in conscious pregnant rats in labor it significantly delayed parturition, in a manner similar to ritodrine. The onset of its action was rapid and the duration was still observed 24h after treatment. In experiments performed in human uterine sections in term pregnancies, SSR-126768A inhibited the response to OT and this effect was observed in a concentration-dependent manner (Serradeil-Le et al., 2004).

Relcovaptan, a vasopressin (V1a) receptor antagonist, was reported to inhibit uterine contractions in women with preterm labor, thus indicating a role for V1a receptors (Steinwall et al., 2005). In a study including 18 women with preterm labor between 32–36 weeks, 12 patients received at random a single oral dose of 400 mg relcovaptan and 6 patients received placebo; uterine contractions were monitored up to 6h after administration. Relcovaptan inhibited uterine contractions and the decrease in the frequency of contractions was significantly higher than the frequency in the placebo-treated group. It has also shown positive initial results when used against Raynaud's disease and dysmenorrhea, although it has not yet been approved for clinical use (Decaux et al., 2008). When relcovaptan was given orally once a day for 7 days in patients with Raynaud's disease, it showed favorable effects compared with placebo on finger systolic pressure and temperature recovery after cold immersion, without inducing side effects (Hayoz et al., 2000). Relcovaptan is administered orally 100 mg or 300 mg daily in women suffering from primary dysmenorrhoea, from 4 hours up to a maximum of 3 days before the onset of bleeding and/or menstrual pain. After the start of dysmenorrhea (defined as the onset of vaginal bleeding or the onset of pain, whichever occurred first), treatment was prolonged for up to 3 days. Relcovaptan showed a therapeutic effect in the prevention of dysmenorrhea (Brouard et al., 2000). Relcovaptan also produced significant neuroprotective actions and reduced ischemic brain edema in an embolic model of stroke in rats when given immediately or 1 hour after middle cerebral artery occlusion, but not when administered at 3 hours after middle cerebral artery occlusion (Shuaib et al., 2002).

As our knowledge on OT/OTR system expands, the development and use of different OTR antagonists becomes an increasingly promising field in the management of preterm labor.

7. Conclusion

OT exerts its myometrial and other actions through a transmembrane receptor that belongs to the G- protein coupled receptor superfamily. Various peptide and non-peptide antagonists have been developed in order to be used as potential tocolytic agents or as research tools in assessing different OT functions. Atosiban is at present the only available OTR antagonist used as a tocolytic agent. Barusiban, L-368,899, SSR-126768A, and

GSK221149A (retosiban) are some other OTR antagonists demonstrating tocolytic properties when tested, but have not so far been approved for clinical use.

8. References

Al-Omari, W.R., Al-Shammaa, H.B., Al-Tikriti, E.M. & Ahmed, K.W. (2006). Atosiban and nifedipine in acute tocolysis: a comparative study. Eur J Obstet Gynecol Reprod Biol, Vol. 128 (1): 129-34.

Boccia, M.L., Goursaud, A.P., Bachevalier, J., Anderson, K.D. & Pedersen, C.A. (2007). Peripherally administered non-peptide oxytocin antagonist, L368,899, accumulates in limbic brain areas: a new pharmacological tool for the study of social motivation in non-human primates. Horm Behav, Vol. 52 (3): 344-51.

Borthwick, A.D. & Liddle, J. (2011). The design of orally bioavailable 2, 5-diketopiperazine oxytocin antagonists: from concept to clinical candidate for premature labor. Med Res Rev, Vol. 31(4): 576-604.

Borthwick, A.D. (2006). Oxytocin antagonists and agonists. Annual Reports in Medicinal Chemistry, Vol. 41: 409-21.

Brouard, R., Bossmar, T., Fournie-Lloret, D., Chassard, D. & Akerlund, M.(2000). Effect of SR49059, an orally active V1a vasopressin receptor antagonist, in the prevention of dysmenorrhoea. BJOG, Vol. 107 (5): 614-19.

Chan, W.Y., Wo, N.C., Cheng, L.L. & Manning, M. (1996). Isosteric substitution of Asn5 in antagonists of oxytocin and vasopressin leads to highly selective and potent oxytocin and V1a receptor antagonists: new approaches for the design of potential tocolytics for preterm labor. J Pharmacol Exp Ther, Vol. 277 (2): 999-1003.

ClinicalTrials.gov. The Safety, Tolerability And Metabolism Of GSK221149A, In Pregnant Women (30-36 Weeks), In Pre-Term Labor. Accessed on July 27, 2011, available from: http://clinicaltrials.gov/ct2/show/study/NCT00404768.

Conti, F., Sertic, S., Reversi, A. &Chini, B. (2009). Intracellular trafficking of the human oxytocin receptor: evidence of receptor recycling via a Rab4/Rab5 "short cycle". Am J Physiol Endocrinol Metab, Vol. 296 (3): E532-42.

Dawood, M.Y. (1995). Novel approach to oxytocin induction-augmentation of labor. Application of oxytocin physiology during pregnancy. Adv Exp Med Biol, Vol. 395: 585-94.

Decaux, G., Soupart, A. & Vassart, G. (2008). Non-peptide arginine-vasopressin antagonists: the vaptans. Lancet, Vol. 371 (9624): 1624-32.

Duckitt, K. & Thornton, S. (2002).Nitric oxide donors for the treatment of preterm labour. Cochrane Database Syst Rev 2002 (3): CD002860.

Freidinger, R.M. & Pettibone, D.J. (1997). Small molecule ligands for oxytocin and vasopressin receptors. Med Res Rev, Vol. 17 (1): 1-16.

Gimpl, G. & Fahrenholz, F. (2001). The oxytocin receptor system: structure, function, and regulation. Physiol Rev, Vol. 81 (2): 629-83.

Hayoz, D., Bizzini, G., Noël, B., Depairon, M., Burnier, M., Fauveau, C., Rouillon, A., Brouard, R., & Brunner, H.R. (2000). Effect of SR 49059, a V1a vasopressin receptor antagonist, in Raynaud's phenomenon. Rheumatology (Oxford), Vol. 39 (10): 1132-38.

King, J., Flenady, V., Cole, S. & Thornton, S. (2005). Cyclo-oxygenase (COX) inhibitors for treating preterm labour. Cochrane Database Syst Rev 2005 (2): CD001992.

Manning, M., Stoev, S., Chini, B., Durroux, T., Mouillac, B., Guillon, G. (2008). Peptide and non-peptide agonists and antagonists for the vasopressin and oxytocin V1a, V1b, V2 and OT receptors: research tools and potential therapeutic agents. Prog Brain Res, Vol.170: 473-512.

McCafferty, G.P., Pullen, M.A., Wu, C., Edwards, R.M., Allen, M.J., Woollard, P.M., Borthwick, A.D., Liddle, J., Hickey, D.M., Brooks, D.P. & Westfall, T.D. (2007). Use of a novel and highly selective oxytocin receptor antagonist to characterize uterine contractions in the rat. Am J Physiol Regul Integr Comp Physiol, Vol. 293 (1): R299-305.

Mirando, M.A., Ott, T.L., Vallet, J.L., Davis, M. & Bazer, F.W. (1990). Oxytocin-stimulated inositol phosphate turnover in endometrium of ewes is influenced by stage of the estrous cycle, pregnancy, and intrauterine infusion of ovine conceptus secretory proteins. Biol Reprod, Vol. 42 (1): 98-105.

Molnar, M. & Hertelendy, F. (1995). Signal transduction in rat myometrial cells: comparison of the actions of endothelin-1, oxytocin and prostaglandin F2 alpha. Eur J Endocrinol, Vol. 133 (4): 467-74.

Papatsonis, D., Flenady, V., Cole, S. & Liley, H. (2005). Oxytocin receptor antagonists for inhibiting preterm labour. Cochrane Database Syst Rev 2005 (3): CD004452.

Papatsonis, D., Flenady, V. & Liley, H. (2009). Maintenance therapy with oxytocin antagonists for inhibiting preterm birth after threatened preterm labour. Cochrane Database Syst Rev 2009 (1): CD005938.

Petraglia, F., Florio, P., Nappi, C.& Genazzani, A.R. (1996). Peptide signaling in human placenta and membranes: autocrine, paracrine, and endocrine mechanisms. Endocr Rev, Vol. 17 (2): 156-86.

Petraglia, F., Imperatore, A. & Challis, J.R. (2010). Neuroendocrine mechanisms in pregnancy and parturition. Endocr Rev, Vol. 31 (6): 783-816.

Pettibone, D.J., Guidotti, M., Harrell, C.M., Jasper, J.R., Lis, E.V., O'Brien, J.A., Reiss, D.R., Woyden, C.J., Bock, M.G., Evans, B.E, et al. (1995). Progress in the development of oxytocin antagonists for use in preterm labor. Adv Exp Med Biol, Vol. 395: 601-12.

Phaneuf, S., Asbóth, G., Carrasco, M.P., Liñares, B.R., Kimura, T., Harris, A. & Bernal, A.L. (1998). Desensitization of oxytocin receptors in human myometrium. Hum Reprod Update, Vol. 4 (5): 625-33.

Phaneuf, S., Liñares, B. R., TambyRaja, R.L., MacKenzie, I.Z. & Bernal A. L. (2000). Loss of myometrial oxytocin receptors during oxytocin-induced and oxytocin-augmented labour. J Reprod Fertil, Vol. 120 (1): 91-7.

Phelan, J.P., Guay, A.T. & Newman, C. (1978). Diabetes insipidus in pregnancy: a case review. Am J Obstet Gynecol , Vol. 130 (3): 365-6.

Pierzynski, P., Lemancewicz, A., Reinheimer, T., Akerlund, M. & Laudanski, T. (2004). Inhibitory effect of barusiban and atosiban on oxytocin-induced contractions of myometrium from preterm and term pregnant women. J Soc Gynecol Investig , Vol. 11 (4): 384-7.

Plested, C.P. & Bernal, A.L. (2001). Desensitisation of the oxytocin receptor and other G-protein coupled receptors in the human myometrium. Exp Physiol , Vol. 86 (2): 303-12.

Rath, W. (2009) Prevention of postpartum haemorrhage with the oxytocin analogue carbetocin.. Eur J Obstet Gynecol Reprod Biol , Vol. 147 (1): 15-20.

Reinheimer, T.M. (2007). Barusiban suppresses oxytocin-induced preterm labour in non-human primates. BMC Pregnancy Childbirth, Vol. 7, Suppl 1: S15.

Ring, R.H., Malberg, J.E., Potestio, L., Ping, J., Boikess, S., Luo, B., Schechter, L.E., Rizzo, S., Rahman, Z. & Rosenzweig-Lipson S. (2006). Anxiolytic-like activity of oxytocin in male mice: behavioral and autonomic evidence, therapeutic implications. Psychopharmacology (Berl), Vol. 185 (2): 218-25.

Ring, R.H., Schechter, L.E., Leonard, S.K., Dwyer, J.M., Platt, B.J., Graf, R., Grauer, S., Pulicicchio, C., Resnick, L., Rahman, Z., Sukoff Rizzo, S.J., Luo, B., Beyer, C.E., Logue, S.F., Marquis, K.L., Hughes, Z.A., Rosenzweig-Lipson, S. (2010). Receptor and behavioral pharmacology of WAY-267464, a non-peptide oxytocin receptor agonist. Neuropharmacology, Vol. 58 (1): 69-77.

Serradeil-Le Gal, C., Valette, G., Foulon, L., Germain, G., Advenier, C., Naline, E., Bardou, M., Martinolle, J.P., Pouzet, B., Raufaste, D., Garcia, C., Double-Cazanave, E., Pauly, M., Pascal, M., Barbier, A., Scatton, B., Maffrand, J.P. & Le Fur, G. (2004). SSR126768A (4-chloro-3-[(3R)-(+)-5-chloro-1-(2,4-dimethoxybenzyl)-3-methyl-2-oxo-2,3-dihydro -1H-indol-3-yl]-N-ethyl-N-(3-pyridylmethyl)-benzamide, hydrochloride): a new selective and orally active oxytocin receptor antagonist for the prevention of preterm labor. J Pharmacol Exp Ther, Vol. 309 (1): 414-24.

Shuaib, A., Xu Wang, C., Yang, T. & Noor, R. (2002). Effects of nonpeptide V(1) vasopressin receptor antagonist SR-49059 on infarction volume and recovery of function in a focal embolic stroke model. Stroke, Vol. 33(1): 3033-7.

Simhan, H.N. & Caritis, S.N. (2007). Prevention of preterm delivery. N Engl J Med, Vol. 357 (5): 477-87.

Soloff, M.S., Jeng, Y.J., Copland, J.A., Strakova, Z. & Hoare, S. (2000). Signal pathways mediating oxytocin stimulation of prostaglandin synthesis in select target cells. Exp Physiol, Vol. 85, Spec No: 51S-58S.

Steinwall, M., Bossmar, T., Brouard, R., Laudanski, T., Olofsson, P., Urban, R., Wolff, K., Le-Fur, G. & Akerlund, M. (2005). The effect of relcovaptan (SR 49059), an orally active vasopressin V1a receptor antagonist, on uterine contractions in preterm labor. Gynecol Endocrinol, Vol. 20: 104-9.

Terzidou, V. (2007).Preterm labour. Biochemical and endocrinological preparation for parturition. Best Pract Res Clin Obstet Gynaecol, Vol. 21: 729-756.

Thornton, S., Goodwin, T.M., Greisen, G., Hedegaard, M. & Arce, J.C. (2009). The effect of barusiban, a selective oxytocin antagonist, in threatened preterm labor at late gestational age: a randomized, double-blind, placebo-controlled trial. Am J Obstet Gynecol, Vol. 200 (6): 627.e1-10.

Viero, C., Shibuya, I., Kitamura, N., Verkhratsky, A., Fujihara, H., Katoh, A., Ueta, Y., Zingg, H.H., Chvatal, A., Sykova, E. & Dayanithi, G. (2010). Oxytocin: Crossing the bridge between basic science and pharmacotherapy. CNS Neurosci Ther, Vol. 16: e138-56.

Wathes, D.C., Mann, G.E., Payne, J.H., Riley, P.R., Stevenson, K.R. & Lamming, G. (1996). Regulation of oxytocin, oestradiol and progesterone receptor concentrations in different uterine regions by oestradiol, progesterone and oxytocin in ovariectomized ewes. J Endocrinol, Vol. 151: 375-93.

The Worldwide Atosiban versus Beta-agonists Study Group. (2001). Effectiveness and safety of the oxytocin antagonist atosiban versus beta-adrenergic agonists in the treatment of preterm labour. BJOG, Vol. 108: 133-42.

Zingg, H.H., Rozen, F., Breton, C., Larcher, A., Neculcea, J., Chu, K., Russo, C. & Arslan, A. (1995). Gonadal steroid regulation of oxytocin and oxytocin receptor gene expression. Adv Exp Med Biol, Vol. 395: 395-404.

15

Lactate Level in Amniotic Fluid, a New Diagnostic Tool

Eva Wiberg-Itzel

Department of Clinical Science and Education, Section of Obstetrics and Gynecology,
Karolinska Institute, South General Hospital, Stockholm,
Sweden

1. Introduction

If exhaustion or muscle fatigue is discussed in a general conversation, usually people will refer lactate accumulation as a primary cause. Lactate accumulates in blood and tissues during exercise, particularly when oxygen is lacking. The concentration is highest at or just following exhaustion. Lactate has historically been considered as a dead-end waste product of anaerobic metabolism due to hypoxia and the primary cause of fatigue (Berzelius 1808; Araki 1891; Hartree & Hill 1921; Hill 1922). Lactate has also been considered as a key factor in acidosis-induced tissue damage; however the role of lactate in metabolism has changed during the last decade (Brooks 1986; Brooks 2002; Brooks 2002) Lactate is no longer considered as a harmful end-product, but mainly one of the central players in cellular and whole body metabolism.

The breakdown of glycogen during anaerobic conditions leads to intracellular accumulation lactic acid. Lactic acid is a strong monocarboxylic acid (Pka 3, 86) and it dissociates easily at physiological pH into lactate and hydrogen ions (H+). The lactate itself has been considered to have little effect on muscle contractions. However, increased production of H+ and reduced pH with acidosis has classically been considered as the cause of muscle fatigue. The role of reduced pH as an important cause of fatigue has been challenged (Karlsson et al. 1975). Present day knowledge is that anaerobic metabolism with the production of lactic acid might also lead to increased production of other factors, like phosphate (Allen et al. 2002; Westerblad & Allen 2002; Westerblad et al. 2002) which is likely to have a more prominent role in muscle fatigue.

One important finding, which has influenced the hypotheses for this thesis, is that the myometrium is a lactate producer (Taggart & Wray 1993; Taggart et al. 1996; Taggart et al. 1997; Taggart & Wray 1998; Wray et al. 2003; Quenby et al. 2004), and the level will increase when there is a lack of oxygen.

The essential function of amniotic fluid (AF) is to cushion the fetus. The fluid gives the fetus space to grow, and allows it to undergo a `physical´ development. The AF function is also to protect the fetus from trauma and to maintain temperature. It also has a minimal nutritive function.

2. Energy metabolism

The main substrate for energy metabolism is glucose (Meyer 1920). Under normal conditions, with sufficient oxygen supply, aerobic metabolism occurs. Here glucose is broken down along the glycolytic pathway, and the resulting pyruvate enters the citric acid cycle (Fig.1). Energy is produced along the glycolytic pathway, together with carbon dioxide (CO_2) and water (H_2O). Nicotinamide adenine dinucleotid (NAD+) is a powerful hydrogen ion acceptor. In the citric acid cycle NAD+ accepts an H+ to produce NADH. In the reaction O_2 is consumed, and a large amount of energy is released (36 ATP).

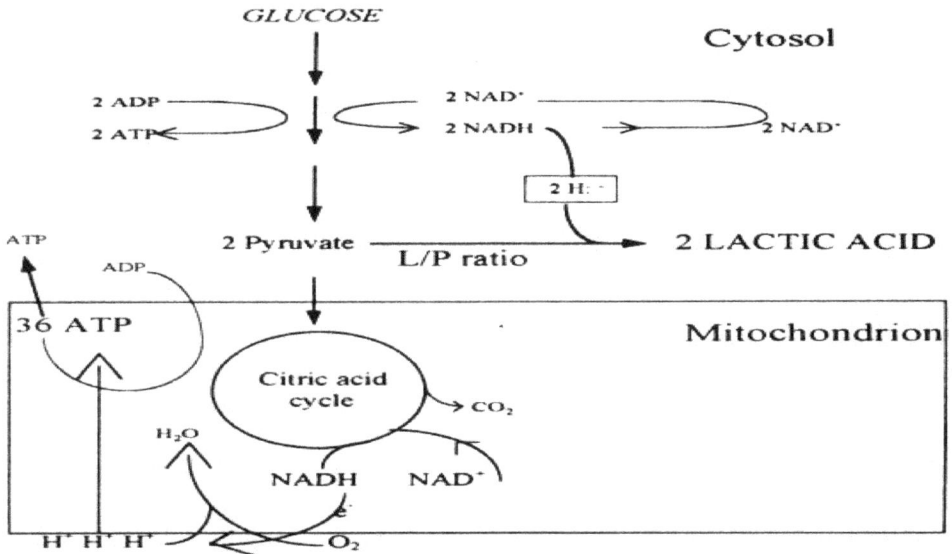

Fig. 1. From: Intrapartum Fetal Hypoxia and Biochemical Markers; a review (Nordstrom & Arulkumaran 1998).

If oxygen supply reaches a critical low level, the metabolism will change to become anaerobic. Here, instead of entering the citric acid cycle, pyruvate is reduced to lactic acid and H+. This reaction is catalyzed by the enzyme lactate- dehydrogenase (LDH), and also involves the oxidation of NADH to NAD+. NADH is generated in glycolysis, and re-oxidised into NAD+. Under anaerobic conditions, this oxidation is impaired, resulting in accumulation of NADH, promoting the conversion of pyruvate to lactate.

In normal conditions there is a steady state relation between lactic acid/pyruvate (L/P). If oxygen supply is limited, a progressive lactate acidemia (metabolic acidosis) develops. Anaerobic metabolism produces less energy (2 ATP/glucose) compared with aerobic conditions (36 ATP/glucose).

2.1 Cellular energy production

With prolonged lack of energy due to anaerobic metabolism, there is difficulty in maintaining cellular integrity. Cellular functions rely on ion gradients across cell membranes. Ion pumps require ATP to function. Regeneration of sufficient amount of ATP can no longer be sustained if anaerobic metabolism continues. In this catabolic situation, the basic cellular functions start to fail. Three different cellular energy statuses are described (Nordstrom & Arulkumaran 1998). The first one is aerobic when there is sufficient amount of oxygen and a lot of energy is produced in the form of ATP. This is an efficient way of energy production. The two others are dependent on the level of oxygen supply, and if the situation is compensated or not. Lack of oxygen forces the cell into an anaerobic metabolism with production of lactate and H+. Energy is produced but to a limited amount. If the demand of energy is still sufficient, the cellular energy status is compensated. This can continue as long as energy demand and production is in balance. If the situation is progressing, regeneration of ATP can no longer be keep up with demands and the cellular energy status will be decompensated

2.2 Buffering systems

In a normal state, the buffering systems of the organism have the capacity to maintain pH within a physiological range. It is important for the organism to maintain stability in pH, i.e. H+ concentrations. A fluctuation of H+ is dangerous for the cell. If the concentration of H+ rises it may disturb cellular function and affect the activity of cellular enzymes.

There are different buffering systems within the organism. The two most important systems are the bicarbonate and the protein buffering systems. These two systems main functions are to neutralize H+ which has been produced through anaerobic metabolism. The role of the bicarbonate buffer is to establish equilibrium between CO2, H2CO3, bicarbonate (HCO3) and hydrogen ions (H+), via the equation shown below (Siggaard-Andersen 1971).

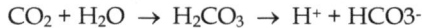

$$CO_2 + H_2O \rightarrow H_2CO_3 \rightarrow H^+ + HCO3^-$$

In this reaction CO2 is passing through and at the end is converted to bicarbonate, which leaves the red blood cells by means of an exchange of chlorides. The equation goes from left to right and back again several times until a steady state condition is established. At steady state total cellular CO2 production equals CO2 elimination.

3. Lactate

Knowledge about lactate is a rapidly changing field, and our understanding of the role of lactate metabolism has changed dramatically from the classical views held in the 19th century. The lactic acid era began in 1808 when Berzelius at the Karolinska Institute in Stockholm, discovered elevated concentrations of lactate in `the muscles of hunted stags´ (Berzelius 1808). Araki showed in 1891 that lactic acid concentration in exhausted animal muscles was proportional to the amount of exercise and was associated to O2 availability (Araki 1891). Some 100 years after Berzelius, Fletcher and Hopkins showed that lactic acid appeared in response to muscle contraction in human muscle (Fletcher & Hopkins 1907).They also showed that accumulated lactate disappeared when oxygen became available. Later on the `lactic-acid-cycle´ was described, and showed two distinct pathways in metabolism, the aerobic and the anaerobic. The coming period was called `the revolution in muscle physiology´. From the 1930's to the early

1970's lactic acid was largely considered to be a `dead-end metabolite of glycolysis after muscle hypoxia´ (Meyerhof 1920; Hill 1922). Lactic acid was also believed to be the major cause of muscle fatigue. Since the early 1970's, a `lactate revolution´ has occurred (Hermansen 1981; Wasserman 1984). At present we are in the midst of a `lactate shuttle era´ with the introduction of the `lactate shuttle hypothesis´ (Brooks GA.1986; Brooks 2000; Brooks 2002).

3.1 Muscle fatigue

It is well known that muscle performance may decline with prolonged or intense muscle activity, especially if there is a shortage of 02 (Allen et al. 1995; Westerblad et al. 2002). This decline is known as muscle fatigue. The causes of fatigue are probably multiple, but the consequence is that the power output may be drastically reduced. The consequence of lost power is obvious during sporting activity, for example, in endurance sports. It is almost impossible to maintain a marathon race if the muscles are exhausted. When a muscle goes from rest to high-intensity exercise a marked acidification occurs because of the shortage of 02. The energy demand exceeds the capacity from available aerobic metabolism. The metabolism will enter the anaerobic pathway and the ATP required will come from anaerobic metabolism. Anaerobic breakdown of glycogen leads to intracellular accumulation of inorganic acids such as, for example, lactic acid. Lactic acid is a strong acid and dissociates easily to lactate and H+ at physiological temperature. Lactate might therefore have limited effect of its own on the muscle contractions. The traditional thinking was that H+ is produced together with lactate, and H+ created the pH change and was the important cause of fatigue.

Recently presented data provide substantial support for that increased inorganic phosphate (Pi) having a key role in muscle fatigue (Westerblad et al. 1991; Westerblad et al. 1998; Westerblad 2002; Westerblad & Allen 2003), especially at physiological temperature (Westerblad et al 1997). For acidosis, on the other hand, most recent data indicate that its depressive effect on muscle contraction is limited. Other studies express doubts about the effect of Pi, and indicate that it is too early to dismiss H+ as an important factor in muscle fatigue (Fitts 2003).

The way in which human uterine smooth muscle cells metabolize and meet the energy demands during labor is still obscure. Energy is produced by glycolysis, ending with the formation of ATP and pyruvate. It has in different studies been demonstrated that the human uterus utilizes glucose as its main energy substrate at term pregnancy. It seems that smooth muscle cells in uterus are capable of producing lactate at a higher rate under aerobic conditions compared with striated muscle cells.

Fatigue has many sources that may be present in different sites in the muscle cells (Taggart & Wray 1998). Many constituents of muscle metabolism change during fatigue and for each of these metabolites we need to know which role they have in the regulation of the muscle contraction. Despite nearly 200 years of muscle function research, the question of muscle fatigue still remains partly unresolved.

3.2 Lactate shuttles

Earlier, lactate was considered to be transported across the membrane only via passive diffusion, depending on a pH gradient, (Crone 1963; Brooks 2002; Philp et al. 2005). Subsequent publications revealed a carrier-mediated transport of lactate across membranes.

An entire family of monocarboxylate transport proteins (MCT), which facilitate the transport of lactate in and out of the cells, has been described (Bonen et al. 1997; Brooks et al. 1999; Bonen 2000; Bonen 2001). During exercise lactate and H+ move in and out of tissue primarily via MCT1 and MCT4, diffusion of undissociated lactate constitutes a smaller component of the transport. It has been proposed that the force of smooth muscle contractions during labor is reduced by hypoxia in uterus, and studies have pointed out that myometrial lactic acidosis is associated with dysfunctional labors.

Lactate exchange is a dynamic process with simultaneous uptake and release between cells at rest and during exercise. At rest muscles slowly release lactate in to the surrounding fluids on a net basis, but cells may also show a small net uptake. During exercise, muscle tissue produces lactate rapidly. This results in an increased intracellular concentration of lactate and an increased net output of lactate from the muscle cells to the surrounding fluids. During recovery there is a net uptake of lactate from the ambient fluid by resting muscles, or other muscles that are exercising at low or moderate intensity. During prolonged exercise of low to moderate intensity, the muscles that originally released lactate on a net basis at the onset of exercise may actually reverse it to net lactate uptake. The conclusion from many recent studies is that lactate is a useful metabolic intermediate which can be exchanged rapidly between tissue compartments (Brooks 2002). Lactate can also be used as a substrate in aerobic condition.

4. The uterus

The uterine muscle has a dualistic function. It has to shelter the growing fetus during pregnancy within the uterine cavity. To fulfil the demand of pregnancy/parturition the human uterus has a unique construction. The uterine cavity is surrounded by smooth muscle where the myocytes are arranged in bundles embedded in connective tissue. This arrangement gives uterus elastic properties and facilitates the transmission of contractile forces generated by individual muscle cells. The uterine muscle has a relatively relaxed state during pregnancy. Second, when labor starts the uterus becomes a strongly coordinated working muscle with a high level of activity.

Blood supply of the uterus is provided by the uterine and ovarian artery. The arteries meet on the surface of the uterus where they are connected. From this connection leaves the radial artery that penetrates the myometrium and supplies both the myometrium and the placenta during pregnancy and labor. During pregnancy the myocytes undergo hypertrophy and hyperplasia resulting in significant size and volume growth of the uterus and increased demand for adequate circulation.

In the last part of pregnancy the uterus in preparation for labor through changes in the ion and hormone balance to optimize the conditions for effective synchronized contractions. The number of gap junctions and calcium concentration in the uterine tissue increases. The relaxing NO decreases. Oxytocin and prostaglandins have an important stimulating role. Oxytocin contributes via oxytocin receptors to increased contractility of the myocytes. Earlier studies of contractile myometrial activity are mostly concerned with the hormonal control. We have knowledge about the effect of oxytocin (Rezapour et al. 1996), gestagens and estrogens (Roy & Arulkumaran 1991; Spencer et al. 2005), as well as the prostaglandins during labor (Challis 1974). Their ultimate effects are assumed to be modified by local factors in the tissue, e.g. metabolites. Extended knowledge about these metabolites seems to be of importance, especially in the light of the clinical expression of labor dystocia (Steingrimsdottir et al. 1995).

During the late 1980's and the 1990's several studies have been published on myometrial activity (Wedenberg et al. 1990; Wedenberg et al. 1991; Ronquist et al. 1993; Steingrimsdottir et al. 1995; Wedenberg et al. 1995). They have shown that the pregnant myometrium has a low energy charge (EC), described as an index of energy status, and compared with striated and cardiac muscles. The difference was considered to be due to the very special demand of the uterine muscle, compared to other muscles. The cardiac muscle has to work continuously, with only short periods of rest (diastole). Striated muscles must work instantly on command. The uterine muscle remains relaxed for long periods of time and then, only for short periods (labor), has to be transferred to a state in which strong contractions are required. This situation demand energy (Steingrimsdottir et al. 1993; Steingrimsdottir et al. 1995; Steingrimsdottir et al. 1997; Steingrimsdottir et al. 1999). Studies have shown an increased content of glucose in the pregnant smooth muscle in term pregnancy, compared with early pregnancy and the non- pregnant uterus. This finding along with a positive artriovenous difference in blood-glucose across the uterus (i.e. net uptake), indicates glucose to be the principal nutritive metabolite for the pregnant uterine muscle (Steingrimsdottir et al. 1999).

The anaerobic pathway seems to be more active in the myometrium than in striated muscles. The Lactate/Pyruvate ratio, an indicator of anaerobic metabolism, is reported to be higher in the pregnant myometrium compared with other muscles (Steingrimsdottir et al. 1995). The lactate content of pregnant uterine muscle has been reported to be doubled compare with the skeletal muscle, probably reflecting a vigorous glycolytic flow when the uterus is active.

The uterus undergoes a general metabolic preparation for a hypoxic condition in late gestation. A significant physiological alkalinisation of the muscle over the last few weeks of pregnancy has been shown (Parratt et al. 1995). This might therefore contribute to the mechanisms ensuring that strong and efficient contractions occur during labor, when acidity is added during normal myometrial contractions.

A number of papers have been published on myometrial acid-base balance, and correlation to inefficient contractions and dysfunctional labor. One finding is that acidification of the myometrium with accumulation of lactate, and a decrease of myometrial pH during contractions, could depress uterine contractions and thereby contribute to dysfunctional labor. It has been shown that lactate concentration of myometrial capillary blood is significantly higher in women having a caesarean delivery due to dystocia than in women having an elective caesarean section or being operatively delivered with normal contractions. Furthermore, reduced pH and raised lactate concentrations in myometrial strips change regular contractions to irregular ones with reduced amplitude in vitro studies. One of the suggested clinical explanations for this process was that during labor blood vessel supply might be occluded while the uterus is contracting. The irregular contractile pattern in dysfunctional labor might lead to extended occlusion of the uterine vessels. Extended occlusion might lead to a lowering of the myometrial oxygen levels and accumulation of lactic acid. Thus, despite the inefficient contractions, there is an inadequate reoxygenation of the uterus. There is a suggestion that that there is a variation in response to intermittent hypoxia in different women. The recovery period from the low oxygen episode after occlusion might differ.

The knowledge that amniotic fluid (AF) contains high concentration of lactate has been published for the first time in the 1970's. Some publications have suggested that the source of lactate in AF is the fetus itself, mainly through urine and lung excretion. Several reports have suggested the myometrium as the most important lactate producer. The lactate concentration in amniotic fluid is reported to be 4 - 6 times higher as compared with fetal and maternal blood. However, from the literature it is not clear from where the high AF lactate concentration is derived.

5. Labor

"*In Africa the sun should never rise twice during labor, then it's dangerous*", an Old African saying was recounted by an African obstetrician at `Federation International Gynecologie Obstetrique´ (FIGO) 2006.

5.1 Normal delivery

Normal childbirth is a retrospective diagnosis that refers to spontaneous delivery starting after a full-term pregnancy, with absence of risk factors and/or complications. The goal of all deliveries is healthy mother, healthy baby and a positive childbirth experience.

In the first stage of labor, uterine contractions increase in frequency and strength. Since Freedman's work in the 1950s, it is considered that normal cervical dilatation during the first stage of labor is 1 cm/hour which gives a mean duration of first stage of 4.5 hours. An opening stage with a 2-3 hours delay is considered as extended or dystosic (Friedman 1955).

5.2 Labor dystocia

Labor dystocia is a common worldwide obstetrical problem, and is one of the main indications for operative intervention during parturition. Labor dystocia is clinically defined as slow/arrest of progress during labor, i.e. cervical dilatation and descent of the presenting part. It is estimated that labor dystocia occurs in about 20% of all deliveries worldwide. However, it is difficult to find a precise definition of the diagnosis of dystocia. The usual method to identifying labor dystocia is to use a partogram with an `alert line´ representing cervical dilation of 1 cm per hour and an `action line´ drawn 2-4 hours to the right of the `alert line´ (Philpot 1972). The clinical method of identifying dystocia is when the graphically plotted rate of progress crosses the action line or if no progress is made over the previous 2 hours (Lavender 2008).

Labor dystocia is associated with increased risks, such as labor abnormalities, increased risk of instrumental/operative intervention, depressed Apgar score at 5´minutes and extended need for newborn care. Dysfunctional labor is also associated with a higher frequency of postpartum infections, higher estimated maternal blood loss and lengthened maternal and newborn hospital stay.

5.3 Partogram

According to World Health Organisation (WHO) every delivery in the world should have a partogram presented during labor (Kwast et al 1994). The partogram detects maternal and fetal complications and the progress of labor. The background of the partogram, the cervicoplot, was constructed by Friedman during the 1950´s. Friedman analyzed the average of cervical dilatation speed during active phase of the 10% women with the slowest labor progress, and estimated a normal progress to be 1 cm /hour. Original curves of the cervical dilation were sigmoid with a clear transition between first and second stage of labor. The partogram has been an important tool in obstetric care since the 1950's.

Some years after Friedman's published work, Philpot and Castle constructed the first partogram. The sigmoid curve was now translated to a straight line with an expected progress of labor with 1 cm/h. This line, which is plotted in most partogram of today, is called the alert line (AL) and corresponds to the expected labor progress. The midwife or the obstetrician in charge should pay attention if labor progress deviate from the expected progress. In the development of the partogram, AL was supplemented with Action Line (ACL). When progress of labor passed ACL a dysfunctional labor was diagnosed. If labor progress crossed the ACL, intervention is recommended primarily with amniotomy and thereafter with oxytocin stimulation. The location of the ACL differs between countries and is usually placed 2-4 hours from the AL. In Sweden the ACL with the 2-hours shift is used.

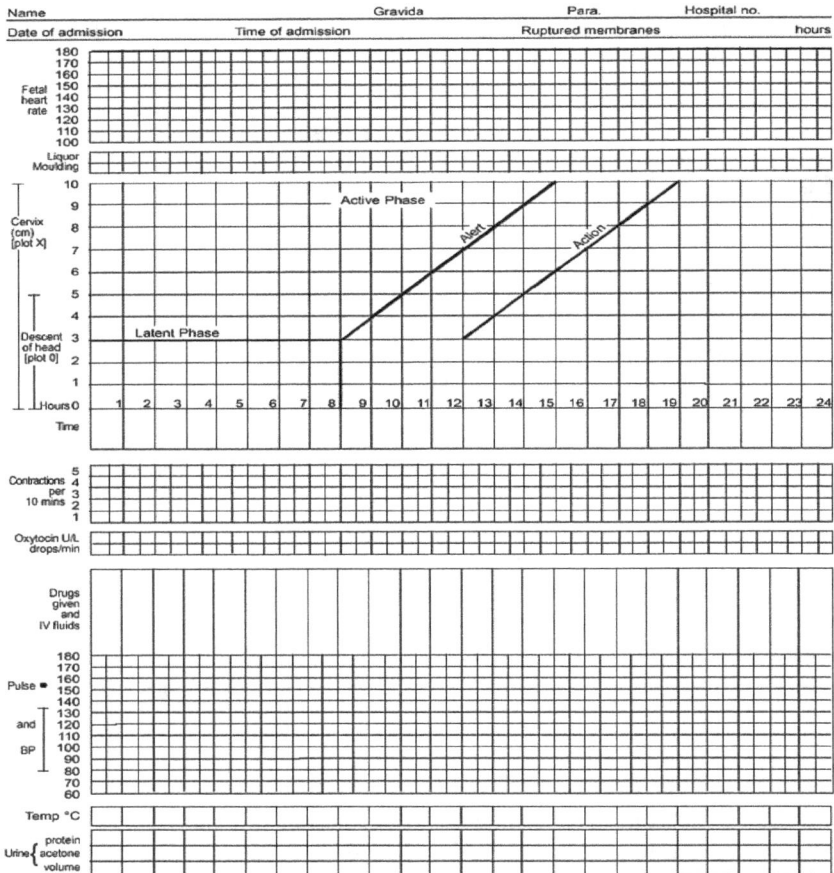

Fig. 2. The WHO Partogram

In early 1990's the WHO partogram was evaluated in a review and it was found that the use of partogram reduces the proportion of deliveries with dystocia, the number of emergency caesarean section and the frequency of stillbirths. Against this background, WHO has recommended an universal use of the partogram since 1994 (Kwast et al 1994).

Nowadays the partogram has been questioned, particularly in terms of design and efficiency. In a Cochrane review the use of partogram was evaluated and a compare with no use of partogram. An evaluation of the partogram with different placement of the ACL was also made. The results were inconclusive and showed that the use of partogram neither decreased the caesarean rates nor gave higher Apgar score at 5 minutes. Four hours displaced ACL lowered the proportion of deliveries stimulated with oxytocin. ACL with 2-hour shift seemed to provide better maternal delivery experience, but no other benefits. In summary, design and use of the partogram is questioned and there is a need for other complementary methods to monitor delivery and to identify slow progress of labor.

5.4 Active management of labor

In the late 1960s O'Driscoll and co-workers at National Maternity Hospital in Dublin, Ireland, carried out some pioneering work on normal/dysfunctional labor (O'Driscoll et al. 1969; O'Driscoll et al. 1973). They approached the management of labor in nulliparas' women, which is nowadays referred to as `active management of labour'. The method includes 1) strict criteria for the diagnosis of labor, 2) early rupture of the membranes, 3) prompt intervention with oxytocin and 4) a commitment to never leave the labouring women unattended during the period of labor. This constitutes `active management of labor'.

Trials have been conducted with some of the strict diagnostic criteria such as early amniotomy, early oxytocin stimulation in the event of abnormal progress of labor (inefficient myometrial contractions), and a commitment to never leave a labouring women unattended during the period of labor. Most of these studies have, however, been based on normal labor and not on dystosic ones. Some criticism has been made of the aggressive approach, and a combination of these interventions. There have only been a few randomised studies with `the total package of management of labor' (Akoury et al 1988; Turner et al. 1988; Boylan et al 1991; Lopez-Zeno et al 1992; Frigoletto et al 1995), and only one of these showed significantly reduction in odds ratio (OR) for caesarean birth associated with active management (Lopez-Zeno et al 1992). In contrast continuous professional support in labor has been shown to reduce the rate of operative interventions.

6. Amniotic fluid

6.1 Amniotic fluid production

The essential function of AF is to cushion the fetus (Williams et al. 1980). The fluid gives the fetus space to grow, and allows it to undergo a `physical' development. The AF function is also to protect the fetus from trauma and to maintain temperature. It also has a minimal nutritive function.

In the first half of pregnancy AF has a composition similar to fetal extra cellular fluid. The volume is closely related to fetal weight, and the skin of the fetus offers no resistant to movement of fluid. AF at this stage may be regarded as an extension of fetal extra cellular fluid. Beyond midpregnancy (about 20 weeks) the fetal skin keratinizes, and continuity between the fetal extra - cellular fluid and AF is lost. AF becomes completely external in the sense that it can now no longer equilibrate with either the fetus or the mother. After keratinisation of the fetal skin, the AF osmolarity decreases. A part of the changing composition reflects the increasing maturity of the fetal kidneys. The fetal kidneys begin to produce urine at about 12 weeks of gestation. Low osmolarity provides a large potential osmotic force for the outward flow of water across the intra- and transmembraneous pathways.

The regulatory mechanisms to achieve an adequate AF volume operate at three levels; placenta control of water and solution, transfer regulation of inflow and outflow by the fetus, and maternal effects of the fetal fluid balance. The most contributing proportion of the AF balance is the fetus and its urine production, and the AF ingested by the fetus through swallowing. A smaller contribution of AF is distributed by the fetal pulmonary fluid production, and fluid filtering through the placenta and the membranes.

The volume of amniotic fluid each week of gestation is quite variable. In healthy pregnancies the AF volume has its maximum at 32-34 weeks, averaging 800 ml. Thereafter it declines, and the decline will be most marked post term.

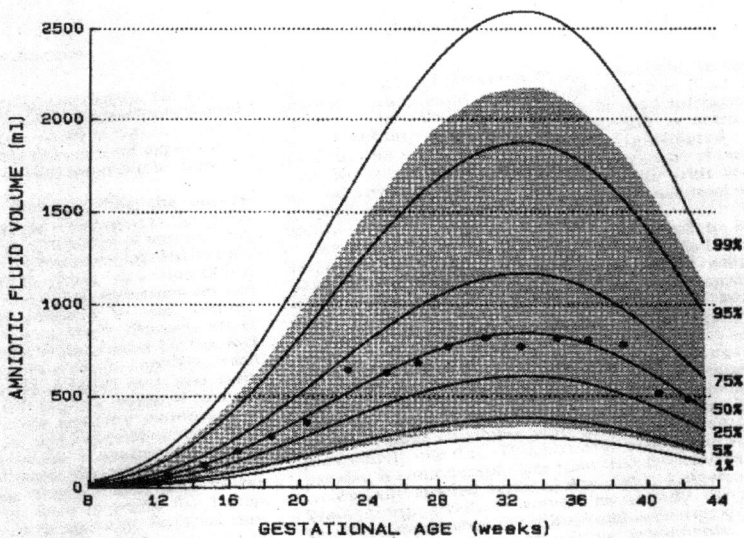

Fig. 3. AF volume as a function of gestational age. Dots represent measured volumes with 2 week intervals (mean) in 705 women. Shaded area represents 95% confidence interval. (From: William's Obstetrics 21st edition, 2001).

7. Lactate in AF, a new diagnostic tool in labor

No major improvement has occurred in the diagnostics of dysfunctional labor since the introduction of the "partogram" by Friedman and Philpot in the 1970´s. Dysfunctional labor is still one of the leading obstetrical problems, worldwide. About 20% of all deliveries have been shown to have an abnormal labor progress.

Dysfunctional labor is according to WHO defined as "a clinical deviation from expected progress" (no dilatation of cervix by 1 cm/hour, or no progress in 2 hours).The partogram is recommended to be used in all deliveries. Dysfunctional labor involves a long and painful delivery. The woman is in active labor, but the delivery progress ceases and the dilation of cervix does not proceed. The fetus does not pass through the birth canal, and the delivery comes to a halt. The reason behind dysfunctional labor is very little known, and several facts are probably due to a dysfunctional labor.

A prospective observational study was performed at Dept of Obstetrics and Gynaecology at South General Hospital, Stockholm, Sweden in 2002-2004 (Wiberg-Itzel et.al 2008). 75 women with a healthy and normal pregnancy and a spontaneous onset of labor were included in the study. AF was collected from an intrauterine pressure catheter and analyzed blinded every 30 minutes during the active phase of labor. The result was then related with the obstetrical outcome (spontaneous vaginal or operative delivery due to dysfunctional labor). The results showed that a high level of lactate in the amniotic fluid (>10.1mmol/l) at two consecutive measure during the active phase of delivery, had a strong association with the diagnosis of dystocia.

A second prospective observational study was carried out at the same hospital in Sweden between 2006-2008 (Wiberg-Itzel et. al 2010). AF from 850 healthy, normal deliveries was collected at every vaginal examination during labor. The samples were analyzed blinded. The purpose of this study was to evaluate if the level of lactate in amniotic fluid, together with the partogram recommended by the WHO could improve the diagnostics of an arrested labor. The study showed that the combination of the level of lactate in amniotic fluid and the partogram gives an improved tool to handling a delivery if there is a halt in labor progress. Among the women who was included in the study and delivered operatively due to dysfunctional labor, over 80% had an increased level of lactate in amniotic fluid (>10.1mmol/l) when labor arrested. The duration of labor was also prolonged within the group of women with an elevated lactate level in AF.

Is there an unknown transport of lactate from the uterine tissue to the AF? Experimental studies with the purpose of finding an explanatory model for the transportation of lactate out of the myometrium and into the amniotic fluid have been performed (Akerud et.al 2009). Biopsies from uterine muscle, amniotic fluid samples, umbilical cord blood and biopsies from placenta of 60 women delivered by caesarean section were collected. The presence of lactate carrying protein was identified by immunohistochemical analysis. The proteins MCT1 and MCT4 were for the first time identified in human uterine tissue. MCT1 was found in all samples but MCT4 was found only in samples from the group of women that were diagnosed as having a dysfunctional labor. The MCT transport proteins bring lactate from uterine tissue to AF, and MCT4 is activated only in dysfunctional labor with a hypoxia of the tissue. Studies are underway to examine whether there are more systems for transport of lactate in myometrial tissue.

Recently a study was published where the association between a high concentration of lactate in amniotic fluid as a possible marker of uterine tissue hypoxia during delivery, pathologic cardiotocography trace (CTG), and adverse neonatal outcome at delivery was shown (Wiberg-Itzel et.al 2011). A sample of AF was collected just before delivery and the lactate concentration was analyzed blinded. An association between high lactate value in amniotic fluid just before delivery and adverse neonatal outcome at birth was confirmed. In the group with AF lactate concentrations greater than 10.1 mmol/L at the last sampling occasion before delivery, significantly more neonates had an adverse neonatal outcome at birth, resuscitation was performed more frequently, and a higher number of newborns were admitted to the neonatal intensive care unit. Two neonates with hypoxic–ischemic encephalopathy grade 2 were found, and both belonged to the group with a high concentration of lactate in amniotic fluid, whereas there were no newborns in the group with lower amniotic fluid lactate that developed hypoxic-ischemic encephalopathy.

In summary, it was found that the use of CTG together with an analysis of the lactate concentration in AF could be a promising and useful predictor of fetal outcome in labor. The method is easy, non-invasive, and safe for the mother and her unborn child. The findings have important clinical implications in view of the fact that children are still born with an unexpected adverse neonatal outcome, even with what is considered to be careful fetal surveillance

7.1 Ongoing study

Currently, a large collaborative prospective project between 10 European and one African clinic is running. In the "Dysfunctional labor study" data, saliva and amniotic fluid from 5000 primiparas and their deliveries is collected. This in a desire to gain more knowledge about the state called dystocia. The study is scheduled to continue until summer 2012.

8. Prelabor rupture of the membranes (PROM)

Prelabor rupture of membranes (PROM) is defined as `spontaneous leakage of AF prior to onset of labor´ with a gestational age of 37 weeks or more (WHO definition). Preterm PROM (PPROM) is ruptured membranes before 37 weeks of gestation. PROM is a relatively common event in obstetric practice, and the prevalence is reported to be 5-19% of all pregnancies (Hannah et al. 1996).

8.1 Clinical management of PROM

The management of PROM has been considered controversy since the 1950's. The modern era of this field began in 1966 with several reports that showed increased risk for both the mother and the fetus, when expectant management of PROM was undertaken. PROM without immediate onset of labor was considered to carry a high potential risk of incurring intrauterine infection (Shubeck et al. 1966; Webb 1967).

In the 1950's the perinatal mortality associated with PROM was estimated to range from 2.6% to 11%, and increased with the duration between PROM and delivery. The maternal mortality related to PROM, was reported to be 0.2‰. On the basis that PROM without immediate onset of labor was considered dangerous an aggressive approach to PROM was advised in the 1970's and 1980's. Early induction and operative intervention were suggested, especially if labor had not started within 24 hours. One problem with this aggressive approach was failed inductions with concomitant increased frequency of caesarean sections.

Studies of women with PROM and unfavourable cervix status have been published (Kappy et al. 1979). A spontaneous onset of labor within 24 hours in 85% of the women with established PROM is presented. They also reported a reduced caesarean section rate with expectant management, and no evidence of increased neonatal infections.

In a large randomised trial of 5041 women with PROM they were randomly assigned to immediate induction of labor or expectant management (Hannah et al. 1996). The women were randomised to induction with oxytocin, vaginal PGE2-gel or expectant management up to four days after PROM. If labor had not started within four days, the women were induced with oxytocin or PGE_2 gel. The primary outcomes were neonatal infection and women's evaluation of their treatment. They found no significant differences between the study groups, and concluded that in both management groups a similar rate of neonatal infections (2-3%) and caesarean sections (10%) were found. Women evaluated early induction of labor more positively than expectant management.

A Swedish PROM study was conducted in the 1990's where 1385 women were included (Ladfors et al. 1996). The result showed a 13% prevalence of PROM after 34 weeks of gestation. They compared obstetric and neonatal outcome between two different expectant management groups, expectancy for 48 or 72 hours. The result showed a higher rate of spontaneous deliveries among nulliparas in the `late´ induction group compared with `early´ induction. The rate of instrumental delivery was lower in the `late´ induction group, but the rate of caesarean sections was similar. They concluded that expectant for 72 hours was to be recommended. Digital vaginal examination before onset of labor was not allowed in this trial. Low frequencies of maternal and fetal infections were found, and there were no differences between the groups.

False negative diagnosis with visual inspection at speculum examination was found to be 12%. No disadvantage, i.e. infections, was found for mother or child if the woman was sent home after a false negative speculum examination. They questioned the value of using biochemical tests in the management of women with suspected PROM. No comments were made on the assumed false positive diagnosis in women with suspect PROM. All women included in the trial had visible AF at examination, but 3.1% of them had intact membranes at delivery.

8.2 Historical review of PROM tests

In 1920's, it was found that vaginal pH turned from acid to neutral or alkaline when contaminated with amniotic fluid. In 1938 the nitrazine test was introduced, which measured pH in vaginal secrete within a narrower range. This method has been widely used all over the world.

The crystallisation pattern of AF was first described in 1950's. The crystallisation phenomenon, also called ferning or arborisation test is dependent on the relative concentration of electrolytes, proteins and hydrocarbonates in AF. The crystallisation test is nowadays still one of the most commonly used methods in clinical practice worldwide.

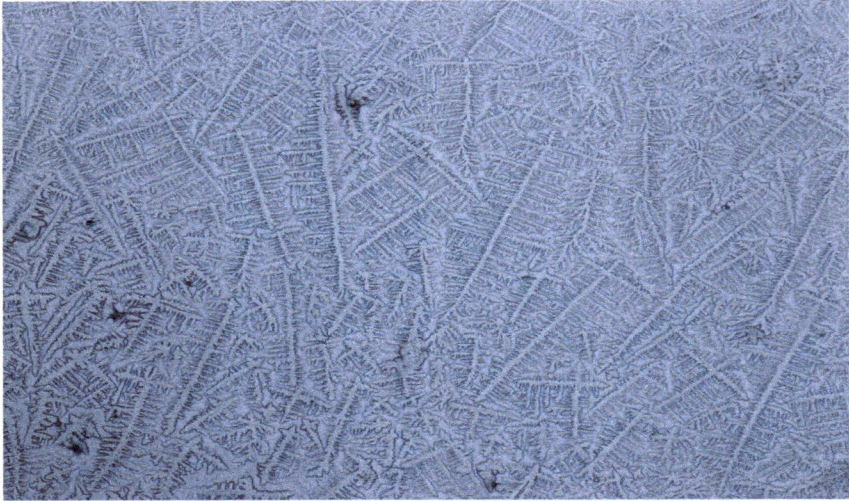

Fig. 4. Photo taken at microscopy (x 40) of AF from one woman included in the "lac-test" study.

Nile blue sulphate staining of the neutral lipid in cells from fetal sebaceous glands was described in 1960's. The cells turn orange as a consequence of the oxazone in Nile blue. The cells are single or grouped in clusters. Other cells, like vaginal squamous, and pus cells or erythrocytes stain blue. A limitation of this test is that these fat-containing cells are only present after 32 weeks of gestation.

In selecting a spectrum of tests to be used in doubtful instances of ruptured membranes, it was determined that a combination of these three tests described above would produce an accuracy of diagnosis approximating 93%.

8.3 Present tests of today

DAO test (DiAmine oxidase activity)

The DAO test was one of the first biochemical tests for PROM, and was developed during the 1970's. DAO is present in high concentrations in AF but is absent in normal vaginal secretions and urine. DAO is produced by placental decidual cells and increases during pregnancy. The method is reported to have a sensitivity of 84-100% and a specificity of 74-100%. The test was carried out with 10 ul of AF absorbed on a paper strip, and the test requires a scintillation counter. This method is not available today because of the toxic chemicals that are used in the analysis.

AFP test (Monoclonal antibody test kit)

AF also contains high concentrations of alpha feto protein (AFP) especially in preterm pregnancy. A monoclonal antibody assay method with high sensitivity and specificity was presented. However, they also reported that a false positive test may occur as AFP may cross weakened membranes in cases with chorioamnionitis or heavy blood contamination. This test is not used in clinical practice any more.

Fetal fibronectin (ROM-check)

Fibronectin is a large plasma glycoprotein. Three sub-types are available, of which one is feta derived. The concentration of fetal fibronectin in amniotic fluid is 5-10 times higher than in maternal plasma. In the 1990's many papers were published about fetal fibronectin and its usefulness to detect AF in women with suspect PROM. To use fetal fibronectin when detecting PROM is a sensitive test (97%) but a test with a very low specificity (27%). Additionally, in patients without rupture of the membranes, the interval between sampling and delivery was shown to be significantly shorter if fetal fibronectin was present. The conclusion was that the presence of fetal fibronectin in cervicovaginal secretions may be a good marker for impending labor rather than a good test for ruptured membranes. Today fetal Fibronectin is used in a combination with ultrasound, to detect the risk of premature delivery.

Insulin-like growth factor binding protein-1 (PROM-test™)

Insulin-like growth factor (IGF) is a peptide and is bound to a binding protein (IGFBP) in the blood circulation. IGFBP-1 is a placental protein and is present in much higher concentrations in AF as compared with serum, cervical mucous, urine or seminal plasma. A commercial kit, with monoclonal antibodies to IGFBP-1 attached to a small wand has been available since 1993 (actim PROM-test™). During the last decade, many papers have been published on the actim PROM-Test™. The sensitivity of the test is reported to be 71-100% and specificity 88-100%. It has been concluded that actim PROM-test™ is one of the most accurate diagnostic tests today in the diagnosis of suspected PROM. However, contamination of maternal blood or leakage of IGFBP-1 through stretched fetal membranes may cause false positive tests. A false negative result may occur if there is an inadequate sampling, intraamniotic infection, vaginal discharge, maternal blood loss, or prolonged time from rupture of membranes to application of the test. Gestatational age should not influence the test.

B-HCG in vaginal washing fluid

B-HCG is a glycoprotein produced exclusively by syncytiotrophoblasts in the placenta. Several studies have investigated β-HCG as a useful test for the diagnosis of PROM in the third trimester. These studies have shown a sensitivity of 68-100% and a specificity of 95-97%.

Amnisure®

In 1975, the placental alpha microglobulin–1 (PAMG-1) protein was isolated from AF. Antibodies were obtained against the protein and Amnisure® is an immunochemical method, used to measure the content of PAMG-1 protein in vaginal fluid, in cases with suspect PROM. Amnisure® has been available on the market since 2005. In a study which included 203 women with suspected PROM, a sensitivity of 98.8% and a specificity of 100% were found.

9. Lactate in AF, a new diagnostic tool when handling a suspect PROM

Lac-test, a good, reliable and useful clinical test for PROM with both a high sensitivity and a high specificity has been presented in several publications. The test is easy to use in the clinical situation with an answer immediately available at the bedside. A vaginal fluid lactate concentration of >4.5 mmol/l in women having a history of suspect PROM is shown to be the best cut-off value to discriminate between visible/non visible AF at speculum examination.

300 Women attending the delivery ward in South General Hospital, Stockholm, with a suspected PROM were included in this prospective study (Wiberg-Itzel E et.al 2005). All women had a singleton pregnancy, a suspected history of PROM (scanty leakage of fluid from the vagina) after 34 weeks gestation and without uterine contractions. Cases with suspected PROM but with obvious pouring water were excluded. A speculum examination was performed, and the clinical management was based on whether AF was visible or not at examination. If AF was observed, induction of labor was planned after two days if labor had not started spontaneously. If AF was not seen and the pregnancy was otherwise uneventful, the woman was sent home with no further follow-up planned. Visible AF at speculum examination was regarded as `true´ ruptured membranes. The lactate concentration in vaginal secretions was analysed and registered by an independent nurse, and the value was concealed from the clinician in charge of the delivery ward.

In most cases, the diagnosis of PROM is obvious. The woman describes having experienced a history of limited water-like secretions from the vagina, and water is seen streaming down the legs or in pads. However, there still remain cases in which the history is strongly suggestive of ruptured membranes but at physical examination no AF can be seen. In these situations a speculum examination is recommended to confirm or exclude ruptured membranes. Studies have shown a false negative diagnosis with visual inspection of speculum examination to be 12% (Ladfors et al 1996). No increased morbidity (i.e. infection) is found in this group. In presented studies where only speculum examination was used, no comments were made on the assumed false positive group i.e. those where AF was thought to be seen but the membranes were obviously not broken. However, 3.1% of the women were reported to have signs of intact membranes at induction of labor, and could represent cases with false positive diagnosis as inspection was used.

When a speculum examination is performed, experience suggests that all ´water seen´ is not always ruptured membranes. Consequently, no visible AF can be a false negative observation, and visible AF can be a false positive one. If the woman has not started labor spontaneously within 48 hours after a diagnosed PROM, she will normally be exposed to induction of labor. 44% intervention rate (instrumental or emergency caesarean delivery) was shown in the induction group in this study. A particularly high frequency of intervention occurred in the group of women with visible AF but low lactate concentration (<=4.5mmol/l). This is an important finding, as reliable diagnosis might prevent unnecessary intervention, the `Lac-test´ is shown to be such a reliable test, which also is simple and handy in the clinical management.

To summarise the `Lac-test´ was found to be a reliable test with both a high sensitivity and a high specificity. Its ease of application makes it attractive in clinical practice.

9.1 Prediction of onset of labor

At term pregnancy PROM is often a part of normal parturition and most of the women with PROM will have a spontaneous onset of labor within a limited period of time. PROM occurs in 5-19% of all patients at term and is followed by spontaneous onset of labor in 60% within

24 hours and in 95% within 72 hours. However, it is crucial to diagnose ruptured membranes. 10% of pregnant women at term attend hospitals with suspected PROM, and to have the possibility to predict those who will start labor spontaneously would clearly simplify management (Wiberg-Itzel et al. 2006). A good prediction is also appreciated by the parturient.

The time to onset of labor was in this work essentially similar among women with lactate concentration of >4.5mmol/l in vaginal fluid. In contrast, women with lactate concentrations <4.5 mmol/l appeared to have longer time to spontaneous onset of labor (median time 54 hours) from the time of examination. These findings lend support to the view that it is the rupture of the membranes (ROM) which is crucial to diagnose, when estimating the probability of spontaneous onset of labor within one or two days.

In clinical practice there is a lack of any adequate predictor to identify women with spontaneous onset of labor within a certain time limit. Transvaginal ultrasonographic measurement of cervical length is one method which is used in clinical practice. However, this method is mainly used in cases with a risk of pre-term labor. No clear, rational and evaluated strategy for daily practical use has emerged.

In this study 54 % of all the women included were in labor within 24 hours. Among those with a lactate concentration > 4.5 mmol/l, 88% had spontaneous onset of labor < 24 hours, compared with 21%among those with lower lactate value. However, in the group where amniotic fluid was not visible and the lactate level was low (<4.5 mmol/l), only 15% had started labor within 24 hours. By using lactate concentration > 4.5 mmol/l as cut-off, a total number of 83%would be correctly classified as to whether they were going to be in labor within 24 hours or not.

Summarising suggests that cases with suspected PROM (not water streaming down the woman's legs) should primarily be correctly diagnosed with the `Lac-test´, to avoid false positive tests at inspection and unnecessary intervention, and to obtain a good prediction of onset of labor.

9.2 PPROM

Preterm prelabor rupture of membrane (PPROM) is defined as 'rupture of the fetal membranes prior to onset of labor in a patient who has a gestational age of less than 37 weeks'. PPROM occurs in approximately 3–5% of all pregnancies and accounts for one-third of all preterm births. PPROM is associated with risks of preterm delivery and with substantially increased risks of perinatal morbidity and mortality.

An accurate diagnosis of PPROM is critical to both long- and short-term health and survival for the baby. The absence of a 'gold standard' for the diagnosis of PPROM has stimulated us to search for a clinically applicable marker of PPROM and a marker to predict onset of preterm labor (Wiberg-Itzel et.al 2009).

We have previously shown that a positive 'LAC test', that is a lactate concentration >4.5 mmol/l in vaginal fluid, is a reliable test for rupture of the membranes in pregnancies of 34 weeks of gestation or more. We have also found a significant association between a positive

LAC test and spontaneous onset of labor within 48 hours in late gestations, that is >34 weeks.

Of the 81 women included in this study, 45 had a gestational age less than 34 weeks at the time of examination. Among these, 11 women (24%) had a lactate concentration of >4.5 mmol/l (positive LAC test), of whom 9 (82%) were in active labor within 48 hours. 'False negatives' (negative LAC test but delivered <48 hours) occurred in 0 of 34 women in this subgroup.

A prediction of spontaneous onset of labor is even more valuable in preterm pregnancies, when antenatal steroids may be administered, and women may be referred to tertiary level of medical care. The publication showed that lactate determination in vaginal fluid seems promising as a tool to predict onset of labor within 48 hours even in women with suspected PPROM. A positive LAC test (>4.5 mmol/l) was more strongly associated with spontaneous onset of labor than visible AF.

10. Conclusion

Failure of progress in labor contributes to the increased frequency of caesarean section worldwide. If we are attempt to address this problem it is necessary to understand the reasons why this occurs, identify the women most likely to develop dystocia in labor and apply timely and appropriate interventions to correct inefficient uterine action when possible, thereby improving outcome for mothers and their babies.

To be able to get a correct diagnose in cases with suspect PROM, to avoid false positive tests, unnecessary intervention and to obtain a good prediction of onset of labor, in term as well as in preterm deliveries, is very appealing.

Our hope is that lactate value in AF will be a new and very useful diagnostic tool in obstetrical care.

11. References

Akoury HA et al. (1988). "Active management of labor and operative delivery in nulliparous women." Am J Obstet Gynecol 158(2): 255-8.

Allen D et al. (1995). "Muscle cell function during prolonged activity: cellular mechanisms of fatigue." Exp Physiol 80(4): 497-527.

Allen D et al. (2002). "Muscle fatigue: the role of intracellular calcium stores." Can J Appl Physiol 27(1): 83-96

Araki T. (1891). Ueber die bildung von milchsaure and glucose im organismmus bei sauerstoffmangel. Zeitschr. Phys.Chem. 15:335-370.

Berzelius JJ (1808). Djurkemien. Stockholm: Marquard.Bonen A et al. (1997). "Lactate transport and lactate transporters in skeletal muscle." Can J Appl Physiol 22(6): 531-52.

Bonen A. (2000). "Lactate transporters (MCT proteins) in heart and skeletal muscles." Med Sci Sports Exerc 32(4): 778-89.

Bonen A. (2001). "The expression of lactate transporters (MCT1 and MCT4) in heart and muscle." Eur J Appl Physiol 86(1): 6-11.

Boylan P et al. (1991). "Effect of active management of labor on the incidence of cesarean section for dystocia in nulliparas." Am J Perinatol 8(6): 373-9.

Brooks GA. (1986). "The lactate shuttle during exercise and recovery." Med Sci Sports Exerc 18(3): 360-8.

Brooks GA. (2000). "Intra- and extra-cellular lactate shuttles." Med Sci Sports Exerc 32(4): 790-9.

Brooks GA. (2002). "Lactate shuttle -- between but not within cells?" J Physiol 541(Pt 2): 333-4.

Challis RG. (1974). "Physiology and pharmacology of PGs in parturition." Popul Rep G (5): 45-53.

Crone C. (1963). "Does "restricted diffusion" occur in muscle capillaries?" Proc Soc Exp Biol Med 112: 453-5.

Fitts RH. (2003). "Effects of regular exercise training on skeletal muscle contractile function." Am J Phys Med Rehabil 82(4): 320-31.

Fletcher WM & Hopkins FG. (1907). Lactic acid in amphibian muscle. J. Physiol. 275:247 309.

Friedman E. A. (1955), 'Primigravid labor; a graphicostatistical analysis', Obstetrics and gynecology, 6 (6), 567-89.

Frigoletto FD et al. (1995). "A clinical trial of active management of labor." N Engl J Med 333(12): 745-50.

Hannah ME et al. (1996)."Induction of labor compared with expectant management for prelabor rupture of the membranes at term. TERM PROM Study Group." N Engl J Med 334(16): 1005-10.

Hartree W & Hill AV. (1921). "The nature of the isometric twitch." J Physiol 55(5-6): 389-411.

Hermansen L. (1981). "Effect of metabolic changes on force generation in skeletal muscle during maximal exercise." Ciba Found Symp 82: 75-88.

Hill AV. (1922). "The maximum work and mechanical efficiency of human muscles, and their most economical speed." J Physiol 56(1-2): 19-41.

Kappy KA et al. (1979). "Premature rupture of the membranes: a conservative approach." Am J Obstet Gynecol 134(6): 655-61

Karlsson J et al. (1975). "Constituents of human muscle in isometric fatigue." J Appl Physiol 38(2): 208-11.

Kwast B. E et al (1994), 'World Health Organization partograph in management of labour. World Health Organization Maternal Health and Safe Motherhood Programme', Lancet, 343 (8910), 1399-404.

Ladfors L et al. (1996). "A randomised trial of two expectant managements of prelabour rupture of the membranes at 34 to 42 weeks." Br J Obstet Gynaecol 103(8): 755-62.

Lavender T et al. (2008), 'Effect of partogram use on outcomes for women in spontaneous labour at term', Cochrane database of systematic reviews, (4), CD005461

Lopez-Zeno JA et al. (1992). "A controlled trial of a program for the active management of labor." N Engl J Med 326(7): 450-4.

Meyerhof O. (1920). Plügers Arch. Gesamte Physiol. Menschen Tiere. 185;11-32.

Nordstrom L & Arulkumaran S. (1998). "Intrapartum fetal hypoxia and biochemical markers: a review." Obstet Gynecol Surv 53(10): 645-57.

O'Driscoll K et al. (1969). "Prevention of prolonged labour." Br Med J 2(5655): 477-80.

O'Driscoll K et al. (1973). "Active management of labour." Br Med J 3(5872): 135- 7.

Parratt JR et al. (1995). "Changes in intracellular pH close to term and their possible significance to labour." Pflugers Arch 430(6): 1012-4.

Philp A et al. (2005). "Lactate--a signal coordinating cell and systemic function." J Exp Biol 208(Pt 24): 4561-75.

Philpott RH. (1972)."Graphic records in labour." Br Med J 4(5833): 163-5.

Rezapour M et al. (1996). "Myometrial steroid concentration and oxytocin receptor density in parturient women at term." Steroids 61(6): 338-44.

Ronquist G et al. (1993). "High adenosine content in human uterine smooth muscle compared with striated skeletal muscle." Clin Chim Acta 223(1-2): 93-102.

Roy AC & Arulkumaran S. (1991). "Pharmacology of parturition." Ann Acad Med Singapore 20(1): 71-7.

Shubeck F et al. (1966). "Fetal hazard after rupture of the membranes. A report from the collaborative project." Obstet Gynecol 28(1): 22-31.

Siggaard-Andersen O. (1971). "An acid-base chart for arterial blood with normal and pathophysiological reference areas." Scand J Clin Lab Invest 27(3): 239-45.

Spencer TE & Hayashi K. (2005). "Comparative developmental biology of the mammalian uterus." Curr Top Dev Biol 68: 85-122.

Steingrimsdottir T et al. (1993). "Energy economy in the pregnant human uterus at term: studies on arteriovenous differences in metabolites of carbohydrate, fat and nucleotides." Eur J Obstet Gynecol Reprod Biol 51(3): 209-15.

Steingrimsdottir T et al. (1995). "Different energy metabolite pattern between uterine smooth muscle and striated rectus muscle in term pregnant women." Eur J Obstet Gynecol Reprod Biol 62(2): 241-5.

Steingrimsdottir T et al. (1997). "Human uterine smooth muscle exhibits a very low phosphocreatine/ATP ratio as assessed by in vitro and in vivo measurements." Eur J Clin Invest 27(9): 743-9.

Steingrimsdottir T et al. (1999). "Low myometrial glycogen content compared with rectus muscle in term pregnant women before labor." Gynecol Obstet Invest 47(3): 166-71.

Taggart M & Wray S. (1993). "Simultaneous measurement of intracellular pH and contraction in uterine smooth muscle." Pflugers Arch 423(5-6): 527-9.

Taggart MJ et al. (1996). "Stimulus-dependent modulation of smooth muscle intracellular calcium and force by altered intracellular pH." Pflugers Arch 432(5): 803- 11.

Taggart MJ et al. (1997). "External alkalinization decreases intracellular Ca++ and spontaneous contractions in pregnant rat myometrium." Am J Obstet Gynecol 177(4): 959-63.

Taggart MJ & Wray S. (1998). "Hypoxia and smooth muscle function: key regulatory regulatory events during metabolic stress." J Physiol 509 (Pt 2): 315-25

Turner MJ et al. (1988). "Active management of labor associated with a decrease in the cesarean section rate in nulliparas." Obstet Gynecol 71(2): 150-4.

Wasserman K. (1984). "The anaerobic threshold measurement to evaluate exercise performance." Am Rev Respir Dis 129(2 Pt 2): S35-40.

Webb GA. (1967). "Maternal death associated with premature rupture of the membranes. An analysis of 54 cases." Am J Obstet Gynecol 98(5): 594-601.

Wedenberg K et al. (1990). "Low energy charge in human uterine muscle." Biochim Biophys Acta 1033(1): 31-4.

Wedenberg K et al. (1991). "Regional differences in energy charge of the pregnant human uterus regardless of functional status in comparison with the non- pregnant uterus." Biochim Biophys Acta 1058(2): 147-51.

Wedenberg K et al. (1995). "Energy economy of human uterine muscle strips under different in vitro conditions and its dependence on tissue redox potential." Eur J Obstet Gynecol Reprod Biol 62(1): 115-9.

Westerblad H et al. (1991). "Cellular mechanisms of fatigue in skeletal muscle." Am J Physiol 261(2 Pt 1): C195-209.

Westerblad H et al. (1997). "The effect of intracellular pH on contractile function of intact, single fibres of mouse muscle declines with increasing temperature." J Physiol 500 (Pt 1): 193-204.

Westerblad H et al. (1998). "Mechanisms underlying the reduction of isometric force in skeletal muscle fatigue." Acta Physiol Scand 162(3): 253-60.

Westerblad H and Allen DG. (2002). "Recent advances in the understanding of skeletal muscle fatigue." Curr Opin Rheumatol 14(6): 648-52

Westerblad H, Allen DG et al. (2002). "Muscle fatigue: lactic acid or inorganic phosphate the major cause?" News Physiol Sci 17: 17-21

Westerblad H and Allen DG (2003). "Cellular mechanisms of skeletal muscle fatigue." Adv Exp Med Biol 538: 563-70; discussion 571.

Wiberg-Itzel et al. (2005). "Lactate determination in vaginal fluids: a new method in the diagnosis of prelabour rupture of membranes." BJOG 112(6): 754-8

Wiberg-Itzel et al. (2006). Association between lactate in vaginal fluid and time to spontaneous onset of labour for women with suspected prelabour rupture of the membranes.BJOG.Dec;113(12):1426-30.

Wiberg-Itzel et al. (2008), 'Association between lactate concentrations in amniotic fluid and dysfunctional labor', Acta obstetricia et gynecologica. Scandinavica, 87 (9), 924-8

Wiberg-Itzel et al. (2009). Prediction of time to spontaneous onset of labour with lactate concentration in vaginal fluid in women with suspected preterm prelabour rupture of the membranes. BJOG Jan; 116(1):62-6.

Wiberg-Itzel et.al (2010), 'Lactate concentration in amniotic fluid: a good predictor of labor outcome', European journal of obstetrics, gynecology, and reproductive biology, 152 (1), 34-8.

Wiberg-Itzel E et al (2011) Association between Adverse Neonatal Outcome and Lactate Concentration in Amniotic Fluid. Obstet Gynecol.Jul;118(1):135-142

Williams et al. (1980). Williams Obstetrics. New York, Appleton-Century-Crofts

Wray S et al. (2003). "Calcium signaling and uterine contractility." J Soc Gynecol Investig 10(5): 252-64.

Quenby S et al. (2004). "Dysfunctional labor and myometrial lactic acidosis." Obstet Gynecol 103(4): 718-23.

Akerud H et al. (2009), 'Lactate distribution in culture medium of human myometrial biopsies incubated under different conditions', American journal of physiology. Endocrinology and metabolism, 297 (6), E1414-9.

16

Operative Vaginal Deliveries in Contemporary Obstetric Practice

Sunday E. Adaji[1] and Charles A. Ameh[2]
[1]Ahmadu Bello University and Ahmadu Bello University Teaching Hospital, Zaria,
[2]Liverpool School of Tropical Medicine, Pembroke Place, Liverpool,
[1]Nigeria
[2]United Kingdom

1. Introduction

The expectation of every pregnant woman is to undergo a spontaneous vaginal delivery with minimal or no resort to operative procedures at the end of pregnancy. For the majority of women this expectation becomes a reality. For some however, assistance is required either in the form of caesarean sections or operative vaginal procedures in order to avert adverse maternal and fetal outcomes. Assisting laboring women to deliver vaginally using specialized instruments is a practice that dates back several centuries. Forceps and ventouse are the most popular of the operative vaginal procedures with comprehensive documentation of their development and use in the lay and medical media. Procedures like symphysiotomy and destructive operations to remove a dead fetus are probably now materials for the waste bins of medical history. However some still argue for a place for them in modern obstetric practices especially in low income countries where the indications for their use may still be found (Maharaj and Moodley, 2002).

Instrumental vaginal delivery is a key element of essential obstetric care, scaling up its use in resource poor countries through training and supply of appropriate equipment is likely to contribute significantly to reduced maternal and newborn morbidity/mortality(Ameh and Weeks, 2009).

2. The obstetrical forceps

'Use only on the most urgent occasions

'Head on the perineum for 6 hours

'If the head advances, no matter how slowly, no interference unless the child be dead

'Use the forceps sparingly –

'Where they save one they murder many'

~A summary of the guidelines for the use forceps in Smellie's time

The obstetrical forceps is probably the earliest instrument designed to assist vaginal delivery. Behind its design, invention and evolvement lies florid and interesting history with ancient Egyptian, Greek, Roman, and Persian texts containing references to the use of forceps to deliver women in cases of intrauterine fetal deaths. The refugee family of William Chamberlain, who facing religious persecution in their home country of France, migrated to London in the 16th Century is widely credited with the development of the obstetrical forceps as is known today. This family takes credit for the design, invention and use of obstetrical forceps to deliver women with obstructed labour for about three generations (Dunn, 1999). The instruments and their use were a well-kept family secret, only revealed nearly 200 years after their invention! Obstetrical forceps have undergone several modifications over time. It is estimated that there may well be over 700 different types of obstetrical forceps in existence, not counting those that did not make it beyond the design stage. The types vary by designer, intended objective of using it, material, place and sometimes the ingenuity of the inventor. Forceps are designed to aid the delivery of the fetal head by the application of traction. To effect a delivery, a pair with each one a mirror image of the other are applied around the fetal head. Each of a pair consists basically of a blade, shank, and a handle (see figure 1 below).

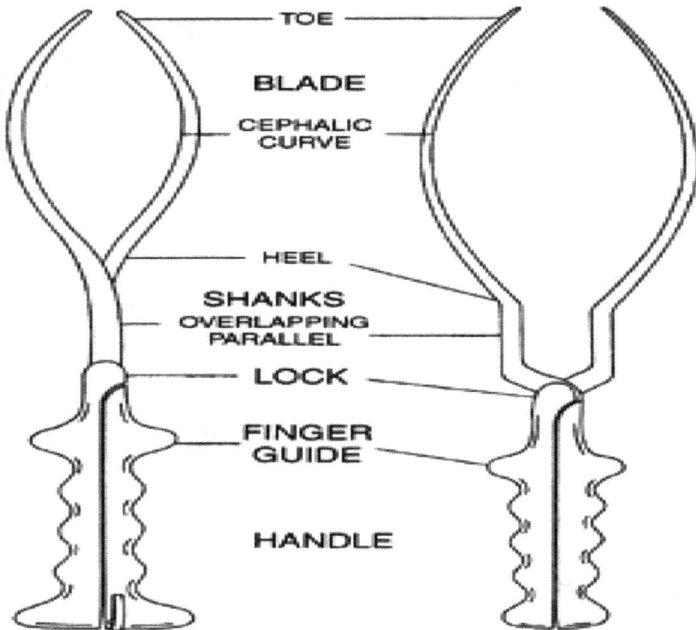

Fig. 1. Parts of the two main types of obstetrical forceps

Based on ability to rotate the fetal head in the birth canal, forceps could be classified into those that can effect traction only and those that can be used to effect rotation and traction. The main difference in the design is in the blades and the lock. An archetype of traction only forceps is the Simpson's forceps with an 'English' lock and pelvic and cephalic curves on the blade while Kielland's forceps is the archetype of traction and rotation forceps with only the cephalic curve and sliding lock (Chiswick and James, 1979).

3. The vacuum extractor

The principle of the vacuum was first applied for the treatment of depressed skull fractures in infants in 1632! That force generated in a closed space (vacuum) can be increased to aid the delivery of a fetus was first reported by James Young, surgeon to the Naval Hospital in Plymouth, England in 1655 (Malmstrom, 1957). About 100 years later Seaman of Jena described his dream of the use of a vacuum device to assist delivery without injury to the mother or baby. "....*an air pump which wherewith one can seize the head of the infant without injury to mother and child. The pump was made of brass and had a covering of rubber with ventilators....*". The European medical and lay literature is replete with such fancies, designs and attempts but none drew international attention and widespread acceptance (Vacca, 2003). Malmstrom's device eventually received international acceptance in the middle of the 20 century. He first introduced his device in 1953 and refined it further by 1957; it was originally used in the first stage of labour to improve uterine action by 'pulling the head down to the cervix'. Malmstrom is therefore credited as the father of the modern vacuum extractor. The unique feature of the Malmstrom's Vacuum Extractor is that the metal cup has an in-curved rounded margin which is of a narrower diameter than the base (see figure 2 below). This design produces a chignon on the fetal scalp thereby minimizing the risk of detachment during traction. Other components include a vacuum pump, a guage, vacuum container and rubber tubing. Malmstrom's device has been modified by other inventors as extensively discussed in the history of vacuum extraction by Baskett (Vacca, 2003).

Bird significantly modified the cup such that the suction port and the traction port are separated; the suction port located close to the rim of the convex surface of the cup and the traction port located at its center. This helps to reduce the leverage on the cup during traction and reduces the risk of detachment. A further advantage of this modification is the improved accessibility to the flexion point in deflexed occipito-transverese and occipito-posterior positions. The Bird modification is also referred to as the 'OP' cup. Over the next 20 years several modifications of the vacuum extractor became popular in Scandanavia, Europe and Africa. This may have been due to a commonly held perception that it required less training for safe use compared to the alternative-obstetric forceps. This view was first suggested about 150 years earlier by Neil Arnott (Vacca, 2003).

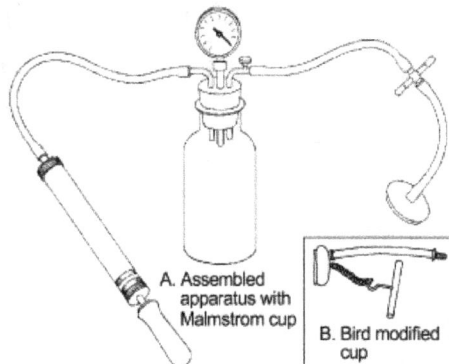

A. Assembled apparatus with Malmstrom cup

B. Bird modified cup

Fig. 2. A Malmstrom's vacuum extractor with its essential components. Inset: Bird's modification of metal cup

4. Types of equipment

4.1 Forceps

Obstetric forceps can be classified based on the depth of the pelvic cavity in which they can be applied to effect delivery (low/outlet, midcavity or high foceps). Worldwide low cavity and outlet forceps delivery are the mostly frequently performed in current practice. High and mid-cavity forceps delivery which could involve rotation of the fetal head are rarely perfomed. At the Ahmadu Bello University Teaching Hospital, only outlet forceps are performed with low-cavity forceps used occasionally (Adaji et al., 2009).

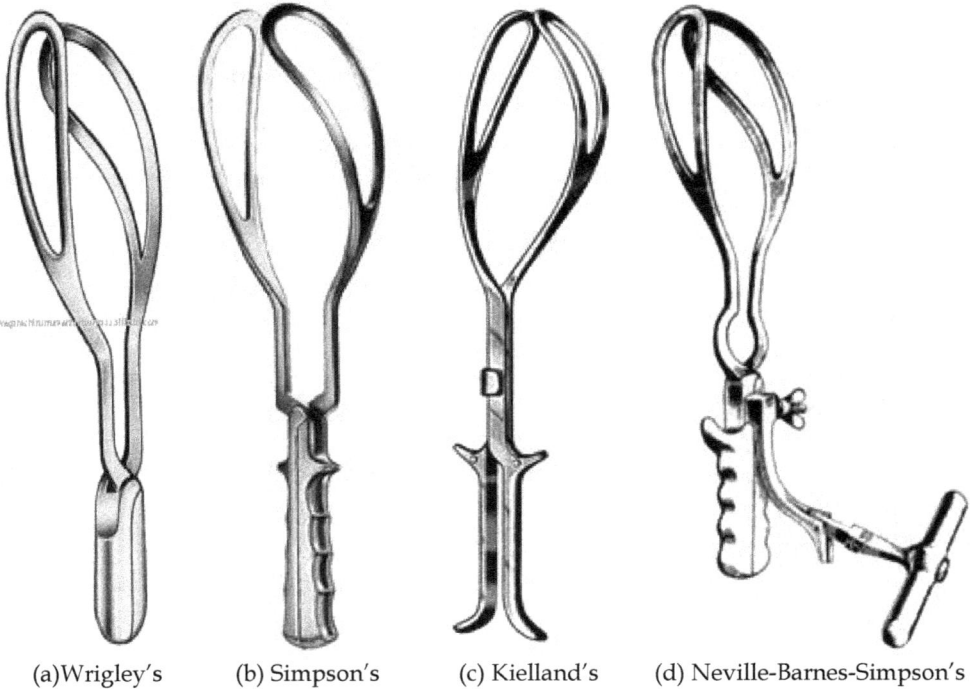

| (a)Wrigley's | (b) Simpson's | (c) Kielland's | (d) Neville-Barnes-Simpson's |

Fig. 3. The common types of obstetric forceps

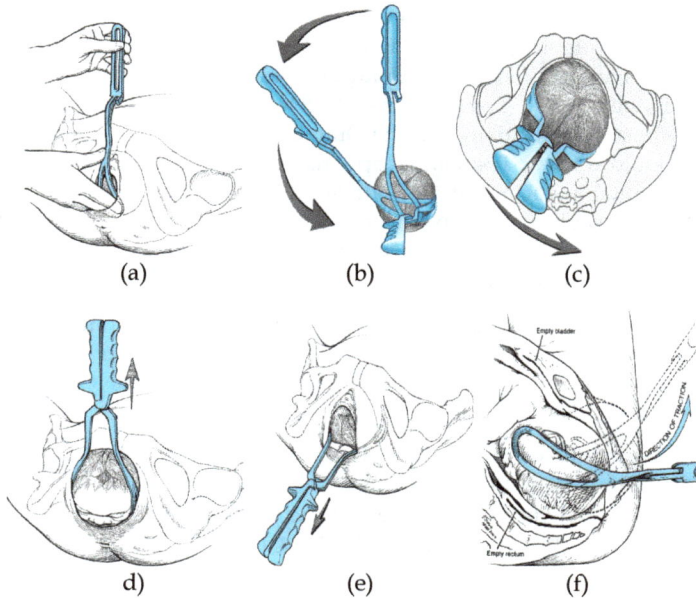

(a)   (b)   (c)

d)   (e)   (f)

Fig. 4. (a-f) – Application and traction on the fetal head using forceps

4.2 Vacuum extractor

There are different types of vacuum extractors, depending on the type of suction mechanism (manual or electrical) and type of cup-rigid or soft (Silc, Malmstrom, Bird, or the OmniCup). The manual suction mechanism which is suitable for resource poor settings due to frequent power outages may be operated via a foot pump, a hand held "bicycle like" pump both operated by an assistant or a hand held pump operated by the birth attendant (Figure 2). The most common and widely available in resource poor settings is the Malmstrom vacuum extractor with rigid or soft cups.

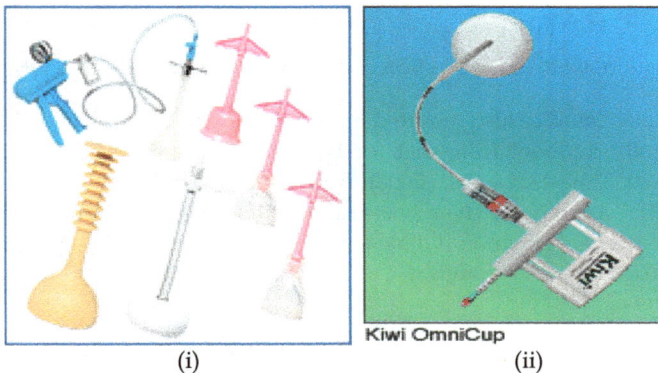

Kiwi OmniCup

(i)   (ii)

Fig. 5. Vacuum extractor soft cups (i) and the Kiwi Omnicup (ii) which has a rigid plastic cup

A more recent design for the vacuum extractor is the rigid plastic cup Kiwi® vacuum assisted fetal delivery device (Clinical Innovations, Murray, UT). It is designed as an integrated unit for complete control without an assistant. The suction for this device is provided by a PalmPump™. The Kiwi has two versions; the ProCup® for low outlet delivery occipito-posterior positions and the OmniCup® for low occipito-posterio asynclitic and lateral fetal malpositions. The OmniCup® has a disposable and a recently developed reusable version suitable for resource poor settings. The cost, portability and ease of maintenance of the reusable OmniCup® makes it attractive for use in resource poor settings. The disposable version on the other hand reduces the potential risk of viral infections between patients (Ismail et al., 2008a).

Metal cups appear to be more suitable for 'occipito-posterior', transverse and difficult 'occipito-anterior' position deliveries because they allow a greater traction force to be applied without cup slip offs. The soft cups seem to be appropriate for straightforward deliveries (Johanson and Menon, 2007).

Several studies have evaluated the effectiveness of the OmniCup compared to the standard vacuum extraction equipment (Malstrom metal rigid cup or Silc cups). Two randomized controlled trials found a higher failure rate: 43% vs. 21% (OR = 1.9; 95%CI = 1.01 – 1.36) (Attilakos et al., 2006) and 30%-19.2%, (RR 1.58; 95% CI = 1.10-2.224) with the OmniCup and one RCT found it to be a suitable alternative to the standard cups (100% delivery rate in both groups) (Ismail et al., 2008b). There was no difference in maternal morbidity between both groups in all 3 RCTs. Only one of the RCTs reported a significant increase in neonatal admission for sub-aponeurotic hemorrhage (p = 0.015, OR = 0.11; 95CI = 0.001 - 0.87).

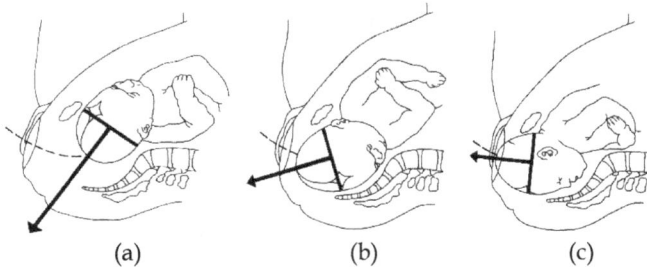

Fig. 6. (a-c) – Position of cup and direction of traction with vacuum extractor

Several observational studies also reported higher rates of successful vaginal delivery which was not statistically different from that for the standard equipment (Ismail et al., 2008a, Hayman et al., 2002, Baskett et al., 2008). Successful vaginal delivery was attributed to familiarity with the equipment. There was also no difference in maternal morbidity in all of these studies. However, Hayman, Gilby and Arulkumaran (2002) reported a significant increase in superficial scalp abrasions in the OmniCup group compared to the standard cup group (Hayman et al., 2002).

The experience from many centers is that nulliparous women with untested pelvis are more likely to need assistance with an operative vaginal delivery procedure. In the Zaria study, more than three-quarters of the parturients who were assisted were nulliparas (Adaji et al., 2009).

5. Epidemiology

Operative vaginal delivery prevalence rates vary from country from country and facility to facility. The rates have however remained fairly stable over the past 3 decades. A recent survey by the World Health Organization (WHO) of method of delivery and pregnancy outcomes in 9 Asian countries analyzed 107, 950 births. Of these births, 3.2 percent were by operative vaginal delivery procedures (Lumbiganon et al., 2010).

Demissie et al comprehensively reviewed operative vaginal delivery rates in US hospitals between 1995 and 1998. Obstetrical forceps were utilized to conduct deliveries in 4.4% of births in 1995, 4% in 1996, 3.6% in 1997 and 3.2% in 1998. The use of ventouse was 7.4%, 7.8%, 7.8% and 7.6% over the same period (Demissie et al., 2004). In the UK, a operative vaginal delivery rates (forceps and ventouse) of between 10 to 15% percent has been estimated (Johanson and Jones, 1999).

Due to weak health systems, national figures for instrumental vaginal deliveries are either unavailable or incomplete from developing countries. Reports from comprehensive emergency obstetric health care facilities may provide the most reliable source of information in such settings. For example, a 5 year review of births at the Ahmadu Bello University Teaching Hospital, Zaria revealed that of 6662 vaginal births between 1997 and 2001, 3.9% were by operative vaginal delivery procedures. Forceps delivery rate was 2.2% while vacuum delivery rate was 1.5%. In addition, fetal destructive operation to deliver confirmed intrauterine fetal deaths was employed in 0.1% of cases (Adaji et al., 2009). This procedure is rarely reported in literature from developed countries suggesting that they are no longer performed. However, in developing countries where moribund mothers, neglected obstructed labour and intrauterine fetal deaths are still seen, fetal destructive operation remains an option [Moody & Maharaj 2002]. Table 1 below shows the situation of operative vaginal procedures based on hospital-based studies in selected countries.

Country	No of births	Year of births	Vacuum (%)	Forceps (%)	All
USA	4,316,233	2007	3.5	0.8	4.3%
England	515,214	2004	7	3	10%
Canada	333,974	2005	10.3	4.6	14.9%
Australia	289,946	2007	7.5	3.6	11.1%
Ireland	71,963	2007	12.3	3.7	16%

Table 1. Operative vaginal deliveries in 5 countries(Gei and Pacheco, 2011)

Assisted vaginal delivery is one of the underutilized and least available emergency obstetric care signal functions in resource poor countries (Kongnyuy et al., 2008, Tsu and Coffe, 2009). Unmet training needs, lack of suitable equipment and human resource shortages are some reasons for this (Bailey, 2005, Fauveau, 2006, Hillier and Johanson, 1994). In many resource poor settings vacuum extraction is performed only by medical doctors who may only be regularly available in large urban hospitals (Fauveau, 2006).

6. Types and classification of operative vaginal delivery procedures

Forceps and vacuum delivery are the most common procedures employed for assisted vaginal delivery. Others like symphysiotomy and fetal destructive operations are rarely if ever performed in developed countries. The ACOG developed a classification system that takes into account the station and position of the fetal head in the maternal pelvis (ACOG, 1992). (Figure 3 and Table 2)

Term	Definition
Outlet	Fetal scalp visible without separating the labia Fetal skull has reached the pelvic floor Sagittal suture is in the antero-posterior diameter or right or left occiput anterior or posterior position (rotation does not exceed 45 degrees) Fetal head is at or on the perineum
Low	Leading point of the skull (not caput) is at station plus 2 cm or more and not on the pelvic floor Two subdivisions: (a) rotation of 45 degrees or less (b) rotation more than 45 degrees
Mid cavity	Fetal head is 1/5 palpable per abdomen Leading point of the skull is above station plus 2 cm but not above the ischial spines Two subdivisions (a) rotation of 45 degrees or less (b) rotation more than 45 degrees
High	Not included in classification

Table 2. Classification for operative vaginal deliveries adapted from ACOG

7. Guidelines and indications

The invention of obstetrical forceps may have been driven by the search for a way to address one of the tragic outcomes of pregnancy of those days; prolonged obstructed labor with a dead fetus. With no luxury of ability to perform a caesarean section, the dilemma faced by the birth accoucheur was undoubtedly formidable. As the tools of the trade grew in number and design, the indications also multiplied. Some institutions like the Royal College of Obstetricians and Gynaecologists (RCOG) UK, The American Congress of Obstetricians and Gynaecologists and the Society of Obstetricians and Gynaecologists of Canada have helped to clearly define the indications for operative vaginal delivery (Table 3). There are several indications for assisted vaginal delivery; these could be due to fetal compromise, maternal indications to avoid Valsalva or inadequate progress in labour. No indication is absolute and each case should be considered individually.

Type	Indication
Fetal	Presumed fetal compromise
Maternal	Medical indications to avoid Valsalva (e.g. cardiac disease Class III or IV*, hypertensive crises, cerebral vascular disease, particularly uncorrected vascular malformations, myasthenia gravis, spinal cord injury)
Inadequate progress	Nulliparous women: Lack of continuing progress for three hours (total of active and passive second stage labour) with regional anaesthesia, or two hours without regional anaesthesia
	Multiparous women: Lack of continuing progress for two hours (total of active and passive second stage labour) with regional anaesthesia, or one hour without regional anaesthesia

*New York Heart Association classification

Table 3. Indications for operative vaginal delivery (no indication is absolute and each case should be considered individually)

The safe use of both the vacuum extractor and obstetric forceps require prerequisites one of which is that "the operator must have the knowledge, experience and skills necessary to use the instrument" (ACOG, 1994). A list of the essential pre-requisites for operative vaginal delivery is presented in Table 4.

Preparation	Essential
Full abdominal and vaginal examination	Head is ≤ 1/5 palpable per abdomen Vertex presentation Cervix is fully dilated and the membranes ruptured Exact position of the head can be determined so proper placement of the instrument can be achieved Pelvis is deemed adequate
Mother	Informed consent must be obtained and clear explanation given Appropriate analgesia is in place, for mid-cavity rotational deliveries this will usually be a regional block A pudendal block may be appropriate, particularly in the context of urgent delivery Maternal bladder has been emptied recently Indwelling catheter should be removed or balloon deflated Aseptic techniques
Staff	Operator must have the knowledge, experience and skills necessary to use the instruments Adequate facilities and back-up personnel are available Back-up plan in place in case of failure to deliver Anticipation of complications that may arise (e.g. shoulder dystocia, postpartum haemorrhage) Personnel present who are trained in neonatal resuscitation

Table 4. Prerequisites for operative vaginal delivery

Facility-based studies from several countries show that indications for operative vaginal delivery procedure fall easily within these categories. Indications for vacuum and forceps delivery in 3 large hospitals in 3 countries are shown in table 5 below.

	Vacuum	Forceps
Nigeria (Zaria)		
Delayed 2nd stage of labour	61 (61)	61 (41.9)
Maternal distress	10 (16.4)	18 (12.3)
Medical illness; PET/eclampsia	20 (32.8)	51 (34.9)
Fetal compromise	9 (9)	12 (8.2)
Fetal prematurity	0 (0)	3 (2.1)
Obstructed labour	0 (0)	1 (0.6)
Total	100 (100)	146 (100)
Cameroon (Yaounde)		
Prolonged 2nd stage	26 (50)	12 (37.5)
Excessive fetal weight	14 (26.9)	10 (31.3)
Acute fetal distress	11 (21.1)	10 (31.3)
Mother with cardiomyopathy	1 (1.9)	0 (0.0)
Total	52 (100)	32 (100)
Greece (Thessaloniki)		
Prolonged 2nd stage	69 (21.5)	9 (18)
Maternal exhaustion	161 (49)	22 (44)
Non re-assuring fetal status	83 (26)	16 (32)
Others	11 (3.5)	3 (6)
Total	324 (100)	50 (100)

Table 5. Indications for vacuum and forceps delivery in health care facilities

7.1 Other indications

- After coming head of a breech presentation. Piper forceps is used to maintain the fetal head in flexion and also enables traction on the fetal head. It has unique features of having only a pelvic curve but no cephalic curve.
- During caesarean section a Kiwi vacuum extractor or Wrigley's obstetric forceps can be used to deliver a 'floating' fetal head.
- Some obstetricians have also used a single forcep blade as an elevator during difficult delivery of an impacted fetal head.

7.2 Contraindications

The following are contraindications to the performance of operative vaginal deliveries.

- Abnormal fetal lie; transverse and oblique
- Abnormal presentation; breech, face or brow presentation, shoulder
- Unengaged vertex

- Incompletely dilated cervix; Forceps (vacuum extractor deliveries at cervical dilatations of 8 and above have been found to be a viable alternative to caesarean section)
- Clinical evidence of CPD
- Gestational age < 34 weeks gestation: vacuum extraction is contraindicated because of the susceptibility of the preterm infant to cephalhaematoma, intracranial haemorrhage, subgaleal haemorrhage, and neonatal jaundice. Some have even suggested that vacuum extractors should not be used at gestations of less than 36 weeks because of the risk of subgaleal and intracranial haemorrhage.
- Need for device rotation *(vacuum)*
- Deflexed attitude of fetal head
- Fetal conditions (e.g. thrombocytopenia)
- Fetal bleeding disorders (e.g., alloimmune thrombocytopenia) or a predisposition to fracture (e.g., osteogenesis imperfecta) are relative contraindications to operative vaginal delivery. However, there may be considerable fetal risk if the head has to be delivered abdominally from deep in the pelvis.

Blood-borne viral infections of the mother e.g HIV are not a contraindication to operative vaginal delivery. However, it is sensible to avoid difficult operative delivery where there is an increased chance of fetal abrasion or scalp trauma and to avoid fetal scalp clips or blood sampling during labour.

8. Complications

While the role of operative vaginal deliveries using instruments like forceps and vacuum extractor has received wide acclaim, complications, sometimes of profound severity have been documented for both mother and child. These undesired outcomes have made operative vaginal delivery an object of great scrutiny by the medical and lay press.

Complication	Vacuum	Forceps
Maternal		
Genital tract laceration	8 (42.1)	16 (44.4)
Postpartum haemorrhage	0 (0)	7 (19.4)
Fetal		
Skin bruises	0 (0)	10 (27.8)
Neonatal jaundice	3 (15.8)	0 (0)
Cephalo haematoma	4 (21.1)	2 (5.6)
Erb's palsy	0 (0)	1 (2.8)
Fetal death	4 (21.1)	0 (0)
Total	20	36

Table 6. Complications observed with instrumental/operative vaginal deliveries in Zaria Nigeria

While a diverse number of complications have been ascribed to these procedures causality has been difficult to establish.

In the Zaria study, maternal/ fetal complication was found in 22.3% of cases of instrumental delivery. Table 6 above provides details of these complications. The most severe of the complications were the fetal deaths recorded for vacuum deliveries. However the deaths may have been due to the severity of the fetal distress that indicated the procedure rather than the procedure itself.

Newborn intracranial injuries and shoulder dystocia were other complications associated with operative vaginal deliveries from large reviews. Intracranial injuries documented include epidural, subdural and subarachnoid haemorrhages. The fetus could also develop sub-galeal (subaponeurotic) haemorrhage (Doumouchtsis).

9. Symphysiotomy

Cutting a parturient's symphysis pubis allows the two halves of her pelvis to separate up to 2.5 cm permitting an otherwise difficult labour to progress and allowing an assisted or spontaneous birth. The procedure is performed by cutting through the fibro-cartilage of the symphysis pubis and the supportive ligaments with a scalpel while ensuring asepsis. At its introduction, symphysiotomy was reputed to play a key role in providing an alternative mode of delivery for mild to moderate cephalo-pelvic disproportion thereby reducing caesarean delivery rates. Cynics however doubt this and worry about the risks to the pelvic bones and the nearby lower urinary tract structures. As a result, this procedure has fallen out of favour and rarely employed in obstetric practice even in least resource parts of the world. In the Zaria study, no single symphysiotomy was performed in 5 years despite the existence of indications for the procedure (Adaji et al., 2009). Moreover the skill to perform the procedure has dwindled among obstetricians over time. However, some still argue for a role for this procedure because it meets women's socio-cultural expectation of a vaginal delivery in areas with dislike and apathy for caesarean sections (Maharaj and Moodley, 2002)

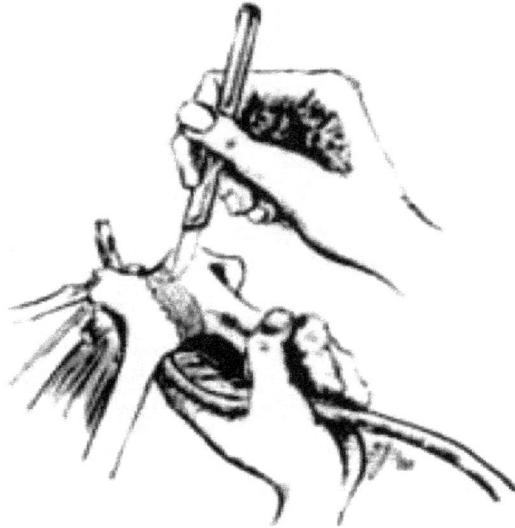

Fig. 7. Performing a symphysiotomy with an instrument placed to protect the urethra

9.1 Fetal destructive operations

These refer to procedures to deliver a dead fetus in the presence of obstructed labour. The value of a caesarean section in this circumstance is low and the maternal situation may even make any resort to an abdominal operation rather dangerous. Craniotomy could be performed to reduce the diameter of the fetal head to allow vaginal delivery, and transverse lie could be relived by decapitation. Cleidotomy could be performed sometimes to reduce bisacromial diameter when the shoulders of a dead fetus are impacted while evisceration or embryotomy could be performed if the dead fetus is large and or the abdomen is swollen due to an intra-abdominal tumor. Destructive operations are no longer performed in developed countries where the indications for it no longer exists. Even in developing countries most obstetricians shy away from performing the procedure. In Zaria, only 0.1% of deliveries were by destructive procedures (Adaji et al., 2009).

10. Conclusion

Operative vaginal procedures, mainly vacuum extraction and obstetric forceps delivery have a long history but both still have a place in contemporary obstetric practice. In competent hands and with strict adherence to guidelines, the outcomes for the mother and child are excellent. There is great gain in ensuring that these arts are not lost to the modern day obstetrician. On the other hand, procedures like symphysiotomy and destructive operations may still have value in obstetric practice in low income settings. However the evidence for their value need to be laid out clearly and the guidelines for their use comprehensively updated.

11. References

ACOG (1992) Operative vaginal delivery. ACOG Technical Bulletin. Number 152--February 1991. *Int J Gynaecol Obstet,* 38, 55-60.

ACOG (1994) Operative vaginal delivery. ACOG Technical Bulletin Number 196-- August 1994 (replaces No. 152, February 1991). *Int J Gynaecol Obstet,* 47, 179-85.

Adaji, S. E., Shittu, S. O. & Sule, S. T. (2009) Operative vaginal deliveries in Zaria, Nigeria. *Ann Afr Med,* 8, 95-9.

Ameh, C. A. & Weeks, A. D. (2009) The role of instrumental vaginal delivery in low resource settings. *BJOG,* 116 Suppl 1, 22-5.

Attilakos, G., Sibanda, T., Winter, C., Johnson, N. & Draycott, T. (2006) A randomised trial of a new handheld vacuum extraction device. *BJOG: An International Journal of Obstetrics and Gynaecology.,* 113, 494-495.

Bailey, P. E. (2005) The disappearing art of instrumental delivery: Time to reverse the trend. *International Journal of Gynecology and Obstetrics,* 91, 89-96.

Baskett, T. F., Fanning, C. A. & Young, D. C. (2008) A prospective observational study of 1000 vacuum assisted deliveries with the OmniCup Device. *J Obstet Gynaecol Can,* 573 580.

Chiswick, M. L. & James, D. K. (1979) Kielland's forceps: association with neonatal morbidity and mortality. *BMJ,* 1, 7-9.

Demissie, K., Rhoads, G. G., Smulian, J. C., Balasubramanian, B. A., Gandhi, K., Joseph, K. S. & Kramer, M. (2004) Operative vaginal delivery and neonatal and infant adverse outcomes: population based retrospective analysis. *BMJ*, 329, 24-9.

Dunn, P. M. (1999) The Chamberlen family (1560-1728) and obstetric forceps. *Arch Dis Child Fetal Neonatal Ed*, 81, F232-4.

Fauveau, V. (2006) Is vacuum extraction still known, taught and practiced? A worldwide KAP survey. *International Journal of Gynecology and Obstetrics*, 94, 185-189.

Gei, A. F. & Pacheco, L. D. (2011) Operative vaginal deliveries: practical aspects. *Obstet Gynecol Clin North Am*, 38, 323-49, xi.

Hayman, R., Gilby, J. & Arulkumaran, S. (2002) Clinical evaluation of a "Hand Pump" vacuum delivery device. *Obstet Gynecol*, 100, 1190-1195.

Hillier, C. E. M. & Johanson, R. B. (1994) Worldwide survey of assisted vaginal delivery. *International Journal of Gynecology and Obstetrics*, 47, 109-114.

Ismail, N. A. M., Saharan, W. S. L., Zaleha, M. A., Jaafar, R., Muhammad, J. A. & Razi, Z. R. M. (2008a) Kiwi Omnicup versus Malmstrom metal cup in vacuum assisted delivery: A randomized comparative trial. *J Obstet Gynaecol Res*, 34, 350-353.

Ismail, N. A. M., Saharan, W. S. L., Zaleha, M. A., Jaafar, R., Muhammad, J. A. & Razi, Z. R. M. (2008b) Kiwi Omnicup versus Malmstrom metal cup in vacuum assisted delivery: A randomized comparative trial. *J Obstet Gynaecol Res. ,* 34, 350-353.

Johanson, R. & Jones, P. (1999) Operative vaginal delivery rates in the United Kingdom. *J Obstet Gynaecol*, 19, 602-3.

Johanson, R. B. & Menon, B. K. (2007) Vacuum extraction versus forceps for assisted vaginal delivery (Review). *The Cochrane Collaboration*. John Wiley & Sons, Ltd.

Kongnyuy, E. J., Leigh, B. & Vandenbroek, N. (2008) Effect of audit and feedback on the availability, utilisation and quality of emergency obstetric care in three districts in Malawi. *Women and Birth*, 21, 149-155.

Lumbiganon, P., Laopaiboon, M., Gulmezoglu, A. M., Souza, J. P., Taneepanichskul, S., Ruyan, P., Attygalle, D. E., Shrestha, N., Mori, R., Nguyen, D. H., Hoang, T. B., Rathavy, T., Chuyun, K., Cheang, K., Festin, M., Udomprasertgul, V., Germar, M. J., Yanqiu, G., Roy, M., Carroli, G., Ba-Thike, K., Filatova, E. & Villar, J. (2010) Method of delivery and pregnancy outcomes in Asia: the WHO global survey on maternal and perinatal health 2007-08. *Lancet*, 375, 490-9.

Maharaj, D. & Moodley, J. (2002) Symphysiotomy and fetal destructive operations. *Best Pract Res Clin Obstet Gynaecol*, 16, 117-31.

Malmstrom, T. (1957) The vacuum extractor, an obstetrical instrument. *Acta Obstetricia at Gynecologica Scandinavica*, 6, 5-50.

Tsu, V. D. & Coffe, P. S. (2009) New and underutilised technologies to reduce maternal mortality and morbidity: What progress have we made since Bellagio 2003? *BJOG: An International Journal of Obstetrics and Gynaecology.*, 116, 247-256.

Vacca, A. (2003) Handbook of vacuum delivery in obstetric practice. Australia, Vacca Research.

17

Bioethics in Obstetrics

Joseph Ifeanyi Brian-D. Adinma
Department of Obstetrics and Gynaecology Nnamdi Azikiwe
University and Teaching Hospital, Nnewi,
Nigeria

1. Introduction

Obstetrics has been defined as the branch of medicine concerned with child birth. This simplistic definition may not entirely represent the plethora of events, many challenging, others contentious that are usually associated with the developmental processes that culminate in the birth of the child. They can therefore be only but a few aspect of clinical practice that are likely to elicit as much bioethical considerations as obstetrics practice. Bioethical questions arise in virtually all aspects of pregnancy and child birth starting from ethical issues involved in genetics and embryo research through the process of assisted reproduction, surrogacy, abortion, the process of normal and abnormal pregnancies, safe motherhood and neonatal care. Cook et al have observed the emerging significant of bio-ethics over the last half a century, at both professional and scholarly levels, and have further highlighted the input of multiple discipline – biology, philosophy, healthcare service, medicine, law, nursing and religious studies in the structuring of modern bioethics. This perhaps has been most profoundly expressed in obstetrics care, and indeed reproductive health as a whole. The medical profession in several cultures has an inherent responsibility to conduct its activities guided by the highest ethical standard. Reproductive healthcare practitioners in particular inevitably face ethical and bioethical challenges, some of which constitute a conflict between the old and new, requiring resolution, for example, the process of super-ovulation with higher multiple pregnancies, associated with assisted reproduction may require the ethically-questionable process of selective reduction foeticide in order to ensure the survival of one or two foetuses and facilitate the success of the procedure. Health professionals looking after woman are more compelled to observe strict ethical principles because they work in areas of women's body that are private and of particular psycho-sexual sensitivity (Ezeani, 2003). The decision to oblige to treatment request, obstetrics care inclusive requires that the reproductive healthcare practitioner appraises and appreciates his or her personal ethical stand-point which is then related to his duty to address the well being of his patients and also the overall character and conscience of the community. The need to include bioethics in the training curriculum of residents in obstetrics and gynaecology has become compelling and over the past two decades been increasingly highlighted (Elkins et al, 1986; Royal College of Physicians and Surgeons of Canada, 1997). As clearly stated by Mckneally and Singer (2001) "Enhancing Clinicians" knowledge and skills in resolving ethical quandaries can increase their ability to deal with issues that cause moral distress and thus enable better team and institutional performance in caring for patients. The Royal College of Physicians and Surgeons of Canada had since the late 1990 insisted that the teaching of bioethics be made a requirement for accreditation of any residency training programme. In furtherance to this, Council on Resident Education in Obstetrics and Gynaecology stated the objectives that residents must demonstrate an understanding of basic ethical concepts and their application to the issues and decisions based in the practice of obstetrics and gynaecology (Royal College of Physicians and Surgeons of Canada, 1997).

This chapter defines bioethics together with a brief account of its historical origin particularly in relation to the development of principles of modern bioethics. It also describes the fundamentals of bioethics – notably bioethical orientation, principles and analytical levels. It further highlights research ethics and reviews key obstetrics issues requiring bio-ethical consideration.

2. Fundamentals of bioethics

The word ethics is derived from the Greek word "ethos" which means customs and habits. Medical ethics has been defined as the principles or norms that regulate the conduct of the relationships between medical practitioners and other groups with whom they come in contact in the course of their practice (COMMAT, 1997). These groups include professional colleagues, other health professionals, the patient, the government and other custodians of healthcare.

Ethical codes are set of principles or rough guides to practice, usually developed following serious breach of ethical standards (Uzodike, 1998). For example, the Nuremberg code of 1947 and Helsinki Declaration of 1964 are guidelines developed on human research, following inhuman experimentation conducted on human subjects (CIOMS, 1993). The Hippocratic Oath of 4th century B.C. in its modified form, sworn to by newly qualified medical doctors, constitutes a component of the ethical codes of most countries of the world.

Bioethics in a narrow sense is a subdivision of ethics that regulates the relationship between the healthcare provider and the beneficiary of healthcare. In a broader sense however, it is regarded as a multidisciplinary filed of inquiry, which addresses ethical issues in clinical practice and healthcare, biomedical research involving humans and animals, health policy and the environment (Cook et al, 2003; Adinma and Adinma, 2009). Bioethics has its roots from the value system developed by ancient Philosophers – Socrates, Aristotle and Plato. The term bioethics was coined by van Rensselaer Potter, an American biochemist at the University of Wisconsin in the 1960's. Although the first institutional use of the word was in 1971 by Kennedy, Institute of Ethics, Georgetown University – Washington DC (Cook et al, 2003). Modern Bioethics is believed to have evolved in the 1960's as a response to various challenges and controversies encumbering health technological development at the time (Callahan, 1997; Rothmans, 1991; Jonsen, 1998). Although Warren Reich opined that the evolution of bioethics in the western countries was a reaction to the tendency of religions to approach developments in medicine through their parochial theological doctrines and perspective.

3. Bioethical orientations

The thinking and end result of bioethical considerations are directed along various set-lines, constituting different bioethical orientations. The ancient Greek value system and philosophy considered to be the origin of bioethics together with the input of various religions notably Christianity and Islam over the years represent the historical orientation of bioethics.

Duty based or deontological bioethical orientation is related to natural laws and reason, distinguishing vice from virtue as an indivisible accompaniment of any action or intention. The Catholic Church is a well known proponent of duty based bioethics and this is evident from the church's stand for instance against the use of condom for prevention of pregnancy or sexually transmitted infection or against artificial forms of contraception, while supporting natural family planning. St. Thomas Aquinas in the 13th century incorporated some natural laws developed and proposed by Aristotle into the doctrine of the Roman Catholic Church. Duty based bioethical orientation is believed to be absolutist and often unbending to the relativity and diversity that characterize ethical considerations. This may have serious implications to reproductive health in general, often replete with bioethical challenges.

Utilitarian or consequentialist bioethical orientation recognizes man's moral responsibility for his or her bioethical choices. Whatever promotes the well-being or happiness of man is considered to be good while whatever causes harm or unhappiness to man is bad. It recognizes man as an important end in himself rather than being a means to an end of whatever form. For example, a woman with an unwanted pregnancy, desirous of termination of the pregnancy should be assisted with safe and un-encumbered induced abortion since this may promote her psychological and social well being.

Feminist bioethical orientation basically aims at incorporating women's social experiences, thinking and behavior into the value system of healthcare and clinical practice. It is also known as ethics of care or connectedness, and constitutes a reaction to the exclusion of women from historical sources of moral authority such as the clergy, top echelons of the military or legislature and other similar position exclusively "restricted" on the basis of sex or gender.

Apart from these bioethical orientations considered to be key towards effective bioethical considerations, there are a few others that have become recognized which include the following:

Virtue – tenets to which biomedical institutions and practitioners should adhere to, such as kindness, trustworthiness, discernment, and integrity, all of which conform to the ethical ideals of Hippocrates.

Communitarianism – bioethical orientation that advances and promotes the good of the community.

Casuistry - proponents of this orientation subscribe to the resolution of issues on the basis of their merit rather than on a resort to universal rules.

4. Principles of bioethics

The development of the principles of modern bioethics is inextricably linked to the contents of the Belmont Report (The Belmont Report, 1978). The Tuskegee Alabama public health service funded syphilis research over the 40 year period, 1932 – 1972, involved inhuman experimentation on 400 indigent black American males (James, 1993). The termination of this research led to American congressional passage of the National Research Act in 1974 and the establishment of the United State's National Commission for the Protection of Human Subjects of Biomedical and Behavioral Research which in 1979 published its findings and recommendations known as the Belmont Report. The Belmont Report provided an analytical frame work to guide the resolution of ethical problems arising from research involving human subjects. Three basic ethical principles contained in the Belmont Report viz: Respect for persons, Beneficence, and Justice, essentially constituted the foundation for the development of the key principle of modern bioethical analysis. Implicit in the principle of beneficence (do good) is non – maleficence (do no harm) which has become recognized as a distinct key principle. These four key principles of bioethical analysis constitute a consensus resolution of different bioethical orientations notably from the works of two American bioethicists - Tom Beauchamp and James Childress and the British expert - Raanan Gillon (Beauchamp and Childress, 2001; Gillon, 1994). In addition to these four key principles, three others have been recognized in modern bioethical analysis – veracity, fidelity and scientific validity.

The principle of respect for person occurs at two levels. The first level refers to autonomy of capable persons which upholds patient's right to voluntary informed consent, and choice based on comprehension of available options, for example, patients right to family size determination. The second level is the protection of persons incapable of autonomy. Three groups of persons are notable in this regard - the unconscious, the mentally sub-normal and the child – all of who require the protection of their autonomy. For example, the decision on the treatment of an unconscious pregnant woman, or the genital mutilation of an infant. This protection requires either the presence of a living will especially in the case of the unconscious patient or the obtaining of consent from the surrogate or where not feasible a clergyman, or the ethical committee of a health institution or as a last resort, the law court. Medical paternalism refers to the overriding of autonomy. Strong paternalism is the overriding of the autonomy of a capable person, and is not ethically permissible. While weak paternalism is the overriding of the autonomy of an incapable person which is permissible if performed for the overall well-being of the person. The principles of Beneficence refer to the ethical responsibility to do and maximize good. It emphasizes what is best to the patient with respect to preventive and curative healthcare. The principles of non–maleficence refers to the ethical duty of the health practitioners to do no harm or cause pain to the patient as in the giving and suturing of episiotomy without local anesthesia in a parturient woman. The principles of Justice refer to the ethical responsibility to uphold fairness and equity in medicare. It refers to the equitable distribution of potential benefits and risks. The ethical principles of veracity enjoins health practitioners to tell the truth - explaining the potential benefits and risks alike involved in whatever treatment being giving to, and procedure being carried out on the patient. The principles of fidelity refers to the ethical responsibility of the health practitioners to carry out whatever promises made to a patient in relation to activities for which he or she has been employed. For example, a pregnant woman used for the purpose of a clinical examination for professional medical students' exams may have been promised free further antenatal care and delivery. The ethical principle of scientific validity enjoins the medical practitioners to ensure professional competence and scientific soundness in the conduct of medicare or research on patient.

5. Analytical levels of bioethics

There are four analytical levels to which bioethical principles are applicable. Each of these has its specific orientation and may or may not be related to the others. Microethical analytical level applies to relationship between individuals and in this case the health care provider and the patient, while the medical practitioner has an ethical obligation to give his patient enough and correct information on all available options to make an informed decision and consent, the patient is obligated to respect his or her medical practitioner's right to conscientious objection to any treatment being requested of him. For example, a medical practitioner's conscientious objection to induced abortion should be respected just as much as the medical practitioner is obligated to refer such patient to where competent treatment can be accessed. Macroethical level of bioethical analysis refers to the relationship between groups or communities – between members of the group of communities themselves, or between them and members of another group or community, for example, the ethical commitment to the provision of healthcare between an urban and rural population, or between different socio-economic classes of people within a group or community. Mesoethical analytical level otherwise known as ethics of intergenerational justice refers to discordance in resource allocation between groups by health managers at both public and private levels. Mesoethics falls between microethical and macroethical levels and implicates the ethical principles of beneficence and distributive justice, for instance contrasting high budgetary allocation to Senators to receive free medicare abroad even for trivial illness treatable locally, to the very low budget allocated to maternal health service delivery, in a developing country with unacceptably high maternal mortality. Megaethical level of bioethical analysis applies to issues operating beyond national boundaries, for example ethical issues related to the treatment of HIV/AIDS with Anti Retroviral Drugs where in the past the drugs are produced at reasonable cost in developed countries and exported to developing countries with a high burden of HIV disease and sold at prohibitive prices. Similar concerns are also manifest in reproductive health issues, and the effect of environmental pollution or degradation.

6. Research ethical review

Ethical considerations are perhaps more profoundly manifest in research than in most other aspect of medicine. Medical research especially those involved with human embryo and stem cell often bring to bear the demands and challenges posed by different bioethical orientations. Deontological bioethicists for their firm adherence to an orientation of natural laws and reasons are unlikely for instance to condone research targeted at exposing life threatening foetal abnormalities that would ordinarily require termination, in a pregnant subject. In the same vein, consequentialist and feminist bioethicists will employ macroethical reasoning to justify the conduct of research on a few human embryo and stem cells for the purpose of obtaining information that will lead to the development of therapy that will benefit many more sick patient (Stephens and Brynner, 2001). Ethical conflicts arise as to the propriety of employing human subject to carry out scientific studies to reveal vital information that will contribute to the successful management of a vast number of patients as was the case with the Tuskegee Syphilis Research which not only unveiled the long term manifestations of syphilis but also heralded the genesis of the developmental framework for the principles of modern bioethics from the Belmont Report. However it has been established that the well-being of human subject should be given priority consideration to the interest of science and the society (WMA, 2000).

It became necessary at a point to develop an acceptable course in bio-medical research involving not only humans but also animals and the environment. Two landmark guidelines emerged over the years concerning the conduct of research on human subjects – the Nuremberg Code of Ethics developed in 1947 following the trial of 23 German Physicians and Administrators for inhuman experimentations on human subjects during the 2nd world war and the Helsinki Declaration of the 18th General Assembly of the World Medical Association which developed recommendations and later ethical principles for medical research involving human subjects (WMA, 2008).

Helsinki consists of 35 principles, the first 30 of which relate to medical research, while the last 5 concern clinical practice. Between 1964 and 2008 Helsinki has been revised 9 times, the 9th of which was at the 59th General Assembly of the World Medical Association in Seoul South Korea in 2008. Helsinki Declaration recognizes the safety, autonomy, confidentiality, and the dignity of human subject in research. It also recognizes that potential benefits that should accrue to research subjects, and that research should be discontinued if the risk out-weighs its benefits. Helsinki Declaration further requires that the protocol of the subject under study be submitted in advance to a Research Ethics Committee that is independent of the investigator or sponsor of the study, for scrutiny, consideration, comments, and ultimate approval or rejection (WMA, 2008). Ethical committee members are multidisciplinary and include not only medical professionals but also a lawyer, a clergy, an ethicists and other notable member of the community all of whom should be familiar with scientific basis of proposals together with the laws and regulations of the country in which the research experiment is performed.

7. Obstetrics issues eliciting ethical attention

The provision of ethical care that respects the sexual and reproductive rights of women is considered fundamental and therefore implicit on professionalism in healthcare of women. The International Federation of Gynaecology and Obstetrics (FIGO) has over the years provided leadership role and direction towards the structuring and promotion of professional ethical standards in women's health and indeed reproductive healthcare as a whole through its committee for the Study of Ethical Aspects of Human Reproduction and Women's Health (FIGO, 2006).

In 2001, FIGO through its Sexual and Reproductive Right Committee carried out a Women's Sexual and Reproductive Right Project, undertaken in six counties:- Nigeria, Ethiopia, India, Pakistan, Sudan and Mexico. This project essentially consisted of advocacy and sensitization of obstetrics and gynaecology professionals on areas of women's sexual and reproductive right infringement and the need to uphold, protect and promote these rights; the development of a human right based code of ethics to guide health professionals caring for women, and also incorporate same into the curriculum of medical education; and advocacy into two key areas of sexual and reproductive right failings of women in each country. The project was conducted in each of the countries by a multidisciplinary steering committee under the auspices of the national FIGO – member society. Ethical guideline developed by each of the participating countries were eventually employed in the development of FIGO professional and ethical responsibility guideline concerning sexual and reproductive rights, at the XVII FIGO World Congress in Santiago Chile in 2006 (Adinma, 2003; FIGO, 2004). These professional ethical guidelines are contained in three basic groupings.

a. **Professional Competence** – which enjoins the health professional to uphold the highest standard of professional practice in the care of his patient, avoid inappropriate relationship with patients or his family members, carry out prompt referral of patients when the expertise to care is lacking or in situation of conscientious objection to care of the patient. The health professional is also obligated to avoid ethical and human right violation in the care of their patient, develop appropriate interpersonal relationship with their patients and others while upholding the highest standard of integrity with colleagues and patients. They should also continuously update their professional knowledge through continuing medical education.

b. **Women's Autonomy and Confidentiality** - which obligates health professionals to inform and educate their patient to facilitate informed consent, ensure their right to privacy and confidentiality and avoid all forms of discrimination. The health professionals will also have an obligation to guide adolescents towards making ethics based reproductive health decisions.

c. **Responsibility to the Community** - which obligates health professionals to advocate for the right of their community members to information, education and means to make appropriate sexual and reproductive rights decision, advocate for the provision of resources and care that will enable women benefit from scientific progress and also promote reproductive health education of community members that will enable them participate in dialogue on health policy decisions concerning them. They should also discourage the patronage of quacks by community members, encourage traditional healers to refer patient, and show compassion to patients with medical emergencies especially with respect to payment of deposit and during industrial actions (FIGO, 2006; Adinma, 2003; FIGO, 2004).

8. Obstetrics care

An unbalance relationship exists between the medical practitioner and his female patient borne out of differences between them in social, cultural and economic circumstances together with inequality in knowledge of medicine. The woman seeking health care is therefore posited on a pedestal of vulnerability. The medical practitioner should address this vulnerability by giving clear information on every available treatment option that will enable the patient decide on her appropriate treatment choice. The woman's autonomy is thereby respected. This situation is no less appropriate to the obstetrics patient than is considered to other patient and this respect for her right to informed decision and consent should be sustained throughout the duration of her pregnancy. Every obstetrics patient has the right to the highest standard of obstetrics care and benefit of scientific progress and should under no circumstances be allowed to go through unnecessary or avoidable pain during the course of the pregnancy. This represents professional commitment to the ethical principles of beneficence, justice and non-maleficence. For example, the giving of episiotomy to a parturient woman to prevent a third degree laceration of the perineum upholds the ethical principles of beneficence, but when the episiotomy is given without prior administration of anesthetic agent, or is repaired without any, or is left un-repaired, this will amount to violation of ethical principles of non – maleficence.

The ethical principles of justice also enjoins that all women should be treated equally and without discrimination in healthcare delivery to them.

9. Genetics, oocyte and embryo research

9.1 Human gene alteration

The application of the knowledge of science to human reproduction falls within the purview of obstetrics and therefore obstetrics and gynaecological professionals should be mindful of the ethical implications of genetic studies, engineering and the application of genetics in disease management.

Gene therapy refers to the alteration of human DNA particularly for the purpose of alleviating disease burden in individual. There are three categories of alteration of human gene viz.

- Genetic alteration of Somatic Cells to treat diseases – which raises ethical issues similar to that in experimental, therapeutic and human research, and therefore requires ethical review, informed consent, and the protection of confidentiality of the subject; If gene therapy studies are successful it is ethically permissible to apply such treatment to the foetus in-utero provided that the safety of the foetus is guaranteed and the autonomy of the woman is respected.
- Germ line genetic alteration - involves the changing of the gamete of the individual which is consequently passed on to subsequent generations. There are presently no safe and reliable means of genetically altering germ cells – sperm, egg or zygotes derived from them, therefore any research proposal targeted at germ cell alteration is ethically not permissible.
- Non – therapeutic genetic alteration (genetic enhancement) - involves insertion of a gene with the aim of improving the genetic makeup of a normal healthy gene. For example, the enhancement of colour, height or beauty. This technology has social implications concerning the weight between its potential risks and benefits to individual subjects. It therefore raises serious ethical questions that prohibit research into its application on human subject.

10. Cloning of human

This involves the asexual reproduction of mammals by the technique of Somatic Cell Nuclear Transfer (SCNT). The birth of the first cloned mammal, sheep Dolly in 1997 using this technique represented a land mark development that unequivocally showed the possibility of replicating this asexual reproduction in man. Somatic cell nuclear transfer technology has however been shown to be associated with a high miscarriage rate and an overall low success rate. It is also fraught with high rate of complications such as the large offspring syndrome and immune system failure. It is generally believed to be unsafe and therefore ethically not permissible for use in human reproduction. However, subject to strict observation of ethical guideline, research on human embryo stem cells from Somatic Cell Nuclear Transfer to produce various cell lines for the purpose of treatment of diseases is permissible.

11. Human embryo and gamete research, sale and donation

Apart from the human embryo, stem cells can be obtained from cord blood, the foetus or adults. It can also be obtained from supernumerary embryos at the blastocyt state, in IVF cycles and embryos created de novo from donated gametes. Stem cell studies may be useful in the treatment of many diseases and also in the improvement of the management of infertility. Ethical questions arise in the use of human embryos produced solely for the purpose of research. This can be permitted only if it is not possible to obtain the information sort for, from research on existing supernumerary embryos. Gametes collection for research must be preceded by specific informed consent. Supernumerary embryos from IVF programmes can be used for research only following the consent of the recipients of the resulting embryo. Women particularly the more vulnerable should not be coerced or induced to donate oocyte or embryo for research. A research ethical review is necessary prior to the employment of human embryo for the purpose of research. Donations of gametes and embryos for the purpose of pregnancy and child birth should be on humanitarian basis rather than on commercial consideration, although reasonable compensation for legitimate expenses is allowable. On no account should genetic materials be sold as a profit making venture (Int. J. Gynecol. Obstet, 1994). The donation of genetic materials - egg, sperm or pre – implantation embryo has been used for the treatment of infertility, ovarian failure, severe rhesus iso-immunization, achievement of post menopausal fertility, habitual abortion etc. Such a donation and accompanying child created from it not only have profound ethical implications but are also associated with legal, cultural, moral and religious questions. The child, the recipient couple and the donor all have interest that need to be taking into consideration as well as protected. Different countries have cultural or legal provisions that determine qualification for donation of genetic materials as well as regulate the relationship between the social and the biological parents, the fate of the genetic material (whether for banking or disposal), the protection of the child's interest, and in particular the record keeping rules. The donation of genetic material should be accompanied with informed and written consent of the donor, the recipient and recipient's lawyer. It must be ensured that genetic material donors are normal, healthy and without diseases such as genetic disorders and sexually transmitted infection. Donors of genetic materials should be anonymous and confidentiality should be maintained except when permission for disclosure has been granted. Members of the recipient team should not be donors, nor should genetic materials be obtained from dead persons unless a written consent had been given prior to death. Genetic materials should not be donated for the purpose of extending natural reproductive life span. Donation from one donor should be limited to avoid the danger of consanguinity or incest in the future.

12. Pregnancy and delivery

12.1 Directed gamete donation for assisted reproduction

Rehmann-Sutter and Wienroth (2009) have identified the influence of reproductive technologies on perceptions and practices related to reproduction and beyond this, even to the cultural and societal imperatives that enable the understanding of the family and in particular motherhood, offspring and other issues related to them.

Ethical considerations arise from gamete donations from known donors as much as is the case with anonymous gamete donation already addressed. The availability of advanced micro-manipulative assisted reproductive technology prohibits the need for request on sperm donations, although such request may still occur for artificial insemination using donor semen (AID). Requests for directed oocyte donation however are common, usually in the treatment of ovarian failure. Directed gamete donations usually take into account various desirable characteristics, of the donor which may include the health status, character, social and cultural background and of course genetic makeup. The confidentiality issues raised in directed donation are more profound in that the identity of all the players, the health professionals, the donor and the recipient is known. Directed donations therefore require confidentiality that is determined by legal, professional ethical standard as well the relationship and understanding of the involved parties. Directed donation requires that the interest of the potential child and the other involved parties, the donor, the recipient and the health professionals be protected with respect to disclosure of identity, written informed consent of the donor and also recognition that the donor is not driven by pressure, coercion or financial consideration in making the decision to donate gamete. The disclosure to the children from directed gamete donation of their genetic origin may serve the purpose of averting consanguinity, or incest, amongst these offspring in the future.

13. Surrogacy

Surrogacy implies the commissioning of a woman to carry a pregnancy whether or not on a commercial basis. It poses ethical challenges having been regarded occasionally the using of one person as a means to the ends of another (Warnock, 1987). Ethics demand that the autonomy of the surrogate mother should be respected and that surrogacy should not be commercialized. Ethical approval is required and the legal requirements for surrogacy in the concerned country should be complied with and duly explained to the concerned parties prior to the surrogate arrangement by the health professional.

14. Multifoetal gestation (multiple pregnancy)

Assisted reproduction requiring the use of ovulation inducing drugs and the need for multiple embryo transfer has been the main factor responsible for the increasing incidence of multiple pregnancies the world over. Multiple pregnancy has grave implications not only for the mother and the foetuses but also for the family, the community, the healthcare provider and the overall health services particularly in respect of the demands of expert on neonatal care, couples seeking for infertility treatment especially by assisted reproductive technology should therefore be adequately informed as to the possibility, and risks that may be associated with multiple pregnancy, particularly of the higher other variety. Obstetrics and gynaecological professionals involved in assisted reproduction should therefore aim at achieving singleton pregnancies and furthermore clearly inform their client and other interest group such as the press that multiple pregnancies arising from assisted reproduction constitute a complication rather than a fit. Where multiple pregnancies especially of the higher order variety occur, it is ethically preferred to reduce the number of foetuses than leave them alone, since this will increase the chances of survival and success of the assisted reproduction.

15. Termination of pregnancy

Termination of pregnancy can occur for variety of reasons. When pregnancy termination occurs before the age of viability of the foetus, it is regarded as abortion. Abortion can occur as a natural process in which case it is regarded as spontaneous abortion or otherwise as a forced procedure regarded as induced abortion. Induced abortion is usually performed for unwanted pregnancy. When performed in countries where the law permits, it is regarded as legal abortion, while it is illegal or criminal if carried out where the law does not permit abortion. In some countries abortion law is restrictive, abortion being allowed under certain circumstances such as for the purpose of saving the life of the mother. In countries where the law does not permit abortion or where the law is restrictive, unsafe abortion is usually of high incidence. Virtually all forms of abortion, but in particular induced abortion are fraught with ethical challenges. A woman with an unwanted pregnancy particularly for strong reasons will go to any length to seek for the termination of such pregnancy – even at the risk of losing her life.

The ethical question is, should her autonomy not be respected by obliging her with a safe termination of the unwanted pregnancy?

A further question that often arises and is capable of throwing the health practitioners into serious ethical dilemma concerns the identity of the foetus that the pregnant woman seeks to abort. Does the foetus not constitute a being albeit incapable of autonomy and therefore vulnerable, whose autonomy needs to be protected, or should the fate of the foetus be allowed to be solely dependent on the decisions of the mother? These ethical questions are applicable to several issues in obstetrics that may constitute danger to the foetus or the mother or both.

16. Prenatal diagnosis and termination of pregnancy following the procedure

Prenatal diagnosis is becoming an increasingly important component of obstetrics care, to identify in –utero, diseases of the foetus and their severity, that may require genetic engineering, future life style adjustment or termination of pregnancy. Prenatal diagnostic procedure requires prior counseling and informed consent of the woman. The woman is also required to state in advance any information that she would not want to be given following the procedure for example the sex of the foetus.

Prenatal diagnosis provides information as to foetal diseases that may permit termination of pregnancy in countries where the law permits. The ethical challenges raised however is related to how one determines the degree of the severity of the disease or abnormality and to what extent this will influence the quality of life of the infant following delivery to justify the termination of the pregnancy.

The decision to terminate a pregnancy following the discovery of foetal abnormality from prenatal diagnosis, is entirely that of the couple and on no account should the couple be coerced into choosing any of the available care option, in fact where abnormality discovered is treatable or compatible with life, termination of pregnancy is discouraged.

17. Interventions for foetal well–being including court-order obstetrical interventions

The majority of pregnant women act in a manner that protects the interest of their foetus. There are few occasions however where the habits or practices of a mother may impair the well-being of her foetus, for example, cigarette smoking, alcohol intake and the use of hard drugs. A mother may also refuse the advice of the health practitioner to carry out procedures such as cesarean section for foetal indication. The healthcare practitioner and indeed the medical team have a responsibility to empathically counsel and fully inform the patient, excising utmost patience in doing so, of the benefits or repercussions of the medical advice. Most of the time, the woman accepts to co-operate if she is adequately informed. Situations however may arise where the pregnant woman emphatically objects to the proposed obstetrics intervention to the extent that judicial mandate is sought for by the hospital authorities. Court order cesarean section, the most common of these interventions has been reviewed by Walden (2007). A 1987 New England Journal of Medicine report indicated that among 21 cases of cesarean sections for which court orders were sought, 86% were obtained; in addition a survey of heads of maternal-foetal medicine departments, revealed that 46% of the respondents supported court ordered cesarean section (Veronika et al, 1987). A more recent study of attendees at the annual meetings of the American College of Obstetricians and Gynecologists and the American Health Lawyers Association found that as high as 51% indicated the likelihood of their supporting forced cesarean section (Samuels et al 2007). The issue of court order (forced cesarean section) and what should constitute the health professionals' approach to it has been summarized in a 2004 American College of Obstetrics and Gynecology (ACOG) guidelines which states as follows:- "if an obstetrician disagrees with a patient's choice and is unable to arrange transfer of care, they must, continue to care for the pregnant woman and not intervene against the patient's wishes, regardless of the consequences." The guideline also states that the use of judicial authority to implement treatment regimens to protect the fetus violates the pregnant woman's autonomy and should be avoided. It further states, "Even in the presence of a court order authorizing intervention, the use of physical force against a resistant, competent woman is not justified. The use of force will substantially increase the risk to the woman, thereby diminishing the ethical justification for such therapy (ACOG, 2007). The position contained in the ACOG guideline concerning court order cesarean section is in tandem with the premise on which the first appellate court vacation of a court order cesarean section was made in 1990. Angela Carder a terminally ill cancer patient at 26 weeks pregnancy had a forced judicial mandate cesarean section at George Washington University Hospital in 1987 – against her wish and that of her doctor and relations. Angela and her child died shortly after the surgery and it was argued that the surgical procedure had accelerated the death.

Angela carder's family and Reproductive Freedom Project (RFP) supported by several other bodies and human rights organizations filed an appeal at the D.C. court of Appeal for the vacation of the court order for that cesarean section and the legal precedents it had set, which was ultimately granted (ACLU, 1997). On no account therefore should a woman be forced or coerced into carrying out a procedure that she is unwilling to accept since this will amount to a violation of her autonomy. It is inappropriate to resort to judicial intervention when a woman has made an informed refusal of a medical or surgical procedure since this is considered to constitute an overriding of her autonomy (strong paternalism). The situation is noteworthy, different when the woman's competence to make decision is impaired as in the unconscious mother or in the mentally sub–normal.

The consent of a surrogate – the woman's spouse or any other member of her family is usually enlisted. It is important however to note that in general the mother should be of prime consideration and therefore decision on her well-being takes precedence over that of the foetus.

18. Interventions for severe congenital malformation of the foetus

A woman carrying a severely malformed foetus has the ethical right of having the pregnancy terminated. In situations where termination of pregnancy is not considered as a management option, for example for legal, religious or other personal reasons, prenatal diagnostic procedures for severe foetal congenital malformations should be preceded by counseling of the woman on the possible findings and ascertaining from her the extent of the findings to be disclosed to her. Pregnancy termination on the basis of the sex of the foetus is un-ethical. In multiple pregnancies involving normal and malformed foetuses prime consideration should be given to survival of the normal foetuses provided the mother's life is not at risk. Where the couple disagrees on the management option in severe foetal malformations, the view of the woman should take precedence over that of spouse. The medical team has the ethical responsibility to encourage the parents, in the case of severe foetal malformation, to seek a second opinion, should they not be satisfied with the medical advice given to them. The decision on the termination of pregnancy for congenital malformation should be made by the parents free from coercion, financial inducement or demographic considerations whether from government or other bodies. Medical practitioner should seek appropriate consent to confirm and appropriately document the nature and extent of foetal malformation following termination and furthermore appropriately inform and counsel parents.

19. Caesaeran section for non-medical reason

Worldwide there has been and increasing incidence in the rate of caesarean section attributable to medical, legal, financial, social and psychological factors. Oftentimes physicians are confronted with request for caesarean section for personal reasons such as the convenience of the patient. Caesarean deliveries are associated with higher risks than vaginal deliveries. Furthermore complications, costs and duration of hospital stay are more following caesarean deliveries compared to vaginal deliveries. It is ethically wrong for medical practitioners to perform caesarean section for indications that are not medical. The health practitioners are therefore obligated to inform adequately and counsel woman against requests for caesarean section for non-medical reasons.

20. Management of pregnancy related to sudden unexpected maternal death

When a pregnant woman is certified dead or is in the danger of imminent death from circulatory or respiratory failure, the life of the foetus is severely endangered and urgent intervention becomes necessary. It is important to maintain the circulation and respiration of the woman while waiting for an urgent decision on the foetus. Pertinent issues requiring considerations includes, the viability, and probable health status of the foetus, any wishes expressed by the mother as well as any views expressed by her family members especially her partner. The management options include immediate caesarean delivery if the foetus is alive and matured, co-ordinating effects to maintain the vital functions of the woman to allow the preterm foetus to mature provided that the informed consent of the woman's partner or family has been obtained, and the deceased had not wished otherwise, and outright discontinuation of support for the respiratory and circulatory function of the woman if the foetus is dead or the two former conditions are not wished by the involved parties. If support for the vital organs of the woman cannot be maintained immediate caesarean section is recommended.

21. HIV infection in pregnancy

HIV infection is a global pandemic. 2008 estimate has if that approximately 33.4 million people worldwide are living with HIV including 2.1 million children under 15years of age (UNAIDS, 2009; WHO, 2009). HIV prevalence rate ranges from as low as less than 0.1% in countries such as Bangladesh, Croatia, and Egypt to as high as 24.8%, and 25.9% in Botswana and Swaziland respectively (UNAIDS, 2010). HIV infection has profound psychological and social implications to the victim, her partner, family, the health worker, and the society at large. Vertical transmission of the infection during pregnancy and breast feeding is the most common source of infant and childhood infection. The disease which runs a chronic course has varying degrees of morbidity and is characterized by social stigmatization of the patient, with discrimination in the work place and societal activities. HIV disease has ethical challenges. The respect for the privacy and confidentiality of the HIV infected person conflict with the need to protect the partner, the health workers and other members of the public that may be placed at risk by virtue of their contact with the infected person. Ethical concerns on the privacy and confidentiality of the infected HIV patient however should be weighed against the need to prevent the disease from getting to epidemic proportions through providing information to the public on the morbidity and mortality statistics of the disease, mandatory screening for antenatal patient, and disclosure of HIV status of patients to partner, health workers and other vulnerable persons. The responsibility of the physician therefore includes the provision of individual counseling, care and treatment for the HIV infected persons and advocacy to the public towards the protection of the patient from stigma and discrimination. The ethical responsibility of the physician to protect persons at risk of being infected by an HIV patient requires proper counseling of the patient together with enough information to enlist the consent for testing, and disclosure to such persons. For example, the partner and the health worker, where informed consent for disclosure is not obtained in spite of adequate counseling of the patient, and the risk of transmission of the disease is high, the physician can after due consultation with relevant bodies such as, the institution's ethical committee, decide to override the patients autonomy of confidentiality.

Vertical transmission of HIV to an infant is averted when breast feeding is avoided. In societies where affordable alternative infant feeding methods are available it is unethical to allow an HIV positive mother to breast feed her infant. In low socio- economically developed societies where infant feeding formula may not be affordable or may be prepared under unhygienic condition with risk of infection to the infant, or in societies with strong cultural ties to breast feeding, it is ethically justified to allow breast feeding provided the countries' protocol for the reduction of the infectivity of the breast milk and increasing its safety to the infant is adhered to. Gamete donation for Assisted Reproduction requires informed consent and screening for HIV. Only donors with sero-negative HIV status are allowed to donate gamete.

22. Safe motherhood

World health organization (WHO) has estimated in a 2007 report that 536, 000 maternal deaths occur annually the world over from causes related to pregnancy and childbirth (WHO, 2007). As high as 99% of these deaths occur in developing countries (WHO, 2001). Maternal and Perinatal mortality statistics are the most important measure of safe motherhood, and their reduction has been recognized in the 5th and 4th component respectively, of the United Nations Millennium Development Goals (UNDP, 2003; UNO, 2003).

Maternal mortality can occur from direct medical causes – obstetrics haemorrhage, sepsis, complications of unsafe abortion, hypertensive disorders in pregnancy and obstructed labour; from indirect medical causes – factors pre –existing or co –existing with pregnancy e:g cardiac diseases and gender based violence; and from non –medical factors – underlying social-cultural, legal, religious, and economic factors, reproductive health factors, health systems and health services factors and delays to access to emergency obstetrics care (Fatusi and Ijadunola, 2003; WHO, 1994; Maine and Wray, 1984).

Most causes of maternal deaths are preventable, such deaths therefore represents a violation of ethical principles and human right of the woman – a situation more marked in the developing countries, lack of access to family planning, abortion services, good antenatal care, delivery by skilled birth attendant, emergency obstetrics care, good neonatal care and postnatal services – all constitute a violation of woman's ethical principles of respect for persons, beneficence, non – maleficence, and justice which may occur both at microethical or macroethical level. Physicians have an ethical responsibility to protect the sexual and reproductive rights of women in other to promote their rights to life, information and education, to decide on whether and when to get married and found a family, to healthcare and protection, to benefit of scientific progress and to be free from ill treatment and torture.

Physicians also have an important role to play in publicity and campaign towards the development of policies and programs that will strengthen the health systems and health service to promote safe motherhood and reduce maternal mortality to the barest minimum.

Governments should work in partnership with non – governmental organizations and communities to provide good roads, acceptable and affordable maternal health services with good health facilities equipped and manned by skilled birth attendants adequately trained on emergency obstetrics care.

23. Cord-blood collection and new born care

Umbilical cord blood is a rich source of haemopoietic stem cells that is used in the treatment of diseases such as leukemia. It can therefore be collected, pooled and stored in core blood bank to be dispensed when required, usually on commercial bases. Maternal consent to the collection of umbilical cord-blood is ethically required. Early clamping of the umbilical cord has been shown to be capable of reducing the new born circulating blood volume by 30% and tripping the newborn into circulatory disturbance. Enlisting maternal consent to cord blood collection should therefore be preceded by the assurance of the mother that the umbilical cord will not be clamped early, to prevent hazard to her new born.

Resuscitation and care of the new born requires that the physician considers the welfare of the individual new born within the context of the ethical principle of respect for persons albeit incapable of autonomy, who should therefore be protected. The parents who constitutes the rightful surrogate of the child should be adequately informed as to the diagnosis and prognosis of the child's condition, for example, the severely preterm infant to enable them make appropriate decision and consent to the treatment of the child.

Gender, religious, ethnic and financial considerations should not influence decisions on the treatment of the new born. The physicians counseling and advice to the parents on treatment decision for the newborn should be based on accurate knowledge of the facts and statistics on the prognosis following the treatment of the condition, and in most circumstances, after due consultations with other members of the health team including a senior obstetrician and gynaecologist. Where there is disagreement between the physician and the parents independent adjudication may be sought for and where necessary, the view of the health facility's ethical committee. Following the death of the infant, permission should be sought from the parents for the conduct of a post mortem examination on the deceased new born, to confirm the definitive cause of death and provide more information for further counseling of the parents particularly for future births.

24. Conclusion

Contemporary global health care has over the years increasingly recognized the need to uphold and promote the sexual and reproductive rights of individuals, especially women, which has been perceived to be an important prerequisite to national development (Adinma and Adinma, 2009; Adinma and Adinma, 2011). It has therefore become absolutely compelling that health professionals caring for women imbibe and observe strict ethical principles in all aspect of reproductive health care of women. In particular, obstetrics care, on account of its exclusiveness for women and the wide range of physical, psychological and social issues, sometimes cross –cutting, that may be associated with the process, from conception to parturition, requires that the health professional be vast with various ethical and human rights challenges associated with every step in obstetrics care.

In countries not already doing so every effort should be made towards including, or broadening the scope, of bioethics in the curriculum of studies of health professionals caring for women, both at under-graduate and post-graduate levels. Furthermore it is necessary to develop human rights based bioethical codes that will guide such health professionals in their day to day obstetrics practice and ensure that the ethical codes are appropriately disseminated for application by health professionals already in obstetrics practice. These health professionals will also benefit from periodic workshops and seminars on bioethics as part of their continuing medical education. Health professionals also have an obligation to guide governments and policy makers towards the development of human rights and ethics - friendly policies and programmes that will invariably promote obstetrics care and overall safe motherhood.

25. References

American College of Obstetricians and Gynecologists. Cesarean delivery on maternal request. ACOG Committee Opinion No. 394. Obstet Gynecol 2007; 110:1501–1504.

Adinma JIB, Adinma ED. Ethical Considerations in Women's Sexual and Reproductive Healthcare: Nigerian Journal of Clinical Practice. 2009; 12(1):92-98.

Adinma JIB, Adinma ED: Impact of Reproductive Health on Socio-economic Development: A Case Study of Nigeria. African Journal of Reproductive health 2011; 15(1): 7

Adinma JIB. International Federation of Gynaecology and Obstetrics / Society of Gynaecology and Obstetrics of Nigeria (FIGO/SOGON) Human Rights Code of Ethics on Women's Sexual and Reproductive Healthcare for health professionals in Nigeria. FIGO/SOGON Women's Sexual and Reproductive Rights Project (WOSRRIP) 2003.

American Civil Liberty Union (ACLU) Coercive and Punitive Governmental Responses to Women's Conduct during Pregnancy September 30, 1997. http://www.aclu.org/reproductive-freedom.

Beauchamp TL, Childress JF. Principles of Biomedical Ethics. Oxford University Press. New York. 2001.

Callahan D. The Social Sciences and the task of bioethics. Daedalus. 1999; 128: 275–294.

Commonwealth Medical Association Trust (COMMAT). Consultation on Medical Ethics and Women's Health, including Sexual and Reproductive Health, as a Human Right. NY, USA, 23–26 January 1997.

Cook RJ, Dickens B, Fathala MF. Reproductive Health and Human Rights. Oxford University Press, 2003.

Council for International Organizations of Medical Sciences (CIOMS). International ethical guidelines for biomedical research involving human subjects. Prepared by CIOMS in collaboration with WHO, Geneva, 1993.

Donation of genetic material for human reproduction, Int. J. Gynecol. Obstet, 1994, 44:185.

Elkins TE, Strong C, Dilts PV Jr. Teaching of Bioethics within a Residency Program in Obstetrics and Gynecology. Obstet Gynecol. 1986 Mar; 67 (3):339-43. Website: http://www.ncbi.nlm.nih.gov/pubmed/3945445

Ethical Issues in Obstetrics and Gynecology by the FIGO Committee for the Study of Ethical Aspects of Human Reproduction and Women's Health. November 2006.

Ezeani CO. Evolving a human rights based code of ethics for medical practitioners caring for women in Nigeria. Trop J Obst Gynae 2002; 19 (Suppl.1): S 26–28.

Fatusi AO, Ijadunola KT. (2003) National study on Emergency obstetrics care facilities in Nigeria, UNFPA/FMOH Abuja.

FIGO Professional and Ethical Responsibilities Concerning Sexual and Reproductive Rights. Dec. 2004. www.figo.org/Codeofethics

Gillon R (Ed). Principles of health care ethics. John Wiley and Sons. Chichester. 1994.

James HJ, Bad Blood: The Tuskegee Syphilis Experiment (New York: Free Press, 1993); Carol A. Heintzelman, "The Tuskegee Syphilis Study and its Implications for the 21st Century" at http/www.socialworker.com/Tuskegee.htm.

Jonsen A. The birth of Bioethics. Oxford University Press. New York. 1998.

Maine D, Wray J (1984) Effects of family planning on maternal and child health. CONTEMPORARY OBS/GYN 1984 O mar. 23(3): 122 – 36.

McKneally MF, Singer PA. Bioethics for clinicians: 25. Teaching bioethics in the clinical setting. *CMAJ* 2001; 164: 1163-1167.

Warnock M (1987). The new Ethical Problems in Infertility. In: Progress in Obstetrics and Gynaecology, edited by Studd J., vol. 6., chapter 13, pp 243 – 251. Edinburgh, Churchill Livingstone.

Rehmann-Sutter C, Wienroth M: Ethical Considerations on new Developments in Reproductive Medicine. Ther Umsch, 2009 Dec, 66 (12): 807 – 11.

Rothmans D. Stranger at the bedside: A history of how Law and Bioethics transformed medical decision making. Basic Books, New York, 1991.

Royal College of Physicians and Surgeons of Canada. General Standards of accreditation. Ottawa: Royal College of Physicians and Surgeons of Canada, 1997. Standard B.V:3:

Samuels TA, Minkoff H, Feldman J, Awonuga A, Wilson TE. "Obstetricians, health attorneys, and court-ordered cesarean sections." *Womens Health Issues*. 2007 Mar-Apr;17(2): 107-14.

Shuster E: Fifty Years Later: The Significance of the Nuremberg Code. NEJM 337.

Stephens T, Brynner R. Dark Remedy (Cambridge, Mass: Perseus Publishing, 2001), on the rehabilitation and therapeutic benefits of Thalidomide.

The National Commission for the Protection of Human Subjects of Biomedical and Behavioral Research. The Belmont Report: Ethical Principles and Guidelines for the Protection of Human Subjects of Research. DHEW Publication No. (OS) 78-0012. Washington, 1978, p. 2.

UNAIDS Global updates of HIV/AIDS. 2009

UNAIDS, Report on the Global AIDS Epidemic, 2010. http://www.unaids.org /Global Report/Global_report. Htm

UNDP. Human DEVELOPMENT Report 2003, MDGs: A compact among nations to end human poverty.

United Nations Millennium Declaration 2000. A/RES/SS/2 18 September, New York. http:/www.un.org/millennium/Declaration/are5552e.pdf. march 2003

Uzodike VO. Ethical codes and statements. In: Uzodike VO, ed. Medical Ethics: Its foundation, philosophy and practice (with special reference to Nigeria and developing countries). Computer Edge Publishers, Enugu, Nigeria, 1998: 21.

Veronika E.B. Kolder, Janet Gallagher, and Michael T. Parsons. "Court-Ordered Obstetrical Interventions." *NEJM* 316.19 (May 7, 1987): 1192-1196.

Walden R. What Do Obstetricians and Lawyers Think About Forced C-Sections? April 7, 2007. http://womenshealthnews.wordpress.com/2007/04/07/.

World Health Organization (WHO): maternal mortality in 2005: estimates developed by WHO, UNICEF, UNFPA, and the World Bank Geneva, WHO,2007

World Health Organization, United Nations Children's Fund, and United Nations Population Fund. Maternal mortality in 1995. Estimates Development by WHO, UNICEF and UNFPA. Geneva 2001. World Health Organization (WHO/RHR/01.9)

World Health organization, United Nations children's fund, UNAIDS (2009) Towards universal access. Scaling up priority HIV/AIDS interventions in the health sector, progress report 2009 Geneva, world Health Organization.

World Health organization. Mother Baby package: implementing safe Motherhood in countries. WHO/FHE/USM/19.11. World Health Organization, 1994.

World Medical Association, Declaration of Helsinki, as amended Oct. 2000, Article 5 (see Pt. III, Ch. 2)

World Medical Association, Declaration of Helsinki, as amended Oct. 2008, Article 5.

18

Umbilical Cord Blood Changes in Neonates from a Preeclamptic Pregnancy

Cristina Catarino[1,2], Irene Rebelo[1,2], Luís Belo[1,2],
Alexandre Quintanilha[2,3] and Alice Santos-Silva[1,2]
[1]*Departamento de Ciências Biológicas, Laboratório de Bioquímica,
Faculdade de Farmácia, Universidade do Porto (FFUP);*
[2]*Instituto de Biologia Molecular e Celular (IBMC), Universidade do Porto;*
[3]*Instituto Ciências Biomédicas Abel Salazar (ICBAS), Universidade do Porto*
Portugal

1. Introduction

During pregnancy, mother's well-being affects directly the newborn development. Some maternal and placental complications, such as gestational diabetes, preeclampsia (PE), preterm delivery and intrauterine growth restriction (IUGR), may contribute to fetal growth deviations or fetal development modifications. Usually the newborn weight correlates positively with placenta weight, showing the interaction between the development of placenta and fetal growth.

Normal human pregnancy is associated with physiological blood changes, namely, neutrophilic leukocytosis, hyperlipidemia and procoagulant, hypofibrinolytic and inflammatory conditions. PE has been associated with an enhancement in these changes and with placental abnormalities, that may condition its perfusion and, therefore, feto-maternal transfer. The placental dysfunction, characterized by a disturbance in the angiogenic/anti-angiogenic factors and in the hypoxia/placental reoxygenation process, seems to trigger a maternal endothelial dysfunction. To this maternal endothelial dysfunction may also contribute the oxidative stress, dyslipidemia and the inflammatory process which are present in maternal circulation.

PE is a maternal pathology involving placental modifications, which is also associated with fetal complications. Prematurity and IUGR, are the most representative complications. In this chapter we will address the impact of the maternal disturbances in the newborns from a normal and a preeclamptic (PEc) gestation. Indeed, there are several studies in literature about changes in maternal circulation, but few studies about fetal blood changes in the presence of PE. Moreover, these studies have shown controversial results. We intend to focus on neonatal consequences of PE, by assessing different biochemical and hematologic parameters in the umbilical cord blood. In this way, we will address the effect of some modifications usually observed in PEc women, such as, in lipid profile, in hematologic profile, inflammatory and antioxidant markers, angiogenic/anti-angiogenic factors and hemostatic disturbances, in umbilical cord blood.

Disturbances in angiogenic/anti-angiogenic factors, in the lipid profile and an enhanced inflammatory response, in the fetal circulation, may cause a short-term effect, such as endothelial dysfunction. However, the impact of these modifications, that are known cardiovascular risk changes, in the future life of these newborn are still unknown and should be clarified. These neonates and their mothers should deserve, therefore, a closer clinical follow-up later in life. This issue will be also addressed in this chapter.

2. Preeclampsia

Hypertensive diseases in pregnancy are the most common causes of mortality and maternal and fetal morbidity (WHO, 2005). PE is a frequent cause for hospitalization, labour induction and dystocic labour, reasons that justify the study of this disease.

Some controversy exists concerning the terminology and the classification of hypertensive disorders; indeed, several reported studies used different classifications. The more consensual, is the classification proposed by the "International Society for the Study of Hypertension in Pregnancy" (ISSHP). The diagnosis of hypertension in pregnancy, according to this classification (Brown et al., 2001) is performed in accordance with the following criteria: an occasional measurement of diastolic blood pressure greater than 110 mmHg, or two or more consecutive measurements equal to or greater than 90 mmHg, with 6 hours or longer intervals between measurements. PE is defined as the onset of hypertension associated with proteinuria after 20 weeks of gestation, in previously normotensive pregnant women (Table 1). Typically, PE is asymptomatic, but in its most severe form it may also present with headache, epigastric pain, visual disturbances and changes in consciousness.

Preeclampsia ISSHP classification:

Hypertension - diastolic blood pressure $\geq$ 110 mmHg (an occasional measurement), or $\geq$ 90 mmHg (two or more consecutive measurements)

Proteinuria ($\geq$ 300 mg/day)

Both present, after 20 weeks of gestation, returning to normal postpartum

Table 1. Preeclampsia ISSHP classification

Eclampsia is the most severe form of pregnancy-induced hypertension. It is characterized by the appearance of seizures, which may occur before, during or within 48 hrs after birth. Eclampsia may appear in pregnant women with moderate increases in blood pressure and mild proteinuria.

2.1 Epidemiology of preeclampsia /risk factors and complications

PE is a pregnancy specific disorder, characterized by an impaired blood perfusion of vital organs, including the fetal-placental unit. The prevalence of PE, although usually reported as 5 to 8%, presents some variations in the literature (Sibai et al., 2005; Maynard et al., 2008), particularly for different populations.

The risk of developing PE seems to be associated with some factors, such as nulliparity (about 2/3 of cases occur in the first pregnancy), multiple pregnancy, change of paternity, age over 40 years, family history of PE and eclampsia, body mass index (BMI) greater than 35 kg/m², diabetes, disease prior to pregnancy (e.g., diabetes mellitus, hypertension, renal disease and thrombophilia) and hydatidiform mole (Duckitt & Harrington, 2005; Magnussen et al., 2007; Jim et al., 2010). According to Magnussen et al. (2007), there is an enhanced risk to develop PE, when cardiovascular risk factors, such as increased triglycerides (TG), total cholesterol and LDLc, are present before pregnancy.

Several studies associate smoking habits with a lower risk of developing PE (Magnussen et al., 2007; Wikström et al., 2010). However, maternal smoking is associated with various maternal and fetal complications (Kalle, 2001; Steyn et al., 2006), including placenta previa, low birth weight, preterm birth, miscarriage and neonatal death.

PE is the main maternal risk factor associated with low birth weight newborns and/or IUGR (Table 2). Intrauterine growth restriction and/or fetal death can occur in about 30% of PEc cases as a direct result of placental insufficiency (Jim et al., 2010). The neonatal complications risk is higher in cases of severe PE and eclampsia (Duley, 2009). IUGR is associated with a high rate of perinatal morbidity and mortality (Rizzo & Arduini, 2009).

Several studies indicate that PE is associated with a higher incidence of newborns with low birth weight (Groom et al., 2007; Duley, 2009; Wu et al., 2009). In addition, there's an increased incidence of newborns with low birth weight in pregnant women who developed PE at an earlier stage of pregnancy, compared with those who later developed PE (Xiong & Fraser, 2004; Groom et al., 2007). Prematurity is the leading cause of perinatal morbidity and mortality (Goldenberg et al., 2008) and PE is often associated with preterm delivery (Sibai et al., 2005; Goldenberg et al., 2008; Duley, 2009; Wu et al., 2009). Some neonatal complications resulting from PEc pregnancy are described, and are associated with prematurity, including jaundice, respiratory distress, apnea, seizures, hypoglycaemia and prolonged hospitalization (Duley, 2009; Wu et al., 2009).

Newborn complications:

Intrauterine growth restriction (IUGR)
Prematurity
Neurologic lesions
Neonatal death
Long term chronic diseases ("fetal programming" or "fetal origins of disease in adult life")

Table 2. Newborn complications in preeclampsia

According to Barker's theory, the origin of some adulthood chronic diseases such as cardiovascular diseases, hypertension and diabetes have their origin in intrauterine life (Barker & Bagby, 2005). This hypothesis, called "fetal programming" or "fetal origins of disease," suggests that the intrauterine environment in which the fetus develops may be the origin of diseases in adult life. Changes that may occur in intrauterine environment and that somehow could disrupt normal development of the fetus can trigger metabolic changes, which may result in the development of long-term disorders (Barker, 2004).

There are studies revealing that children of PEc women present in adolescence, higher blood pressure levels with increased risk of developing hypertension, compared to children of normotensive pregnant women (Vatten et al., 2003; Tenhola et al., 2006, Kajantie et al., 2009). In another study, adolescents with low birth weight also presented blood pressure values higher than adolescents who were born with adequate weight (Covelli et al., 2007).

Low birth weight appears to be associated with an increased risk of developing type 2 Diabetes mellitus(Whincup et al., 2008), cardiovascular disease (Barker & Bagby, 2005) and hypertension (Lenfant, 2008) in adult life. This risk appears to be even greater if, in addition to low birth weight, further develop a marked increase in BMI (Eriksson et al., 2007; Barker et al., 2009). In a recent study, Raghupathy et al. (2010) mentioned that individuals who were underweight at birth and during infancy, followed by a sharp increase in BMI during adolescence, were associated with a reduction in glucose tolerance and development of type 2 Diabetes mellitus.

2.2 Etiology and pathophysiology of preeclampsia

PE is considered a multisystem disorder, affecting several organs and maternal systems, including the vascular system, liver, kidney and brain. Despite the intensive research in this area, the etiology of PE remains unknown. PE seems to have a multifactorial cause and is also known as the "disease of theories". In fact, there are several hypotheses raised to explain its etiology. Some those theories propose modifications in the trophoblastic invasion, immunologic intolerance between maternal and fetoplacental tissue, inflammatory changes in pregnancy and genetic modifications, underlying PE development.

Although its unknown cause, it is consensual that there are modifications occurring at different levels, like changes in placental perfusion, increased inflammatory response with changes in leukocyte activation, activation of the coagulation system, endothelial dysfunction and changes in lipid metabolism. The most accepted theory describes two stages for PE (Roberts & Gammil, 2005; Steegers et al., 2010): stage 1 - reduced placental perfusion; stage 2 - multisystem maternal syndrome.

According to this theory, the first pathological change in PE occurs in the uteroplacental circulation, resulting in an inadequate vascular remodelling and/or placental ischemia. In the second phase, the damaged placenta (ischemic placenta) secretes factors that cause endothelial dysfunction, followed by the appearance of maternal clinical symptoms.

The event(s) that trigger(s) the change in the trophoblastic invasion remains unknown; however, genetic, immunological and environmental factors (nutritional deficiencies and hypoxia environment) seem to have some contribution.

The remodelling of spiral arteries takes place at the end of the 1st trimester of pregnancy, and is very important, because it allows an increasing blood flow, in response to higher feto-maternal exchanges. A failure in this process may result in reduced placental blood flow, causing the formation of a hypoxic environment that may trigger PE, which might be associated or not with IUGR. In this case, the spiral arteries have a reduction in its lumen and may be linked to inadequate placentation and acute atherosis, or both.

The placenta seems to play a key role in the pathogenesis of PE, since the clinical symptoms disappear only after placental expulsion. PE seems to develop after a partial failure in the process of placentation, a process that occurs between 6-18 weeks of gestation. In this condition, only some of the spiral arteries of the placental circulation are invaded by trophoblasts. In the myometrial spiral arteries the muscular-elastic layer is not replaced; therefore, vascular resistance is higher and uteroplacental flow is reduced, as compared to what occurs in a normal pregnancy. This decrease in placental perfusion may significantly affect oxygenation, nutrition and fetal development. The reduction in placental perfusion in PE is usually accompanied by a reduction in fetal weight for gestational age (Catarino et al., 2008a).

The first observations on this phenomenon have been published for over three decades (Brosens et al., 1972), but several authors have confirmed these observations and attempted to clarify the mechanisms involved (Chaddha et al., 2004; Burton et al., 2009). Doppler fluxometry applied to the uterine arteries allowed the confirmation of the hemodynamic disturbances underlying placental insufficiency, and demonstrated that in PE occurs an increased (circulatory) resistance of placental vascular territory (Papageorghiou & Leslie, 2007; Boukerrou et al., 2009). As changes in placental blood flow are observed in PE before the onset of symptoms (Papageorghiou & Leslie, 2007), uterine artery Doppler, is performed early in the second trimester of pregnancy, in order to predict PE.

In PE an acute atherosis in the myometrial spiral arteries may also develop. The acute atherosis is an injury similar to the atherosclerotic lesion, characterized by the presence of fibrin deposits, accumulation of foam cells and infiltration of mononuclear leukocytes. This type of injury leads to a reduction of the arteries lumen, and, thus, to a decrease in placental perfusion, even in the absence of an inadequate placentation (Pijnenborg et al., 2006). The atherosis may progress to acute vascular obstruction of the spiral arteries, reducing blood flow to the placenta and causing placental infarction. In a study involving 400 placentas from PEc women, the vascular lesions in the placenta correlated with the severity of this pathology (Ghidini et al., 1997).

2.2.1 Maternal syndrome of preeclampsia

Placenta has the ability to synthesize several molecules, including mediators of inflammation and angiogenic factors, whose expression appears to be regulated by oxygen pressure and by the presence of oxidative stress (Rusterholz et al., 2007; Redman & Sargent, 2009). The expression of these molecules appears to be affected in PE; placental hypoxia/reperfusion and placental oxidative stress seems to be involved in this regulation, however, other modulators may contribute to that expression, such as genetic and immunological factors.

Some studies state that PE induces changes in the placental expression of tumor necrosis factor (TNF)-α, increasing this and other pro-inflammatory cytokines (Hung et al., 2004), and interleukin (IL)-6 (Bowen et al., 2005); however, there are conflicting results (Rusterholz et al., 2007).

Placenta seems to be the main source of placental growth factor (PlGF) and soluble vascular endothelial growth factor receptor (sVEGFR)-1, during pregnancy. A change in placental function may, therefore, interfere with the synthesis of these angiogenic/anti-angiogenic factors. It has been shown that PEc placentas present an increased expression of sFlt1 (Gu et al., 2008), and a decreased expression of PlGF (Gu et al., 2008). These placental factors and cytokines appear to be released in maternal circulation, resulting in a generalized endothelial dysfunction, causing the multisystem complications of a PEc pregnancy (Rusterholz et al., 2007; Maynard et al., 2008) (Fig. 1).

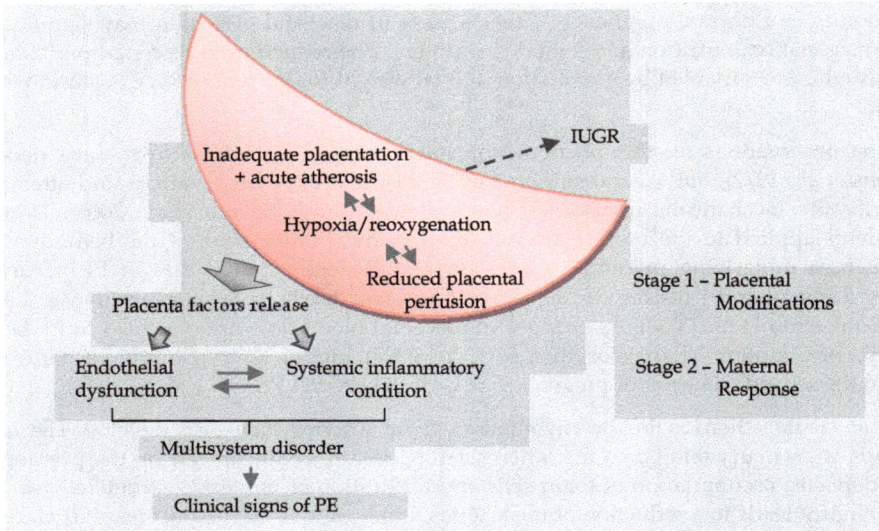

Fig. 1. Possible mechanisms involved in the pathogenesis of preeclampsia

3. Maternal and umbilical cord blood modifications

PE is a disorder involving maternal and placental changes. It involves fetal complications, such as, prematurity and IUGR, which are the most representative. Newborns, whose mothers develop PE, usually present a lower birth weight than infants born from mothers with a normal pregnancy (Catarino et al., 2008a). Moreover, newborns small for gestational age, as well as newborns with Apgar score below 7, are frequently observed in PE (Catarino et al., 2008a).

There are several studies concerning maternal modifications in PE, but there are few studies carried out in umbilical cord blood. We will address the effect of some modifications usually observed in PEc women, such as, in lipid profile, in hematologic profile, inflammatory and antioxidant markers, angiogenic/anti-angiogenic factors and hemostatic disturbances, in umbilical cord blood.

3.1 Angiogenic/anti-angiogenic factors

A normal placental development is essential for adequate feto-maternal nutrients and gas exchanges. In addition, placenta is an important endocrine organ that synthesizes various hormones, cytokines and angiogenic growth factors. These factors are released into the maternal circulation, and may contribute to changes in endothelial function. It is recognized that placenta has an important role in the protection and development of the fetus, promoting feto-maternal exchanges which are essential to a normal pregnancy. On the other hand, it is also recognized that in PE there are changes in placental development (Pijnenborg et al., 2006; Young et al., 2010), which can compromise the feto-maternal exchange, limiting fetal development, and trigger a maternal and fetal response to adapt to these changes.

Angiogenic factors have been subject of intensive research in recent years, as they appear to be involved in the aetiology of PE. Several studies show a decrease in the concentration of PlGF (Polliotti et al., 2003; Levine et al., 2004) and an increase in circulating levels of sVEGFR-1 (McKeeman et al., 2004; Levine et al., 2004) in PEc women. Nevertheless, there is some controversy regarding the concentration of VEGF in pregnant women with PE (Simmons et al., 2000; McKeeman et al., 2004). Since sVEGFR-1 is an antagonist of PlGF and VEGF, there is a reduction of the effects of these factors, i.e., a change in angiogenesis and in endothelial function (Luttun & Carmeliet, 2003). The anti-angiogenic effect in pregnant women with PE seems to disappear after delivery (Maynard et al., 2008; Myatt & Webster, 2009), strengthening the involvement of placental factors in PE. VEGF plays an important role in vascular development, especially at placenta level, but also induces NO and prostaglandins synthesis, which are mediators of vasodilation (Myatt & Webster, 2009).

The processes of vasculogenesis/angiogenesis are crucial for the development of uteroplacental circulation and placenta. In a study performed by our group (Catarino et al., 2009a), we observed a disturbance of the angiogenic/anti-angiogenic factors in the maternal circulation in PE. PEc women had significantly higher levels of sVEGFR-1 (Fig. 2B) and VEGF values and significantly lower PlGF levels (Fig. 2A). This disruption in angiogenesis factors seems to be associated with placental dysfunction, since these factors are mainly produced by the placenta (Kaufmann et al., 2004), during pregnancy.

We also observed a positive correlation between levels of PlGF and maternal placental weight, in PEc pregnancy, which highlights the importance of PlGF in placental development (Catarino et al., 2009a). It is worthy to note that sVEGFR-1, an inhibitor of PlGF and VEGF, was significantly correlated with the amount of proteinuria, a marker of PE severity, suggesting an important role of sVEGFR-1 in the pathogenesis of PE (Catarino et al., 2009a). The abnormal development of the placenta in PE, reduces the placenta perfusion and may also contribute to the observed increase in the amounts of sVEGFR-1 and VEGF, since the tissue hypoxia regulates its production, stimulating it.

In cord blood samples of PEc cases, we observed a significant decrease in PlGF (Fig. 2C) and VEGF concentrations and a significant increase in the levels of sVEGFR-1 (Fig. 2D) (Catarino et al., 2009a). This disruption, particularly at values of PlGF and sVEGFR-1, seems to be an indirect indicator of the involvement of placental dysfunction in PE, since both are produced primarily in the placenta.

The observed correlation between mother and child for sVEGFR-1 seems to indicate that the release of these factors by placenta, occurs both for the maternal and fetal circulation. However, the levels of sVEGFR-1 are higher in the blood of mothers, when compared with cord blood levels, which allows us to suppose that decidua, since it is able to secrete sVEGFR-1 (Lockwood et al., 2007), may also contribute for maternal levels of sVEGFR-1.

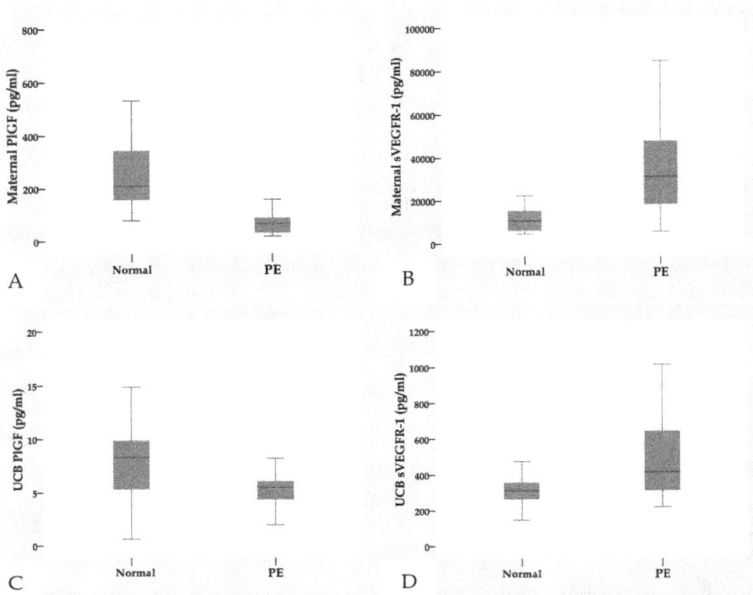

Fig. 2. Concentrations of PlGF in maternal blood (A) and cord blood (C), and sVEGFR-1 levels in maternal blood (B) and cord blood (D) from women with preeclampsia (PE) or with normal pregnancy (N). (Adapted from Catarino et al., 2009a)

3.2 Endothelial dysfunction

Several investigators support the hypothesis that in PE endothelial dysfunction occurs, what contributes to the onset of maternal clinical manifestations. Furthermore, this dysfunction seems to be the link between changes in placental and multisystem complications (Roberts & Gammil, 2005; Young et al., 2010).

In literature, a large number of studies describing changes in endothelial function markers in PE can be found, in particular, an increase of plasma endothelin-1 (Baksu et al., 2005a; Bernardi et al., 2008a), soluble vascular cell adhesion molecule (sVCAM), plasma fibronectin (Aydin et al., 2006; Dane et al., 2009) and tissue fibronectin (Powers et al., 2008), a decrease of plasma and urinary nitric oxide (NO) levels (Baksu et al., 2005a; Mao et al., 2009).

PE is thus associated with a decrease in vasodilatory mediators such as NO and prostacyclin, and an increase in vasoconstrictive mediators such as endothelin-1, angiotensin II and thromboxane A2 (Myatt & Webster, 2009). There are also markers related with hemostasis that are altered in PE and can also be considered as markers of endothelial dysfunction (see Hemostasis section).

In PE, there are several entities that may induce or contribute to injury and/or endothelial dysfunction. These include changes at the level of angiogenic factors/anti-angiogenic, the presence of oxidative stress, exacerbation of the inflammatory process, changes in lipid profile and also a hypoxic environment (Myatt & Webster, 2009).

3.3 Hemostasis

The hemostatic system is altered in PE, which may increase the incidence of maternal and fetal complications. In PEc women, a decrease in the number of platelets compared with normal pregnancy is frequently described (Howarth et al., 1999; Osmanağaoğlu et al., 2005), and thrombocytopenia may occur. Maternal thrombocytopenia is usually associated with more severe pathology, including the HELLP syndrome. Harlow et al. (2002) stated that the decrease in the platelets value is the result of an increase in consumption, as they observed intense platelet activation in patients with PE compared with other pregnancy hypertensive diseases and normal pregnancy. On the other hand, the increase in the mean platelet volume (increased younger platelets, with larger size) (Howarth et al., 1999) and the higher thrombopoietin circulating levels (specific growth factor that promotes thrombocytopoiesis) in women with PE (Johnson et al., 2001), reflect an increase in platelet production. Thus, the reduction of platelet count in PE seems to be due to a higher consumption.

The fibrinolytic system is usually disturbed in PE, due to increased plasminogen activator inhibitor (PAI)-1 and PAI-2. Several studies describe a significant increase in plasma levels of PAI-1 in cases of PE compared to normal pregnancy (Belo et al., 2002a; Tanjung et al., 2005; Sartori et al., 2008; Hunt et al., 2009). The expression of PAI-1 is also elevated in placentas from PEc pregnant women, and PAI-1 plasma levels seem to be positively correlated with the severity of placental damage (Estelles et al., 1998). PAI-2 can be considered a marker of placental function, as it is mainly synthesized at trophoblastic tissue. In PE a decrease in plasma PAI-2 seems to occur (Roes et al., 2002; Tanjung et al., 2005; Sartori et al., 2008), suggesting a modification of placental function. Considering the increased PAI-1 and the decrease of PAI-2, some authors suggest that the rise in the ratio PAI-1/PAI-2 in maternal plasma may be considered a marker of PE (Chappell et al., 2002; Hunt et al., 2009). Several authors report that tissue plasminogen activator (tPA), one of the physiological plasminogen activators, is increased in PE (Belo et al., 2002a; Tanjung et al., 2005; Hunt et al., 2009). Increased levels of D-dimers (fragments of fibrin degradation products) were also reported in PE (Belo et al., 2002a; Hunt et al., 2009), reflecting an increase in the activation process of coagulation and fibrinolysis. The production of D-dimer depends on the formation of thrombin, resulting from activation of the coagulation and fibrinolytic systems. At hemostatic level changes in other parameters, such as a decrease in antithrombin III (Osmanağaoğlu et al., 2005; Tanjung et al., 2005) and an increase in thrombin-antithrombin complex (TAT) in PE (Hunt et al., 2009) were described.

In order to clarify the involvement of hemostatic abnormalities in PE, we assessed fibrinolytic markers, in particular, tPA and PAI antigens and fibrin degradation products (D-dimers). We found that the values of tPA (Fig. 3A) and PAI-1 were significantly higher in PE, without changes in D-dimers (Catarino et al., 2008b). The high levels of tPA and PAI-1 suggest endothelial dysfunction in this syndrome, as both substances are produced by the endothelial cell and exert antagonic roles in the fibrinolytic process. In addition, both PAI-1 and tPA present positive correlations with proteinuria, suggesting that the severity of PE is associated with increased activation/endothelial dysfunction (Catarino et al., 2008b). Furthermore, the maternal endothelial (dys)function, appears to be related to placental (dys)function, considering the positive correlation that we observed between tPA and sVEGFR-1 values in normal and PEc pregnancy (Catarino et al., 2009a).

As already mentioned, different hemostatic modifications are recognized in normal and in PEc pregnancy; however, the exact pattern of these changes in the fetus is still poorly understood. Some authors have reported a decrease in fibrinogen levels, but there were no differences in tPA, PAI-1 and D-dimer (Zanardo et al., 2005), while others reported an increase in PAI-1, however with no differences in tPA values (Roes et al., 2002). Higgins et al. (2000) suggest that infants are somehow protected, at hemostatic system level, since no differences in D-dimers were observed in newborns whose mothers developed PE (Higgins et al., 2000). In a study performed by our group (Catarino et al., 2008b), we also observed similar values of D-dimers. However, and similarly to what we observed in PEc mothers, significantly increased tPA values were found in the newborns of these women (Fig. 3B). Our results suggest that these changes do not arise in response to activation of coagulation, but as a result of endothelial cell dysfunction. Furthermore, we observed a relationship between placental dysfunction and endothelial dysfunction in fetal circulation in PE, suggested by the positive significant correlation that we identified between the levels of tPA and sVEGFR-1 in umbilical cord blood (Catarino et al., 2009a).

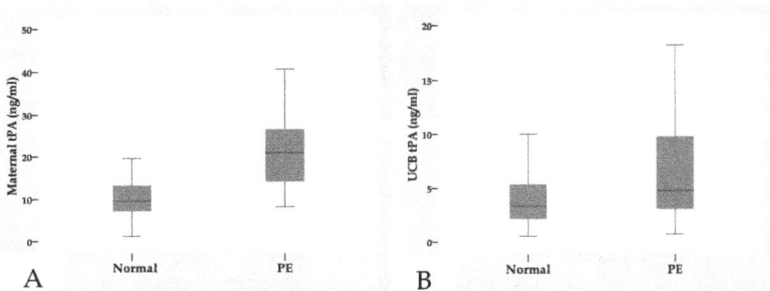

Fig. 3. Maternal (A) and fetal (B) tPA levels in PE and normal pregnancy. (Adapted from Catarino et al., 2008b)

3.4 Oxidative stress

In PE there is evidence of oxidative stress that results from an increased production of oxidizing agents that is not counteracted by antioxidant activity. In fact, an increase in reactive oxygen species, namely in superoxide anion, and a decrease in superoxide dismutase (SOD) activity is observed in trophoblast cells from PEc women (Wang & Walsh, 2001). Different studies demonstrate the development of oxidative stress in PE (Raijmakers et al., 2004; Roberts & Gammil, 2005); either by decreased concentrations of antioxidants, or indirectly by increased lipid peroxidation in maternal circulation, that results from the action of oxygen metabolites, provided by leukocyte activation and/or increased cellular metabolism. The oxidative stress can also take place at the placenta, as a result of the hypoxia/reoxygenation mechanism (intermittent placental perfusion) observed in placentas of pregnant women with PE (Hung & Burton, 2006).

The preterm infants have a lower antioxidant capacity and are therefore more susceptible to oxidative stress triggered at birth, which appears to be associated with complications, including retinopathy and bronchopulmonary dysplasia (Saugstad, 2003). However, there are conflicting results considering oxidative stress in newborns. Some studies describe an increase of lipid peroxidation (MDA), followed by decreased total antioxidant capacity and ascorbic acid levels in newborns whose mothers developed PE (Mehendale et al., 2008; Howlader et al., 2009), while other studies report no difference in lipid peroxidation (Tastekin et al., 2005; Braekke et al., 2006).

Experimental studies (Poston et al., 2006; Rahimi et al., 2009; Xu et al., 2010), performed in pregnant women at risk, showed no beneficial effect on the antioxidant consumption such as vitamins E and C, in preventing the development of PE, despite the evidence for the involvement of a state of oxidative stress in PE. In fact, according to these trials, antioxidant therapy does not appear to be sufficient to prevent the development of the PE, further increasing the risk of neonatal complications, including increased rate of newborns with low birth weight (Poston et al., 2006; Rahimi et al., 2009).

3.5 Inflammation

There are various mechanisms by which oxidative stress is linked to the inflammatory process. During the inflammatory response production and release of reactive oxygen metabolites occurs leading to oxidative stress. On the other hand, products of oxidative stress, such as those resulting from lipid peroxidation, are considered pro-inflammatory.

PE may be considered as an exacerbated inflammatory condition compared with physiological pregnancy, which appears to contribute to endothelial dysfunction. Initially, there is a localized inflammatory response within the placenta, while in a second phase predominates a systemic inflammatory response. Numerous studies have reported an increase of pro-inflammatory cytokines such as IL-6 and TNF-α (Bernardi et al., 2008b; Guven et al., 2009; Ouyang et al., 2009) in pregnant women with PE, when compared with normotensive pregnant women.

Concerning acute phase proteins, C-reactive protein (CRP) is probably the most studied one, mainly due to its sensibility in detecting inflammation, with a significant increase being observed in PEc pregnancy (Belo et al., 2003; Tjoa et al., 2003; Guven et al., 2009). Tjoa et al. reported an increase in plasma concentration of CRP between 10 and 14 weeks of gestation in pregnant women who subsequently developed PE and gave birth to newborns with growth restriction (Tjoa et al., 2003).

Cell adhesion molecules (CAM), necessary for the adhesion of leukocytes to vascular endothelium, are also altered in PE. Despite some contradictory results, plasma levels of (sICAM)-1, soluble vascular cell adhesion molecule (sVCAM)-1, soluble platelet endothelial cell adhesion molecule (sPECAM)-1 and soluble E-selectin are raised in PEc pregnant women (Kim et al., 2004; Chavarrva et al., 2008).

The neutrophil activation also seems to be associated with PE, as some studies mentioned an increase in circulating levels of myeloperoxidase (Mellembakken et al., 2001; Gandley et al., 2008) and elastase (Belo et al., 2003; Gupta et al., 2006), both released during the degranulation of neutrophils in the inflammatory process.

The increase in inflammatory markers in the maternal circulation could result from the release of substances from the placenta (local inflammation), then triggering a systemically inflammatory response. Some authors have suggested that tissue hypoxia resulting from reduced placental perfusion, determines an unregulated production of different cytokines, including TNF-α, which is reflected in an increase in the maternal circulation (Rusterholz et al., 2007; Redman & Sargent, 2009).

There is little information for the assessment of inflammatory markers in newborns. Braekke et al. (2005) found no evidence of inflammation in cord blood of newborns from pregnant women with PE, because no differences in CRP or in calprotectin where detected. For studies addressing CAM, the existing information is somewhat contradictory, as is the case for oxidative stress. Some authors have reported an increased expression of L-selectin and integrins on the surface of neutrophils (Mellembakken et al., 2001; Saini et al., 2004) in the fetal circulation in PEc pregnancy, demonstrating an activation of neutrophils. It was also described a decrease in sL-selectin and sE-selectin in the fetal circulation of PEc pregnancy. However, other researchers found no differences between the fetal circulation to a normal pregnancy and PE on levels of sICAM, sVCAM and sE-selectin (Kraus et al., 1998).

The marked inflammatory response in maternal circulation, in the case of PE, seems to be also accompanied by increased inflammatory markers at umbilical cord blood level. Both CRP and α1-antitrypsin are elevated in cord blood, suggesting the presence of an inflammatory response, although less intense than in the maternal circulation (unpublished data).

3.6 Lipid profile

The physiological hyperlipidemia observed in healthy pregnant women is further exacerbated in PE. PE is characterized by intense changes of lipid profile (Ray et al., 2006) similar to what happens in atherosclerosis. Several studies indicate a significant increase in serum triglycerides (TG) in PEc pregnancy, compared with normal pregnancy (Belo et al., 2002b; Baksu et al., 2005b; Bayhan et al., 2005). This is probably the most consistent finding in lipid profile. In a study performed by our group the most pronounced lipid modification that we found was for TG levels (Fig. 4A), which doubled its value in PE in relation to normal pregnancy (Catarino et al., 2008a). Furthermore, TG levels correlated positively and significantly with proteinuria, a known marker of PE severity (Catarino et al., 2008a). In agreement with this, free fatty acids also appear to be higher in PE (Villa et al., 2009).

It is also referred an increase in LDLc (Bayhan et al., 2005) and total cholesterol (Bayhan et al., 2005) and a decrease in hight HDLc (Belo et al., 2002b; Baksu et al., 2005b; Bayhan et al., 2005) in PE compared with normal pregnancy. However, these parameters are not always altered in PE (Baksu et al., 2005b; Manten et al., 2005) and, when they do, the extent of modification is not so pronounced as with TG.

Another biochemical parameter also subject to some controversy is the lipoprotein (a) [Lp(a)]; some studies reported no significant differences in Lp(a) levels in PEc pregnancy (Belo et al., 2002c; Baksu et al., 2005b), while others described an elevation of Lp(a) in PE (Bar et al., 2002; Bayhan et al., 2005). Moreover, Mori et al. described a positive correlation between maternal Lp(a) levels and the severity of PE (Mori et al., 2003).

In PE there is a change in the lipoprotein subclasses profile, particularly a predominance of small and dense LDL (Sattar et al., 1997). The increase of small, dense LDL fraction is especially important, since this is considered the most atherogenic and also more susceptible to oxidation (Wakatsuki et al., 2000), resulting in the formation of oxidized LDL. The oxidized LDL appears to play a crucial role in endothelial (dys)function observed in PE and some authors report that PE is associated with an increase in oxidized LDL levels (Uzun et al., 2005; Kim et al., 2007). However, other articles referred that there are no significant differences in relation to normal pregnancy (Belo et al., 2005; Qiu et al., 2006). Since oxidized LDL is immunogenic, the formation of autoantibodies to oxidized LDL occurs in circulation; some authors also confirm the increase of autoantibodies to oxidized LDL in the circulation of PEc pregnant women (Uotila et al., 1998). In contrast, other study report no changes (Jain et al., 2004). Additionally, it was proposed that pregnant women who present an increase in oxidized LDL plasma levels are associated with increased risk of developing PE (Qiu et al., 2006). Most changes found in lipid profile, including increased plasma TG and VLDL (TG-rich), decreased HDLc and an increase in small, dense LDL subfraction represent a risk profile similar to that predisposing to atherosclerosis and cardiovascular disease (Crowther, 2005). Some authors also propose that changes in lipid metabolism may contribute to the endothelial dysfunction, a key step in the atherosclerotic process (Bayhan et al., 2005; Ray et al., 2006).

Hypertriglyceridemia may contribute to endothelial dysfunction, but may also reflect placental dysfunction, since, unlike free fatty acids and cholesterol, TG does not cross the placenta and have no receptors in the placenta (unlike what happens with lipoproteins). For this, it is necessary that the lipoprotein lipase, which is abundant in the placenta, ensures the TG hydrolysis to be transferred in the form of free fatty acids to the fetus. It is possible that this hydrolysis is impaired in PE, causing a TG accumulation in maternal blood and a reduction in the nutrients uptake by the fetus. On the other hand, the significant increase of TG in maternal blood can be regarded as a physiological mechanism to increase the nutrients supply to the fetus, take into consideration the greater difficulty of nutrients transfer through the placenta.

Considering that in PE also occurs a change in placental perfusion, fetal lipid profile may also be affected due to disturbances in placental transfer of lipids. Rodie et al. (2004) reported an increase in TG levels, total cholesterol and total cholesterol/HDLc ratio in newborns of pregnant women who developed PE, although no correlation between the lipid and lipoprotein levels between mothers and newborns was observed. In turn, Ophir et al. (2006) found no differences in TG or total cholesterol, only observed an increase of LDLc in umbilical cord blood from PEc pregnancy. In our previous study, newborns of mothers with PE showed decreased levels of lipids and lipoproteins (exception for HDLc), but a significant increase in TG (Fig. 4B) (Catarino et al., 2008a).

As already noted, the increase of TG in maternal blood can result from a physiological mechanism of compensation. The high levels of TG in newborns of mothers with PE may, therefore, be a reflection of increased values in the maternal circulation.

Some authors argue that to compensate the difficulty of transferring these nutrients will notice an increased expression of a particular type of receptor, for example to LDL. Other authors propose that there is an increased blood flow to overcome the difficulty in transferring nutrients and/or gas and that this adaptation is that justifies the increase in maternal blood pressure characteristic of PE.

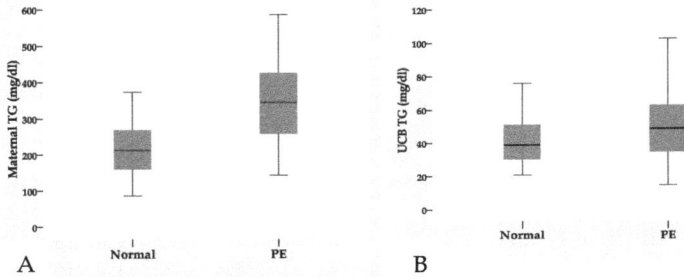

Fig. 4. Maternal (A) and UCB (B) TG levels in PE and normal pregnancy (N). (Adapted from Catarino et al., 2008a)

The impact of the changes in lipid profile in the future of newborns from PEc mothers is uncertain. However, the increase in TG, the ratio LDLc/HDLc and Apo B/Apo AI, suggest that these infants present an increment in their cardiovascular risk.

3.7 Hematologic system

When compared with normal pregnancy PE presents an exacerbation of inflammatory and oxidative stress markers. The release of mediators resulting from inflammatory cell activation can trigger changes in surrounding cells. These cell activation products may contribute to erythrocyte damage, accelerating their aging process and its premature removal. This hypothesis can be tested by evaluating markers of erythrocyte production, damage/aging and removal.

3.7.1 Plasma volume/erythrocyte number

Throughout pregnancy, plasma volume increases gradually, reaching its maximum at about 30 weeks of gestation. This increase would correspond to about 50% of the average plasma volume in non-pregnant woman (Gordon, 2002) and is essential to face the decrease in vascular resistance within the feto-placental unit, protecting the mother and the fetus from hypotension. It is also important in case of bleeding during the delivery (Gordon, 2002). The erythrocyte number increases progressively until the end of pregnancy. This increase may reach 18% in pregnant women without iron supplementation or 30% when diet is accompanied by iron supplements (Gordon, 2002).

Since plasma volume increases at an earlier stage of pregnancy and more rapidly than the increase in the erythrocyte number, the hematocrit decreases until the end of the second trimester. This hemodilution leads to anemia, commonly known as "physiologic anaemia of pregnancy". Therefore, only when pregnant women present a hematocrit below 0.33 l/l and hemoglobin below 11g/dL, there is a true anemia. From the third trimester, when the increase in plasma volume is accompanied by an equivalent increase in erythrocyte number, the hematocrit stabilizes or increases slightly until the end of pregnancy. During pregnancy, in response to the increased "turnover" of hemoglobin, due to the increased demand of oxygen consumption, there is an increased synthesis of erythropoietin (Gordon, 2002) - a specific erythropoiesis growth factor. Erythropoietin acts at bone marrow, stimulating the erythrocyte differentiation, proliferation and the early release of reticulocytes in peripheral blood. The decreased affinity for oxygen of maternal hemoglobin, caused by increased 2,3-diphosphoglycerate within erythrocytes, represents a compensation mechanism for the increased oxygen consumption needed for oxygen transfer to fetus. This transfer is also favoured by the higher oxygen affinity of fetal hemoglobin, which is the predominant form of fetal hemoglobin.

To respond to the erythropoietic stimulation, there is a mobilization of maternal iron stores and an increase in intestinal iron absorption (Gordon, 2002). To overcome this increase in iron demands during pregnancy, iron supplements are usually given to maintain maternal iron stores, usually after 20 weeks of gestation (Cunningham et al., 2005). During normal pregnancy there is an increase of younger erythrocytes, as shown by an increased number of circulating reticulocytes and, consequently, an increase in "red cell distribution width" (RDW) (Shebat et al., 1998). Tissue hypoxia that occurs physiologically during pregnancy appears to stimulate erythropoietin production, resulting in reticulocyte release from bone marrow into the bloodstream (Lurie & Mamet, 2000).

3.7.2 Erythrocyte membrane protein band 3

The human erythrocyte has a lifespan of about 120 days, being removed from the circulation, mainly, by the spleen. Mature erythrocyte has no nuclei and organelles, and presents a very limited biosynthetic capacity, accumulating physical and/or chemical changes throughout its life span. Several modifications occur with cell aging, namely, reduction in cell volume, enzyme activity, antioxidant capacity and deformability.

The erythrocyte membrane protein band 3 is a transmembrane protein, also known as an anion channel, as it mediates the exchange of HCO_3^- and Cl^- ions, which is important for the transport of CO_2 from the tissues to the lungs. Band 3 links the cytoskeleton to the membrane lipid bilayer, participating in the maintenance of cell morphology. Band 3 is also involved in the removal of senescent/damaged erythrocytes (Wang, 1994).

The development of oxidative stress may occur when exogenous oxygen metabolites diffuse through the membrane or when oxygen metabolites result from autoxidation of hemoglobin, and the red blood cell (RBC) is unable to detoxify the cell, due to depletion in antioxidant defenses. Accumulation of oxygen metabolites can cause hemoglobin oxidation that has a high affinity for the cytoplasmic domain of band 3 (Fig. 5) (Low et al., 1985). This linkage causes band 3 oligomerization and/or aggregation (Waugh et al., 1987), which is recognized by natural autoantibodies anti-band 3 IgG (Fig. 5). The autoantibodies anti-band 3 have a higher affinity for Band 3 oligomers than for band 3 monomers (Lutz, 1992). The band 3 aggregates will act as a neoantigen on the erythrocyte membrane surface, marking the aged or injured erythrocyte for removal by macrophages of the reticulo-endothlial system. Thus, an increase in membrane-bound hemoglobin (MBH) (Santos-Silva et al., 1998) and in band 3 aggregation are good markers of erythrocyte senescence and/or damage.

Changes in band 3 profile (% of band 3 monomers, aggregates and proteolytic fragments), besides that associated to erythrocyte aging, were also reports in different inflammatory models, namely, in myocardial infarction (Santos-Silva et al., 1995), ischemic stroke (Santos-Silva et al., 2002) and in high competition physical exercise (Santos-Silva et al., 2001). In vitro studies showed that neutrophil activation and elastase, a leukocyte activation product, trigger changes in band 3 profile that are similar to those found in inflammatory conditions and senescent erythrocyte (Santos-Silva et al., 1998). Senescent and/or damaged erythrocyte show an increase in band 3 aggregates and a decrease in band 3 monomers and fragments.

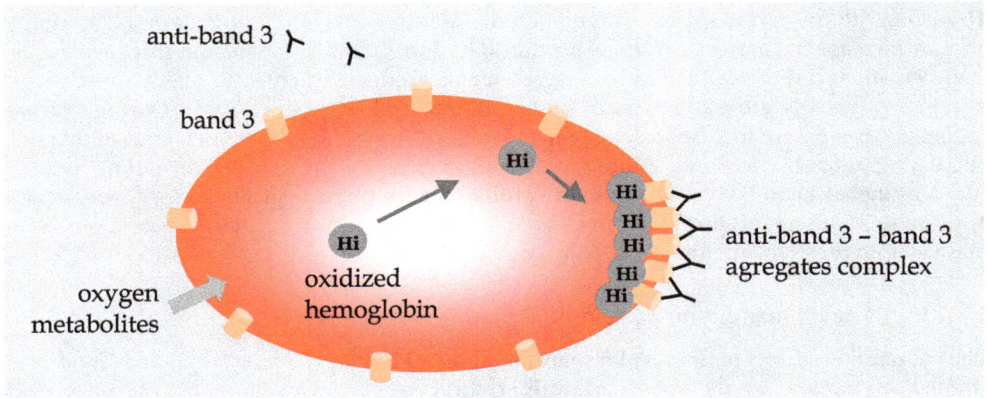

Fig. 5. Illustration of erythrocyte removal mechanism, mediated by band 3 aggregation.

Belo et al. (2002d) reported changes in band 3 profile, in pregnancy and in puerperium. In the first trimester, pregnant women, when compared with non-pregnant women, showed decreased aggregates of band 3 and increased total fragments. During pregnancy, an increase of total fragments was also observed, suggesting a rise in younger erythrocytes (Belo et al., 2002d).

The exacerbated inflammatory process of pregnancy (which can limit the absorption and mobilization of iron for erythropoiesis), the development of oxidative stress (triggering cumulative oxidative damages in erythrocytes) and the changes in placental perfusion (reduction of feto-maternal oxygen transfer and placental hypoxia), all observed in PE, seems to cause oxidative modifications in erythrocytes and disturbances in the erythropoietic process. In a study by our group, PEc mothers showed an increase in erythrocyte number, reticulocyte number and reticulocyte production index (RPI), reflecting an erythropoietic stimulus, which may be triggered by an accelerated removal of aged/damaged erythrocytes (Catarino et al., 2009b). In fact, in PEc women, an increase in MBH and changes in band 3 profile (with an increase in band 3 aggregates) were observed (Fig. 6) (Catarino et al., 2009b). The increase in bilirubin levels, suggests that these lesions led to the early removal of damaged erythrocytes. In fact, high MBH levels are consistent with increased oxidative stress and inflammation associated with PE. The band 3 profile, observed in PE, seems to reflect the existence of a heterogeneous erythrocyte population, ie, a senescent erythrocyte subpopulation (more band 3 aggregates) and a younger erythrocyte subpopulation (reticulocyte, less band 3 aggregates). This reflects a stimulation of the erythropoietic response that seems to mask the erythrocyte injury.

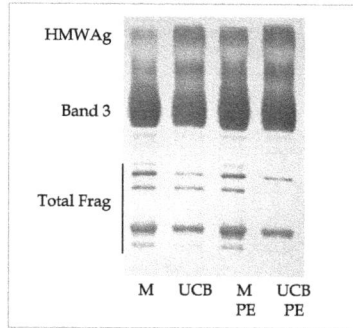

Fig. 6. Erythrocyte band 3 profile in maternal (M) blood and umbilical cord blood (UCB), in normal pregnancy and preeclampsia (PE) (Adapted from Catarino et al., 2009b)

As was observed in PEc mothers, their newborns had significantly higher MBH and evidences of an erythropoietic stimulation, with an increase in erythrocytes, in nucleated red blood cell (NRBC), reticulocyte count and RPI (Catarino et al., 2009b). This erythropoietic stimulation can occur in response to tissue hypoxia, due to the reduced placental perfusion, with lower oxygen transfer to fetal erythrocytes. Erythropoietic stimulation may also be triggered by tissue hypoxia resulting from increased erythrocyte removal, due to increased RBC injury and/or aging. There were no significant differences in the band 3 profile (Fig. 6) (Catarino et al., 2009b). As already mentioned, the increase of NRBC and reticulocytes, a younger erythroid population, prominent in the fetal circulation, may mask the injury observed in the mature erythrocyte population. The increase in MBH in PEc cases, shows an increase of oxidative stress in erythrocytes, as a result in raised hemoglobin oxidation with subsequent membrane binding.

4. Concluding remarks

PE is a hypertensive disorder of pregnancy that affects several organs and systems. Although important quantitative information exists regarding maternal blood modifications in PE, few studies have addressed the influence of this syndrome in newborns from PEc mothers. Moreover, many of the results available in the literature are controversial. The main changes that our group observed in biochemical and hematological umbilical cord blood of newborns from PEc pregnancy when compared with the newborn from normal pregnancy are described in table 3.

The placental dysfunction associated with hypoxia/reoxygenation of the placenta in PE, in the maternal circulation appears to trigger endothelial dysfunction (Fig. 7). To this dysfunction may contribute the hypertriglyceridemia, oxidative stress and the exacerbation of the inflammatory condition. Placental dysfunction, associated with the changes observed in maternal blood, seem to limit the transfer of oxygen and nutrients and, eventually, an abnormal release of products synthesized by the placenta to the fetal circulation; these changes seem to trigger a fetal response in order to adapt to this condition, with the development of endothelial dysfunction, dyslipidemia, and inflammatory response, similar to what occurs in the mother, although less intense. The reduction of oxygen transfer to the fetus associated with oxidative stress, determines oxidative damage in erythrocytes and an erythropoietic stimulation (Fig. 7).

Placental dysfunction	↓↓↓PlGF	↑↑sVEGFR-1	↓VEGF	
Endothelial dysfunction	↑tPA	↓↓PAI-1/tPA		
Lipid profile	↑TG	↓↓↓HDLc	↓↓Apo A-I	↑↑↑LDLc/HDLc
Inflammation	↑α1- antitrypsin	↑CRP		
Leukocyte activation	↑sVCAM	↓↓sL-Selectin		
Oxidative stress	↑↑↑Uric acid			
Erythrocyte	↑↑↑MCV	↑↑↑MCH	↑NRBC	
(damage/remove/production)	↑Reticulocytes	↑RPI	↑↑↑MBH	

PlGF, placental growth factor; sVEGFR-1, soluble vascular endothelial growth factor receptor type 1; VEGF, vascular endothelial growth factor; tPA, tissue plasminogen activator; PAI-1, plasminogen activator inhibitor; TG, triglycerides; HDLc, HDL cholesterol; LDLc, LDL cholesterol; Apo, apolipoprotein; CRP, c-reactive protein; sVCAM, soluble vascular cell adhesion molecule; MCV, mean cell volume; MCH, mean cell hemoglobin; NRBC, nucleated red blood cell; RPI, reticulocyte production index; MBH, membrane-bound hemoglobin ↑↑↑ - P<0.001; ↑↑ - P<0.01; ↑ - P<0.05

Table 3. Main changes observed in biochemical and hematological umbilical cord blood of newborns from PEc pregnancy when compared with the newborn in normal pregnancy.

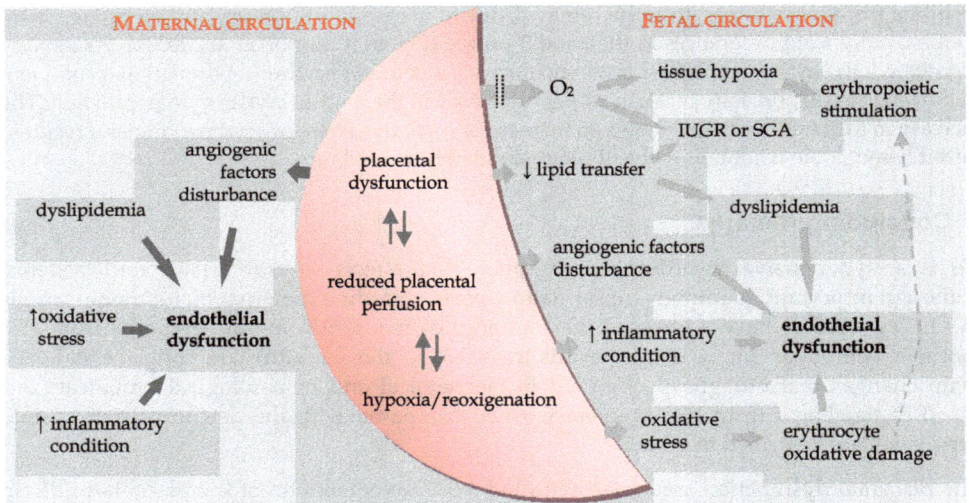

Fig. 7. Schematic of some modifications observed in maternal and cord blood. IUGR, intrauterine growth restriction; SGA, small for gestational age.

In summary, most of the changes observed in the maternal circulation in PE women are also present in the cord blood of their newborns, although these changes are less pronounced.

PE shares several similarities with atherosclerosis, such as modifications in the lipid profile, amplification of the inflammatory process and increased oxidative stress. These changes may contribute to disturbe cell activation with subsequent endothelial dysfunction. Some studies have suggested that pregnant women who developed PE have a predisposition to develop, at long term, cardiovascular diseases. Changes in the inflammatory response and endothelial dysfunction observed in umbilical cord blood of newborns from mothers with PE, may also have an increased risk to develop cardiovascular diseases in the future.

It would be especially interesting to study these and other parameters associated with cardiovascular risk in children born from mothers who developed PE during pregnancy at different stages of its growth and also to study in women with a history of PE.

5. Acknowledgements

The authors are grateful to the nursery group of Obstetrics Service of Hospital S. João, in particular to nurse Célia Ribeiro for her generous help in the maternal and cord blood collection. This work was supported by FCT and FSE for PhD grant (SFRH/BD/7056/2001).

6. References

Aydin T., Varol F. & Sayin N. (2006). Third trimester maternal plasma total fibronectin levels in pregnancy-induced hypertension: results of a tertiary center. *Clin Appl Thromb Hemost*, Vol. 12, No. 1, pp. 33-9, ISSN 1076-0296

Baksu B., Davas I., Baksu A., Akyol A. & Gulbaba G. (2005a). Plasma nitric oxide, endothelin-1 and urinary nitric oxide and cyclic guanosine monophosphate levels in hypertensive pregnant women. *Int J Gynaecol Obstet*, Vol. 90, No. 2, pp. 112-7, ISSN 0020-7292

Baksu B., Baksu A., Davas I., Akyol A. & Gulbaba G. (2005b) Lipoprotein(a) levels in women with pre-eclampsia and in normotensive pregnant women. *J Obstet Gynaecol Res*, Vol. 31, No. 3, pp. 277-282, ISSN 1341-8076

Bar J., Harell D., Bardin R., Pardo J., Chen R., Hod M. & Sullivan M. (2002). The elevated plasma lipoprotein(a) concentrations in preeclampsia do not precede the development of the disorder. *Thrombosis Research*, Vol. 105, pp. 19–23, ISSN 0049-3848

Barker D. (2004). The Developmental Origins of Adult Disease. *J Am Coll Nutr*, Vol. 23, No. 6, 588S–595S, ISSN 0731-5724

Barker D. & Bagby S. (2005). Developmental antecedents of cardiovascular disease: a historical perspective. *J Am Soc Nephrol*, Vol. 16, No. 9, pp. 2537-44, ISSN 1046-6673

Barker D., Osmond C., Kajantie E. & Eriksson J. (2009). Growth and chronic disease: findings in the Helsinki Birth Cohort. *Ann Hum Biol*, Vol. 36, No. 5, pp. 445-58, ISSN 0301-4460

Bayhan G., Konyigit Y., Atamer A., Atamer Y. & Akkus Z. (2005). Potential atherogenic roles of lipids, lipoprotein(a) and lipid peroxidation in preeclampsia. *Gynecol Endocrinol*, Vol. 21, No. 1, pp. 1-6, ISSN 0951-3590

Belo L., Caslake M., Gaffney D., Santos-Silva A., Pereira Leite L., Quintanilha A. & Rebelo I. (2002a). Changes in LDL size and HDL concentration in normal and preeclamptic pregnancies. *Atherosclerosis*, Vol. 162, pp. 425-432, ISSN 0021-9150

Belo, L.; Rebelo, I.; Castro, E.; Catarino, C.; Pereira-Leite, L.; Quintanilha, A. & Santos-Silva A. (2002b). Band 3 as a marker of erythrocyte changes in pregnancy. *Eur J Haematol*, Vol. 69, No. 3, pp. 145-51, ISSN 0902-4441

Belo L., Santos-Silva A., Rumley A., Lowe G., Pereira Leite L., Quintanilha A. & Rebelo I. (2002c). Elevated tissue plasminogen activator as a potential marker of endothelial dysfunction in pre-eclampsia: correlation with proteinuria. *BJOG*, Vol. 109, pp. 1250-1255, ISSN 0028-4793

Belo L., Caslake M., Santos-Silva A., Pereira Leite L., Quintanilha A. & Rebelo I. (2002d) Lipoprotein(a): a longitudinal versus a cross-sectional study in normal pregnancy and its levels in preeclampsia. *Atherosclerosis*, Vol. 165, pp. 393-395, ISSN 0021-9150

Belo L., Santos-Silva A., Caslake M., Cooney J., Pereira Leite L., Quintanilha A. & Rebelo I. (2003). Neutrophil activation and c-reactive protein concentration in preeclampsia. *Hypertens Pregnancy*, Vol. 22, No. 2, pp. 129-141, ISSN 1064-1955

Belo L., Santos-Silva A., Caslake M., Pereira Leite L., Quintanilha A. & Rebelo I. (2005) Oxidized-LDL levels in normal and pre-eclamptic pregnancies: Contribution of LDL particle size. *Atherosclerosis*, Vol. 183, pp. 185-186, ISSN 0021-9150

Bernardi F., Constantino L., Machado R., Petronilho F. & Dal-Pizzol F. (2008a). Plasma nitric oxide, endothelin-1, arginase and superoxide dismutase in pre-eclamptic women. *J Obstet Gynaecol Res*, Vol. 34, No. 6, pp. 957-63, ISSN 1341-8076

Bernardi F., Guolo F., Bortolin T., Petronilho F. & Dal-Pizzol F. (2008b). Oxidative stress and inflammatory markers in normal pregnancy and preeclampsia. *J Obstet Gynaecol Res*, Vol. 34, No. 6, pp. 948-51, ISSN 1341-8076

Boukerrou M., Bresson S., Collinet P., Delelis A., Deruelle P., Houfflin-Debarge V., Dufour P, Subtil D. (2009). Factors associated with uterine artery Doppler anomalies in patients with preeclampsia. *Hypertens Pregnancy*, Vol. 28, No. 2, pp. 178-89, ISSN 1064-1955

Bowen R., Gu Y., Zhang Y., Lewis D. & Wang Y. (2005). Hypoxia promotes interleukin-6 and -8 but reduces interleukin-10 production by placental trophoblast cells from preeclamptic pregnancies. *J Soc Gynecol Investig*, Vol. 12, No. 6, pp. 428-32, ISSN 1071-5576

Braekke K., Holthe M., Harsem N., Fagerhol M. & Staff A. (2005). Calprotectin, a marker of inflammation, is elevated in the maternal but not in the fetal circulation in preeclampsia. *Am J Obstet Gynecol*, Vol. 193, pp. 227-33, ISSN 0002-9378

Braekke K., Harsem N. & Staff A. (2006). Oxidative stress and antioxidant status in fetal circulation in preeclampsia. *Pediatr Res*, Vol. 60, No. 5, pp. 560-4, ISSN 0031-3998

Brosens I., Robertson W. & Dixon H. (1972). The role of the spiral arteries in the pathogenesis of preeclampsia. *Obstet Gynecol Annu*, Vol. 1, pp. 177-91, ISSN 0091-3332

Brown M., Lindheimer M., Swiet M., Assche A. & Moutquin J. (2001) The classification and diagnosis of the hypertensive disorders of pregnancy: statement from the international society for the study of hypertension in pregnancy (ISSHP). *Hypertens Pregnancy*, Vol. 20, No. 1, pp. ix-xiv, ISSN 1064-1955

Burton G., Woods A., Jauniaux E. & Kingdom J. (2009). Rheological and physiological consequences of conversion of the maternal spiral arteries for uteroplacental blood flow during human pregnancy. *Placenta*, Vol. 30, No. 6, pp. 473-82, ISSN 0143-4004

Catarino, C.; Rebelo, I.; Belo, L.; Rocha-Pereira, P.; Rocha, S.; Castro, E.; Patrício, B.; Quintanilha, A. & Santos-Silva, A. (2008a). Fetal lipoprotein changes in pre-eclampsia. *Acta Obstet Gynecol Scand*, Vol. 87, No. 6, pp. 628-34, ISSN 0001-6349

Catarino, C.; Rebelo, I.; Belo, L.; Rocha, S.; Castro, E.; Patricio, B.; Quintanilha, A. & Santos-Silva, A. (2008b). Relationship between maternal and cord blood hemostatic disturbances in preeclamptic pregnancies. *Thromb Res*, Vol. 123, No. 2, pp. 219-24, ISSN 0049-3848

Catarino, C.; Rebelo, I.; Belo, L.; Rocha, S.; Castro, E.; Patrício, B.; Quintanilha, A. & Santos-Silva, A. (2009a). Fetal and maternal angiogenic/anti-angiogenic factors in normal and preeclamptic pregnancy. *Growth Factors*, Vol. 27, No. 6, pp. 345-51, ISSN 0897-7194

Catarino, C.; Rebelo, I.; Belo, L.; Rocha-Pereira, P.; Rocha, S.; Castro, E., Patrício, B.; Quintanilha, A. & Santos-Silva, A. (2009b). Erythrocyte changes in preeclampsia: relationship between maternal and cord blood erythrocyte damage. *J Perinat Med*, Vol. 37, No. 1, pp. 19-27, ISSN 0300-5577

Chaddha V., Viero S., Huppertz B. & Kingdom J. (2004). Developmental biology of the placenta and the origins of placental insufficiency. *Semin Fetal Neonatal Med*, Vol. 9, pp. 357-69, ISSN 1744-165X

Chappell L., Seed P., Briley A., Kelly F., Hunt B., Charnock–Jones S., Mallet A. & Poston L. (2002). A longitudinal study of biochemical variables in women at risk of preeclampsia. *Am J Obstet Gynecol*, Vol. 187, pp. 127-36, ISSN 0002-9378

Chavarría M., Lara-González L., García-Paleta Y., Vital-Reyes V. & Reyes A. (2008). Adhesion molecules changes at 20 gestation weeks in pregnancies complicated by preeclampsia. *Eur J Obstet Gynecol Reprod Biol*, Vol. 137, No. 2, pp. 157-64, ISSN 0301-2115

Covelli M., Wood C. & Yarandi H. (2007). The Association of Low Birth Weight and Physiological Risk Factors of Hypertension in African American Adolescents. *J Cardiovasc Nursing*, Vol. 22, No. 6, pp. 440-447, ISSN 0889-4655

Crowther M. (2005). Pathogenesis of atherosclerosis. *Hematology Am Soc Hematol Educ Program*, pp. 436-41, ISSN 1520-4391

Cunningham F., Hauth J., Leveno K., Gilstrap L., Bloom S. & Wenstrom K (Eds.). (2005). Williams Obstetrics, twenty-second edition, McGraw-Hill, New-York.

Dane C., Buyukasik H., Dane B. & Yayla M. (2009). Maternal plasma fibronectin and advanced oxidative protein products for the prediction of preeclampsia in high risk pregnancies: a prospective cohort study. *Fetal Diagn Ther*, Vol. 26, No. 4, pp. 189-94, ISSN 1015-3837

Duckitt K. & Harrington D. (2005). Risk factors for pre-eclampsia at antenatal booking: systematic review of controlled studies. *BMJ*, Vol. 12, No. 330, pp. 7491, ISSN 0959-8138

Duley L. (2009). The Global Impact of Pre-eclampsia and Eclampsia. *Semin Perinatol*, Vol. 33, pp. 130-137, ISSN 0146-0005

Eriksson J., Forsén T., Kajantie E., Osmond C. & Barker D. (2007). Childhood growth and hypertension in later life. *Hypertension*, Vol. 49, No. 6, pp. 1415-21, ISSN 0194-911X

Estelles A., Gilabert J., Grancha S., Yamamoto K., Thinnes T., Espana F., Aznar J., Loskutoff D. (1998). Abnormal expression of type 1 plasminogen activator inhibitor and tissue factor in severe preeclampsia. *Thromb Haemost*, Vol. 79, pp. 500-8, ISSN 0340-6245

Gandley R., Rohland J., Zhou Y., Shibata E., Harger G., Rajakumar A., *et al.* (2008). Increased myeloperoxidase in the placenta and circulation of women with preeclampsia. *Hypertension*, Vol. 52, No. 2, pp. 387-93, ISSN 0194-911X

Ghidini A., Salafia C. & Pezzullo J. (1997). Placental vascular lesions and likelihood of diagnosis of preeclampsia. *Obstet Gynecol*, Vol. 90, pp. 542-5, ISSN 0029-7844

Goldenberg R., Culhane J., Iams J. & Romero R. (2008). Epidemiology and causes of preterm birth. *Lancet*, Vol. 371, pp. 75-84, ISSN 0140-6736

Gordon M. Maternal physiology in pregnancy, pp 63-91. *In* Gabbe S, Niebyl J, Simpson J [eds.]. Obstetrics: Normal and Problem Pregnancies. 2002, 4th edition, Churchill Livingstone, Philadelphia

Groom K., North R., Poppe K., Sadler L. & McCowan L. (2007). The association between customised small for gestational age infants and preeclampsia or gestational hypertension varies with gestation at delivery. *BJOG*, Vol. 114, pp. 478–484, ISSN 1470-0328

Gu Y., Lewis D. & Wang Y. (2008). Placental productions and expressions of soluble endoglin, soluble fms-like tyrosine kinase receptor-1, and placental growth factor in normal and preeclamptic pregnancies. *J Clin Endocrinol Metab*, Vol. 93, No. 1, pp. 260-6, ISSN 0021-972X

Gupta A., Gebhardt S., Hillermann R., Holzgreve W. & Hahn S. (2006). Analysis of plasma elastase levels in early and late onset preeclampsia. *Arch Gynecol Obstet*, Vol. 273, pp. 239–242, ISSN 0932-0067

Guven M., Coskun A., Ertas I., Aral M., Zencirci B. & Oksuz H. (2009). Association of maternal serum CRP, IL-6, TNF-alpha, homocysteine, folic acid and vitamin B12 levels with the severity of preeclampsia and fetal birth weight. *Hypertens Pregnancy*, Vol. 28, No. 2, pp. 190-200, ISSN 1064-1955

Harlow F., Brown M., Brighton T., Smith S., Trickett A., Kwan Y. & Davis G. (2002). Platelet activation in the hypertensive disorders of pregnancy. *Am J Obstet Gynecol*, Vol. 187, pp. 688-95, ISSN 0002-9378

Higgins J., Bonnar J., Norris L., Darling M. & Walshe J. (2000). The effect of pre-eclampsia on coagulation and fibrinolytic activation in the neonate. *Thromb Res*, Vol. 99, No. 6, pp. 567-70, ISSN 0049-3848

Howarth S., Marshall L., Barr A., Evans S., Pontre M. & Ryan N. (1999). Platelet indices during normal pregnancy and pre-eclampsia. *Br J Biomed Sci*, Vol. 56, No.1, pp. 20-2, ISSN 0967-4845

Howlader M., Parveen S., Tamanna S., Khan T. & Begum F. (2009). Oxidative stress and antioxidant status in neonates born to pre-eclamptic mother. *J Trop Pediatr*, Vol. 55, No. 6, pp. 363-7, ISSN 0142-6338

Hung T., Charnock-Jones D., Skepper J. & Burton G. (2004). Secretion of tumor necrosis factor-alpha from human placental tissues induced by hypoxia-reoxygenation causes endothelial cell activation in vitro: a potential mediator of the inflammatory response in preeclampsia. *Am J Pathol*, Vol. 164, No. 3, pp. 1049-61, ISSN 0002-9440

Hung T. & Burton G. (2006). Hypoxia and reoxygenation: a possible mechanism for placental oxidative stress in preeclampsia. *Taiwan J Obstet Gynecol*, Vol. 45, No. 3, pp. 189-200, ISSN 1028-4559

Hunt B., Missfelder-Lobos H., Parra-Cordero M., Fletcher O., Parmar K., Lefkou E. & Lees C. (2009). Pregnancy outcome and fibrinolytic, endothelial and coagulation markers in women undergoing uterine artery Doppler screening at 23 weeks. *J Thromb Haemost*, Vol. 7, pp. 955–61, ISSN 1538-7933

Jain M., Sawhney H., Aggarwal N., Vashistha K. & Majumdhar S. (2004). Auto antibodies against oxidized low density lipoprotein in severe preeclampsia. *J Obstet Gynaecol Res*, Vol. 30, No. 188 –192, ISSN 1341-8076

Jim B., Sharma S., Kebede T. & Acharya A. (2010). Hypertension in pregnancy: a comprehensive update. *Cardiol Rev*, Vol. 18, No. 4, pp. 178-89, ISSN 1061-5377

Johnson J., Kniss D. & Samuels P. (2001). Thrombopoietin in pre-eclampsia and HELLP syndrome. *Am J Obstet Gynecol*, Vol. 185, No. 6, pp. S83, ISSN 0002-9378

Kajantie E., Eriksson J., Osmond C., Thornburg K. & Barker D. (2009). Pre-eclampsia is associated with increased risk of stroke in the adult offspring: the Helsinki birth cohort study. *Stroke*, Vol. 40, No. 4, pp. 1176-80, ISSN 0039-2499

Kalle K. (2001). The impact of maternal smoking during pregnancy on delivery outcome. *Europ J Pub Health*, Vol. 11, pp. 329-33, ISSN 1101-1262

Kaufmann P., Mayhew T. & Charnock-Jones D. (2004). Aspects of human fetoplacental vasculogenesis and angiogenesis. II Changes during normal pregnancy. *Placenta*, Vol. 25, pp. 114-126, ISSN 0143-4004

Kim S., Ryu H., Yang J., Kim M., Ahn H., Lim H., et al. (2004). Maternal serum levels of VCAM-1, ICAM-1 and E-selectin in preeclampsia. *J Korean Med Sci*, Vol. 19, No. 5, pp. 688-92, ISSN 1011-8934

Kim Y., Park H., Lee H., Ahn Y., Ha E., Suh S., & Pang M. (2007). Paraoxonase gene polymorphism, serum lipid, and oxidized low-density lipoprotein in preeclampsia. *Eur J Obstet Gynecol Reprod Biol*, Vol. 133, No. 1, pp. 47-52, ISSN 0301-2115

Krauss T., Azab H., Dietrich M. & Augustin H. (1998). Fetal plasma levels of circulating endothelial cell adhesion molecules in normal and preeclamptic pregnancies. *Eur J Obstet Gynecol Reprod Biol*, Vol. 78, No. 1, pp. 41-5, ISSN 0301-2115

Lenfant C. (2008). Low birth weight and blood pressure. *Metabolism*, Vol. 57, No. 2, pp. S32–S35, ISSN 0026-0495

Levine R, Maynard S, Qian C, Lim K, England L, Yu K, et al. (2004). Circulating Angiogenic factors and the risk of preeclampsia. *N Engl J Med*, Vol. 350, pp. 672-83, ISSN 0028-4793

Lockwood C., Toti P., Arcuri F., Norwitz E., Funai E., Huang S., Buchwalder L., Krikun G. & Schatz F. (2007). Thrombin regulates soluble fms-like tyrosine kinase-1 (sFlt-1) expression in first trimester decidua: implications for preeclampsia. *Am J Pathol*, Vol. 170, No. 4, pp. 1398-405, ISSN 0002-9440

Low P., Waugh S., Zinke K. & Drenckhahn D. (1985). The role of hemoglobin denaturation and band 3 clustering in red blood cell aging. *Science*, Vol. 227, No. 4686, pp. 531-3, ISSN 0036-8075

Lurie S. & Mamet Y. (2000). Red blood cell survival and kinetics during pregnancy. *Eur J Obstet Gynecol Reprod Biol*, Vol. 93, pp. 185-192, ISSN 0301-2115

Luttun A. & Carmeliet P. (2003). Soluble VEGF receptor Flt1: the elusive preeclampsia factor discovered? *J Clin Invest*, Vol. 111, No. 5, pp. 600-2, ISSN 0021-9738

Lutz H. (1992). Naturally occurring anti-band 3 antibodies. *Transfus Med Rev*, Vol. 6, No. 3, pp. 201-11, ISSN 0887-7963

Magnussen E., Vatten L., Lund-Nilsen T., Salvesen K., Davey Smith G & Romundstad P. (2007). Prepregnancy cardiovascular risk factors as predictors of pre-eclampsia: population based cohort study. *BMJ*, Vol. 10, No. 335, pp. 7627, ISSN 0959-8138

Manten G., van der Hoek Y., Sikkema J., Voorbij H., Hameeteman T., Visser G. & Franx A. (2005). The role of lipoprotein (a) in pregnancies complicated by pre-eclampsia. *Med Hypotheses*, Vol. 64, pp. 162-169, ISSN 0306-9877

Mao D., Che J., Li K., Han S., Yue Q., Zhu L., Zhang W. & Li L. (2010). Association of homocysteine, asymmetric dimethylarginine, and nitric oxide with preeclampsia. *Arch Gynecol Obstet*, Vol. 282, No. 4, pp. 371-5, ISSN 0932-0067

Maynard S., Epstein F. & Karumanchi A. (2008). Preeclampsia and Angiogenic Imbalance. *Annu Rev Med*, Vol. 59, pp. 437–54, ISSN 0066-4219

McKeeman G., Ardill J., Caldwell C., Hunter A. & McClure N. (2004). Soluble vascular endothelial growth factor receptor-1 (sFlt-1) is increased throughout gestation in patients who have preeclampsia develop. *Am J Obstet Gynecol*, Vol. 191, pp. 1240-6, ISSN 0002-9378

Mehendale S., Kilari A., Dangat K., Taralekar V., Mahadik S. & Joshi S. (2008). Fatty acids, antioxidants, and oxidative stress in pre-eclampsia. *Int J Gynaecol Obstet* Vol. 100, No. 3, pp. 234-8, ISSN 0020-7292

Mellembakken J., Høgåsen K., Mollnes T., Hack C., Abyholm T. & Videm V. (2001). Increased systemic activation of neutrophils but not complement in preeclampsia. *Obstet Gynecol*, Vol. 97, No. 3, pp. 371-4, ISSN 0029-7844

Mori M., Mori A., Saburi Y., Sida M. & Ohta H. (2003). Levels of lipoprotein(a) in normal and compromised pregnancy. *J Perinat Med*, Vol. 31, pp. 23–28, ISSN 0300-5577

Myatt L. & Webster R. (2009). Vascular biology of preeclampsia. *J Thromb Haemost* Vol. 7, No. 3, pp. 375-84, ISSN 1538-7933

Ophir E., Dourleshter G., Hirsh Y., Fait V., German L. & Bornstein J. (2006). Newborns of pre-eclamptic women: a biochemical difference present in utero. *Acta Obstet Gynecol Scand*, Vol. 85, No. 10, pp. 1172-8, ISSN 0001-6349

Osmanaпaoпlu M., Topпuoпlu K., Фzeren M. & Bozkaya H. (2005). Coagulation inhibitors in preeclamptic pregnant women. *Arch Gynecol Obstet*, Vol. 271, pp. 227–230, ISSN 0932-0067

Ouyang Y., Li S., Zhang Q., Cai H. & Chen H. (2009). Interactions between inflammatory and oxidative stress in preeclampsia. *Hypertens Pregnancy*, Vol. 28, No. 1, pp. 56-62, ISSN 1064-1955

Papageorghiou A. & Leslie K. (2007). Uterine artery Doppler in the prediction of adverse pregnancy outcome. *Curr Opin Obstet Gynecol*, Vol. 19, No. 2, pp. 103-9, ISSN 1040-872X

Pijnenborg R., Vercruysse L. & Hanssens M. (2006). The uterine spiral arteries in human pregnancy: facts and controversies. *Placenta*, Vol. 27, No. 9-10, pp. 939-58, ISSN 0143-4004

Polliotti B., Fry A., Saller D., Mooney R., Cox C. & Miller R. (2003). Second-trimester maternal serum placental growth factor and vascular endothelial growth factor for predicting severe, early-onset preeclampsia. *Obstet Gynecol*, Vol. 101, No. 6, pp. 266-74, ISSN 0029-7844

Poston L., Briley A., Seed P., Kelly F. & Shennan A. (2006). Vitamin C and vitamin E in pregnant women at risk for pre-eclampsia (VIP trial): randomised placebo-controlled trial. *Lancet*, Vol. 367, pp. 1145–54, ISSN 0140-6736

Powers R., Catov J., Bodnar L., Gallaher M., Lain K. & Roberts J. (2008). Evidence of Endothelial Dysfunction in Preeclampsia and Risk of Adverse Pregnancy Outcome. *Reprod Sci*, Vol. 15, No. 4, pp. 374–381, ISSN 1933-7191

Qiu C., Phung T., Vadachkoria S., Muy-Rivera M., Sanchez S. & Williams M. (2006). Oxidized Low-Density Lipoprotein (Oxidized LDL) and the Risk of Preeclampsia. *Physiol Res*, Vol. 55, pp. 491-500, ISSN 0862-8408

Raghupathy P., Antonisamy B., Geethanjali F., Saperia J., Leary S., Priya G., Richard J., Barker D. & Fall C. (2010). Glucose tolerance, insulin resistance and insulin secretion in young south Indian adults: Relationships to parental size, neonatal size and childhood body mass index. *Diabetes Res Clin Pract*, Vol. 87, No. 2, pp. 283-92, ISSN 0168-8227

Rahimi R., Nikfar S., Rezaie A. & Abdollahi M. (2009). A meta-analysis on the efficacy and safety of combined vitamin C and E supplementation in preeclamptic women. *Hypertens Pregnancy*, Vol. 28, No. 4, pp. 417-34, ISSN 1064-1955

Raijmakers M., Dechend R. & Poston L. (2004). Oxidative stress and preeclampsia. *Hypertension*, Vol. 44, pp. 374-380, ISSN 0194-911X

Ray J., Diamond P., Singh G. & Bell C. (2006). Brief overview of maternal triglycerides as a risk factor for pre-eclampsia. *BJOG*, Vol. 113, pp. 379-386, ISSN 1470-0328

Redman C. & Sargent I. Placental stress and pre-eclampsia: a revised view. (2009). *Placenta*, Vol. 30, Suppl 1, pp. 38-42, ISSN 0143-4004

Rizzo G. & Arduini D. (2009) Intrauterine growth restriction: diagnosis and management. A review. *Minerva Ginecol*, Vol. 61, No. 5, pp. 411-20, ISSN 0026-4784

Roberts J. & Gammil H. (2005). Preeclampsia - recent insights. *Hypertension*, Vol. 46, pp. 1243-1249, ISSN 0194-911X

Rodie V., Caslake M., Stewartt F., Sattar N., Ramsay J., Greer I. & Freeman D. (2004). Fetal cord plasma lipoprotein status in uncomplicated human pregnancies complicated. *Atherosclerosis*, Vol. 176, pp. 181-187, ISSN 0021-9150

Roes E., Sweep F., Thomas C., Zusterzeel P., Geurts-Moespot A., Peters W. & Steegers E. (2002). Levels of plasminogen activators and their inhibitors in maternal and umbilical cord plasma in severe preeclampsia. *Am J Obstet Gynecol*, Vol. 187, pp. 1019-25, ISSN 0002-9378

Rusterholz C., Hahn S. & Holzgreve W. (2007). Role of placentally produced inflammatory and regulatory cytokines in pregnancy and the etiology of preeclampsia. *Semin Immunopathol*, Vol. 29, No. 2, pp. 151-62, ISSN 1863-2297

Saini H., Puppala B., Angst D., Gilman-Sachs A. & Costello M. (2004). Upregulation of neutrophil surface adhesion molecules in infants of pre-eclamptic women. *J Perinatol*, Vol. 24, pp. 208-212, ISSN 0743-8346

Santos-Silva A., Castro E., Teixeira N., Guerra F. & Quintanilha A. (1995). Altered erythrocyte membrane band 3 profile as a marker in patients at risk for cardiovascular disease. *Atherosclerosis*, Vol. 116, No. 2, pp. 199-209, ISSN 0021-9150

Santos-Silva A., Castro E., Teixeira N., Guerra C. & Quintanilha A. (1998). Erytrocyte membrane band 3 profile imposed by cellular aging, by activated neutrophils and by neutrophilic elastase. *Clin Chim Acta*, Vol. 275, pp. 185-96, ISSN 0009-8981

Santos-Silva A., Rebelo I., Castro E., Belo L., Guerra A., Rego C. & Quintanilha A. (2001). Leukocyte activation, erythrocyte damage, lipid profile and oxidative stress imposed by high competition physical exercise in adolescents. *Clin Chim Acta*, Vol. 306, pp. 119-126, ISSN 0009-8981

Santos-Silva A., Rebelo I., Castro E., Belo L., Catarino C., Monteiro I., Almeida M. & Quintanilha A. (2002). Erytrocyte damage and leukocyte activation in ischemic stroke. *Clin Chim Acta*, Vol. 320, pp. 29-35, ISSN 0009-8981

Sartori M., Serena A., Saggiorato G., Campei S., Faggian D., Pagnan A. & Paternoster D. (2008). Variations in fibrinolytic parameters and inhibin-A in pregnancy: related hypertensive disorders. *J Thromb Haemost*, Vol. 6, No. 2, pp. 352-8, ISSN 1538-7933

Sattar N., Bendomir A., Berry C., Shepherd J., Greer I. & Packard C. (1997). Lipoprotein subfraction concentrations in preeclampsia: pathogenic parallels to atherosclerosis. *Obstet Gynecol*, Vol. 89, pp. 403–408, ISSN 0029-7844

Saugstad O. (2003). Bronchopulmonary dysplasia-oxidative stress and antioxidants. *Semin Neonatol*, Vol. 8, No. 1, pp. 39-49, ISSN 1084-2756

Sibai B., Dekker G. & Kupferminc M. (2005). Pre-eclampsia. *Lancet*, Vol. 365, pp. 785–99, ISSN 0140-6736

Simmons L., Hennessy A., Gillin A. & Jeremy R. (2000). Uteroplacental blood flow and placental vascular endothelial growth factor in normotensive and pre-eclamptic pregnancy. *BJOG*, Vol. 107, No. 5, pp. 678-85, ISSN 1470-0328

Steegers E., von Dadelszen P., Duvekot J. & Pijnenborg R. (2010). Pre-eclampsia. *Lancet*, Vol. 376, No. 9741, pp. 631-44, ISSN 0140-6736

Steyn K., de Wet T., Saloojee Y., Nel H. & Yach D. (2006). The influence of maternal cigarette smoking, snuff use and passive smoking on pregnancy outcomes: the Birth To Ten Study. *Paediatr Perinat Epidemiol*, Vol. 20, No. 2, pp. 90-9, ISSN 0269-5022

Tanjung M., Siddik H., Hariman H. & Koh S. (2005). Coagulation and fibrinolysis in preeclampsia and neonates. *Clin Appl Thromb Hemost*, Vol. 11, No. 4, pp. 467-73, ISSN 1076-0296

Tastekin A., Ors R., Demircan B., Saricam Z., Ingec M. & Akcay F. (2005). Oxidative stress in infants born to preeclamptic mothers. *Pediatr Int*, Vol. 47, No. 6, pp. 658-62, ISSN 1328-8067

Tenhola S., Rahiala E., Halonen P., Vanninen E. & Voutilainen R. (2006). Maternal preeclampsia predicts elevated blood pressure in 12-year-old children: evaluation by ambulatory blood pressure monitoring. *Pediatr Rev*, Vol. 59, pp. 320 324, ISSN 0191-9601

Tjoa M., Vugt J., Go A., Blankenstein M., Oudejans C. & Wijk I. (2003). Elevated c-reactive protein levels during first trimester of pregnancy are indicative of preeclampsia and intrauterine growth restriction. *J Reprod Immunol*, Vol. 59, pp. 29-37, ISSN 0165-0378

Uotila J., Solakivi T., Jaakkola O., Tuimala R. & Lehtimäki T. (1998). Antibodies against copper-oxidised and malondialdehyde-modified low density lipoproteins in pre-eclampsia pregnancies. *BJOG*, Vol. 105, No. 10, pp. 1113-7, ISSN 1470-0328

Uzun H., Benian A., Madazli R., Topçuoğlu M., Aydin S. & Albayrak M. (2005). Circulating oxidized low-density lipoprotein and paraoxonase activity in preeclampsia. *Gynecol Obstet Invest*, Vol. 60, No. 4, pp. 195-200, ISSN 0378-7346

Vatten L., Romundstad P., Holmen T., Hsieh C., Trichopoulos D. & Stuver S. (2003). Intrauterine exposure to preeclampsia and adolescent blood pressure, body size, and age at menarche in female offspring. *Obstet Gynecol*, Vol. 101, pp. 529-533, ISSN 0029-7844

Villa P., Laivuori H., Kajantie E. & Kaaja R. (2009). Free fatty acid profiles in preeclampsia. *Prostaglandins Leukot Essent Fatty Acids*, Vol. 81, pp. 17–21, ISSN 0952-3278

Wakatsuki A., Ikenoue N., Okatani Y., Shinohara K. & Fukaya T. (2000). Lipoprotein particles in preeclampsia: susceptibility to oxidative modification. *Obstet Gynecol*, Vol. 96, pp. 55–59, ISSN 0029-7844

Wang D. (1994). Band 3 protein: structure, flexibility and function. *FEBS Lett*, Vol. 346, No. 1, pp. 26-31, ISSN 0014-5793

Wang Y. & Walsh S. (2001). Increased superoxide generation is associated with decreased superoxide dismutase activity and mRNA expression in placental trophoblast cells in pre-eclampsia. *Placenta*, Vol. 22, No. 2-3, pp. 206-12, ISSN 0143-4004

Waugh S., Walder J. & Low P. (1987). Partial characterization of the copolymerization reaction of erythrocyte membrane band 3 with hemichromes. *Biochemistry*, Vol. 26, No. 6, pp. 1777-83, ISSN 0006-2960

Whincup P., Kaye S., Owen C., Huxley R., Cook D., Anazawa S., et al. (2008). Birth weight and risk of type 2 diabetes: a systematic review. *JAMA*, Vol. 300, No. 24, pp. 2886-97, ISSN 0098-7484

WHO. (2005). World Health Report: make every mother and child count. Geneva: World Health Org

Wikström A., Stephansson O. & Cnattingius S. (2010). Tobacco use during pregnancy and preeclampsia risk: effects of cigarette smoking and snuff. *Hypertension*, Vol. 55, No. 5, pp. 1254-9, ISSN 0194-911X

Wu C., Nohr E., Bech B., Vestergaard M., Catov J. & Olsen J. (2009). Health of children born to mothers who had preeclampsia: a population-based cohort study. *Am J Obstet Gynecol*, Vol. 201, No. 3, pp. 269.e1-269.e10, ISSN 0002-9378

Xiong X. & Fraser W. (2004) Impact of pregnancy-induced hypertension on birthweight by gestational age. *Paediatr Perinat Epidemiol*, Vol. 18, pp. 186–9, ISSN 0269-5022

Xu H, Perez-Cuevas R, Xiong X, Reyes H, Roy C, Julien P, *et al.* (2010). An international trial of antioxidants in the prevention of preeclampsia (INTAPP). *Am J Obstet Gynecol,* Vol. 202, No. 3, pp. 239.e1-239.e10, ISSN 0002-9378

Young B., Levine R. & Karumanchi A. (2010). Pathogenesis of preeclampsia. *Annu Rev Pathol,* Vol. 5, pp. 173-92, ISSN 1553-4006

Zanardo V., Savio V., Sabrina G., Franzoi M., Zerbinati P., Fadin M., Tognin G., Tormene D., Pagnan A. & Simioni P. (2005). The effect of pre-eclampsia on the levels of coagulation and fibrinolysis factors in umbilical cord blood of newborns. *Blood Coagul Fibrinolysis* Vol. 16, No. 3, pp. 177-81, ISSN 0957-5235

Permissions

The contributors of this book come from diverse backgrounds, making this book a truly international effort. This book will bring forth new frontiers with its revolutionizing research information and detailed analysis of the nascent developments around the world.

We would like to thank Stavros Sifakis, MD, PhD and Nikos Vrachnis, MD, DFFP, PCME, for lending their expertise to make the book truly unique. They have played a crucial role in the development of this book. Without their invaluable contribution this book wouldn't have been possible. They have made vital efforts to compile up to date information on the varied aspects of this subject to make this book a valuable addition to the collection of many professionals and students.

This book was conceptualized with the vision of imparting up-to-date information and advanced data in this field. To ensure the same, a matchless editorial board was set up. Every individual on the board went through rigorous rounds of assessment to prove their worth. After which they invested a large part of their time researching and compiling the most relevant data for our readers. Conferences and sessions were held from time to time between the editorial board and the contributing authors to present the data in the most comprehensible form. The editorial team has worked tirelessly to provide valuable and valid information to help people across the globe.

Every chapter published in this book has been scrutinized by our experts. Their significance has been extensively debated. The topics covered herein carry significant findings which will fuel the growth of the discipline. They may even be implemented as practical applications or may be referred to as a beginning point for another development. Chapters in this book were first published by InTech; hereby published with permission under the Creative Commons Attribution License or equivalent.

The editorial board has been involved in producing this book since its inception. They have spent rigorous hours researching and exploring the diverse topics which have resulted in the successful publishing of this book. They have passed on their knowledge of decades through this book. To expedite this challenging task, the publisher supported the team at every step. A small team of assistant editors was also appointed to further simplify the editing procedure and attain best results for the readers.

Our editorial team has been hand-picked from every corner of the world. Their multi-ethnicity adds dynamic inputs to the discussions which result in innovative outcomes. These outcomes are then further discussed with the researchers and contributors who give their valuable feedback and opinion regarding the same. The feedback is then collaborated with the researches and they are edited in a comprehensive manner to aid the understanding of the subject.

Apart from the editorial board, the designing team has also invested a significant amount of their time in understanding the subject and creating the most relevant covers. They scrutinized every image to scout for the most suitable representation of the subject and create an appropriate cover for the book.

The publishing team has been involved in this book since its early stages. They were actively engaged in every process, be it collecting the data, connecting with the contributors or procuring relevant information. The team has been an ardent support to the editorial, designing and production team. Their endless efforts to recruit the best for this project, has resulted in the accomplishment of this book. They are a veteran in the field of academics and their pool of knowledge is as vast as their experience in printing. Their expertise and guidance has proved useful at every step. Their uncompromising quality standards have made this book an exceptional effort. Their encouragement from time to time has been an inspiration for everyone.

The publisher and the editorial board hope that this book will prove to be a valuable piece of knowledge for researchers, students, practitioners and scholars across the globe.

List of Contributors

Bruce W. Newton
University of Arkansas for Medical Sciences, USA

Alexander B. Poletaev
P.K. Anokhin Research Institute of Normal Physiology Russian Acad. Med. Sci., Medical Research Ctr. "Immunculus", Moscow, Russia

Leila Roshangar and Jafar Soleimani Rad
Tabriz University of Medical Sciences, Tabriz, Iran

Batool Mutar Mahdi
Al-Kindy College of Medicine - Baghdad University, Iraq

Hiroko Watanabe
Department of Clinical Nursing, Shiga University of Medical Science, Japan

Echendu Dolly Adinma
Department Of Community Medicine, Faculty Of Medicine, College Of Health Sciences, Nnamdi Azikiwe University, Nnewi Campus, Nnewi, Anambra State, Nigeria

Dennis G. Chambers
Queen Elizabeth Hospital Pregnancy Advisory Centre, Adelaide, Australia

Mats Fagerquist
North Elfsborg County Hospital, Trollhattan, Sweden

Dimitra Kappou and Stavros Sifakis
Department of Obstetrics-Gynecology, University Hospital of Heraklion, Crete, Greece

Nikos Vrachnis
2nd Department of Obstetrics & Gynecology, Aretaieion Hospital, University of Athens, Athens, Greece

Victor Gourvas
Department of Pathology, General Hospital "G. Genimatas", Thessaloniki, Greece

Efterpi Dalpa
Department of Pediatrics, General Hospital "G. Papageorgiou", Thessaloniki, Greece

Stavros Sifakis
Department of Obstetrics & Gynecology, University Hospital of Heraklion, Crete, Greece

Esther Fandiño García
Hospital de Jerez de la Frontera, Spain

Juan Carlos Delgado Herrero
Hospital Juan Grande, Spain

Chantal Bon, Françoise Poloce and Jean Pichot
Department of Biochemistry, Hospital Croix-Rousse, Lyon, France

Daniel Raudrant, Fabienne Champion and François Golfier
Department of Gynecology – Obstetrics, Hospital Lyon-Sud, Pierre-Bénite Cedex, France

André Revol
Department of Biochemistry, Hospital Lyon-Sud, Pierre-Bénite Cedex, France

Julia Unterscheider
Royal College of Surgeons in Ireland, Rotunda Hospital Dublin, Ireland

Keelin O'Donoghue
Anu Research Centre, University College Cork, Cork University Maternity Hospital, Ireland

N. Vrachnis, Z. Iliodromiti, D. Botsis and G. Creatsas
2nd Department of Obstetrics and Gynecology, University of Athens Medical School, Aretaieio Hospital, Athens, Greece

F.M. Malamas
1st Department of Obstetrics and Gynecology, University of Athens Medical School, Alexandra Hospital, Athens, Greece

S. Sifakis
Department of Obstetrics and Gynaecology, University Hospital of Heraklion, Crete, Greece

A. Parashaki
Health Center of Thira, Thira, Greece

Eva Wiberg-Itzel
Department of Clinical Science and Education, Section of Obstetrics and Gynecology, Karolinska Institute, South General Hospital, Stockholm, Sweden

Sunday E. Adaji
Ahmadu Bello University and Ahmadu Bello University Teaching Hospital, Zaria, Nigeria

Charles A. Ameh
Liverpool School of Tropical Medicine, Pembroke Place, Liverpool, United Kingdom

Joseph Ifeanyi Brian-D. Adinma
Department of Obstetrics and Gynaecology Nnamdi Azikiwe University and Teaching Hospital, Nnewi, Nigeria

Cristina Catarino, Irene Rebelo, Luís Belo and Alice Santos-Silva
Departamento de Ciências Biológicas, Laboratório de Bioquímica, Faculdade de Farmácia, Universidade do Porto (FFUP), Portugal
Instituto de Biologia Molecular e Celular (IBMC), Universidade do Porto, Portugal

Alexandre Quintanilha
Instituto Ciências Biomédicas Abel Salazar (ICBAS), Universidade do Porto, Portugal